Enemy in the Blood

To Susan,

Thanks for inspiring
this book!

All the best,

[signature]

8/2/13

ENEMY IN THE BLOOD

Malaria, Environment, and Development in Argentina

Eric D. Carter

THE UNIVERSITY OF ALABAMA PRESS

Tuscaloosa

Copyright © 2012
The University of Alabama Press
Tuscaloosa, Alabama 35487-0380
All rights reserved
Manufactured in the United States of America

Typeface: Bembo

∞
The paper on which this book is printed meets the minimum requirements of
American National Standard for Information Sciences—Permanence of Paper for
Printed Library Materials, ANSI Z39.48-1984.

Library of Congress Cataloging-in-Publication Data

Carter, Eric D.
    Enemy in the blood : malaria, environment, and development in Argentina / Eric D.
Carter.
        p. cm.
    Includes bibliographical references and index.
    ISBN 978-0-8173-1760-7 (cloth : alk. paper) — ISBN 978-0-8173-8595-8
(electronic : alk. paper) 1. Malaria—Argentina—History. 2. Malaria—Argentina—
Prevention. 3. Public health—Argentina—History. I. Title.
    RC162.A7C37 2012
    616.9′36200982—dc23
                                                                                                    2011022669

Cover art: "Drainage canal for malarious marshes" [Canal de desagüe para pantanos
palúdicos]. From "La campaña contra el paludismo," *Caras y Caretas,* December 23,
1911.

To my parents, Dale and Virginia Carter

Contents

Illustrations

Acknowledgments

No work of scholarship is ever a solo effort, so I have many people to thank for their contributions to this book, over a decade in the making.

In Argentina, three scholars were key facilitators of this research, especially in its earliest and most precarious stages. The late Dr. Alfredo G. Kohn Loncarica oriented me, intellectually and socially, when I started this project in 2001. Despite being extremely busy with his responsibilities as an administrator at the Facultad de Medicina at the Universidad de Buenos Aires, he always made time for me. With his death in January 2005, we lost a scholar, a friend, and a great man. Although we met in person only once, the late Dr. Jobino P. Sierra Iglesias, of San Pedro, Jujuy, provided invaluable resources on the history of medicine in Northwest Argentina. I hope in some way that this book carries on the legacy of the Northwest's regional scientists, whose work he celebrated. Dr. Susana Curto, a medical geographer, has been a fount of information and opinion, particularly on the epidemiology of vector-borne diseases in Argentina. I cherish our conversations over the years on matters relating not just to malaria and medical geography, but also to national politics, society, and culture.

A special thanks goes to Karina Ramacciotti, whose insights into the history of public health in Argentina, especially during the Juan D. Perón era, have helped add texture and depth to the latter chapters of this book.

Other scholars and researchers in Argentina—mainly historians, geographers, and medical scientists—deserve my thanks: Abel L. Agüero, Rolando Boffi, Romina Plastina, Carlos Reboratti, Héctor Recalde, Hilda Sábato, Norma Isabel Sánchez, Abraham Sonis, and José Trujillo in Buenos Aires; Susana Belmartino in Rosario; and Alfredo Bolsi, Horacio Madariaga, and Daniel Campi in Tucumán.

There is plenty of gratitude to be spread among the librarians and archivists of Argentina for their dedication and kindness. In Buenos Aires, I thank the staffs of the Academia Nacional de Historia, the Universidad de Buenos

Aires-Facultad de Medicina, the Academia Nacional de Medicina, the Archivo General de la Nación (especially the photo archives), the Asociación Médica Argentina, the Biblioteca Nacional, the Biblioteca Tornquist, the Instituto Geográfico Militar (map library), INDEC, Sociedad Científica Argentina, and the Universidad de Buenos Aires-Instituto de Estudios Geográficos. In the interior, I got to know the librarians a little better, so I have more personal thanks. In Salta, I offer my sincere thanks to Gregorio Caro Figueroa for granting me access to his vast private library at his home in Cerrillos. At the Archivo y Biblioteca Históricos of Salta, head librarian Carolina Linares granted me special access to the registry logs of El Milagro Hospital, demonstrating her passion to preserve and share the documents that form the history of Salta. I also thank Liliana Arenas at the Biblioteca Dr. Atilio Cornejo and the librarians of the periodical room of the Biblioteca Provincial Dr. Victorino de la Plaza.

In Tucumán, Susana Cuezzo, Eduardo Carranza, and Constanza Fernández Murga at the Casa Histórica de la Independencia helped me gain access to some unique archival sources; Mercedes Porcel and Alicia Ferrari made the library at the Universidad Nacional de Tucumán-Instituto de Estudios Geográficos feel like home; Carlos Lobo and José María Vera at the Delegación Sanitaria Federal gave me access to the abandoned but still-intact library of the old Malaria Service; and Mario Rodríguez generously allowed the reproduction of photographs from the archives of *La Gaceta* newspaper. At the Archivo Histórico de Tucumán, Celina Correa Uriburu and Marcela Magliani, as well as regular clients Ingeniero Medina and María Lenis, assisted me with searches through dusty old volumes of local newspapers.

Susana Curto, Horacio Madariaga, and the Instituto Geográfico Militar provided some of the geospatial data that I used to create the maps in this book.

Outside of Argentina, thanks are also due to the staffs of the Rockefeller Archive Center in New York, especially Michele Hiltzik and Charlotte Sturm; the archives of the London School of Hygiene and Tropical Medicine, especially Richard Meunier; and the National Library of Medicine in Bethesda, Maryland.

Another valuable learning experience took place outside of the libraries, through my affiliation with the current and former personnel of Argentina's Malaria Service, today known as the Programa Nacional de Control de Vectores. Dr. Mario Zaidenberg, the director of the agency's headquarters in Salta, made it possible for me to work and travel with the service's personnel. I thank the chief of the base in Tartagal, Héctor Janutolo, and other personnel there for the opportunity to see dengue fever control in action. I spent much more time with the Malaria Service in Orán, and there I'd like to thank

Federico Vianconi Sr., Bernardo Carrazan, Enrique Laci, and Carlos Medina for their help and friendship. Special thanks to Federico (Nery) Vianconi Jr., who took me to the remotest reaches of the Malaria Service's jurisdiction, accompanied me on interviews, explained local history, and welcomed me into his home. I could never have gotten to know the great people of Orán and its vicinity as well as I did without his assistance. Dr. Néstor Taranto gave me special insight into the local epidemiology of the Orán area. María Julia Dantur, of Tucumán, accompanied me on most of my forays around Orán and Tartagal, and I thank her for teaching me about field methods in entomology and the biology of the *Anopheles pseudopunctipennis* mosquito. The assistance of Ariel Zorrilla and Gabriela Quintana, and all of the other researchers who passed through the Fundación Proyungas in Orán, was invaluable.

Many people shared their memories of the old malaria campaign or local history with me in interviews and tours. They include Serafín Fernando Vera, Francisco Sotelo, and José Guanco, of Tucumán; Tulio Ottonello, José Luis Albarracín, and Regino Racedo, of Monteros, Tucumán; Rodolfo Carcavallo, of Buenos Aires; Miguel Angel Cáseres, of Salta; and Pedro "Peter" Alvarado, of Jujuy. Three research assistants in Argentina, David Lenis, Sandra Lico, and Gabriel Linares, helped me with data collection.

At the University of Wisconsin, Madison, fellow graduate students helped me tremendously in my research and many have become great friends as well. Special thanks go to Christian Brannstrom, Mike Benedetti, Mike Daniels and Jane Rosecky, Kristin Gunther, Jonathan Haws, Noah and Michelle Rost, Jeff Stone, Rob Rose, Alex Diener, Bill Gartner, Zoltán Grossman, Blake Harrison, Morgan Robertson, Christopher Rosin, Antoinette WinklerPrins, Kendra Smith-Howard, Dawn Biehler, and Tom Robertson.

At the University of Wisconsin, Steve Stern, Judy Leavitt, Bill Cronon, and Matt Turner offered invaluable advice about my research and teaching and helped enormously to sharpen my ideas and my prose. Other faculty in the Geography Department, especially Jim Knox, Jim Burt, Bob Sack, Bob Kaiser, Yi-Fu Tuan, Lisa Naughton, A-Xing Zhu, Tom Vale, and the late David Woodward, were also a great help to me. Faculty in other departments, such as Nancy Langston, Florencia Mallon, Gregg Mitman, and Arnie Alanen, also contributed to the development of this book. Very special thanks are reserved for Karl Zimmerer for his generous spirit, scholarly engagement, and attention to detail.

Through exchanges at conferences and by letter and e-mail, many scholars have offered advice and encouragement: Conevery Bolton Valencius, David Keeling, Andrew Sluyter, Kent Mathewson, Dan Gade, David Robinson, Paul Robbins, Marcos Cueto, Diego Armus, Gilberto Hochman, Simone Kropf, Randall Packard, Paul Sutter, Jaime Benchimol, and Hugh Prince. Portions of this book were presented in lectures at University College, London, and the University of Manchester in 2009, and I thank both Federico Caprotti and Matthias vom Hau for organizing these events and for their insightful comments on my work. Margaret Humphreys offered excellent comments on the complete manuscript of this book, and I also appreciate her longstanding support for me, a geographer doing research in the history of medicine.

Colleagues at Grinnell College have been supportive of my research. Thanks especially to Mike Guenther, Elizabeth Prevost, David Cook-Martin, David Harrison, Dan Reynolds, and Dan Kaiser. Student Kathryn Vanney helped with copyediting in the later stages, and I am grateful for her careful attention to detail.

Major funding for the research that ultimately led to this book was provided by the National Science Foundation (D.D.I. Award No. BCS-0117381); the Rockefeller Archive Center in New York; the University of Wisconsin–Madison Latin American, Caribbean, and Iberian Studies Program (Nave Summer Field Research Grant); and the UW–Madison International Institute (Global Studies Fellowship). A grant from Millersville University allowed me to consult the Fred L. Soper papers at the National Library of Medicine, and Grinnell College supported follow-up research in Argentina in 2007.

I'd like to thank the following institutions for generously allowing me to reproduce original photographs and maps for this book: the Rockefeller Archive Center, *La Gaceta* newspaper (Tucumán), and the Archivo General de la Nación in Buenos Aires. Content from my article " 'God Bless General Perón': DDT and the Endgame of Malaria Eradication in Argentina in the 1940s" from the *Journal of the History of Medicine and Allied Sciences* (vol. 64, 2009) comprises the bulk of chapter 5, so I'd like to thank Oxford University Press for permission to reprint it here. Thanks also to Elsevier Press for permission to use parts of my article "Development Narratives and the Uses of Ecology: Malaria Control in Northwest Argentina, 1890–1940" from the *Journal of Historical Geography* (vol. 33, 2007).

My family is the main reason that I've come this far in life. Thanks always to my parents, Dale and Virginia Carter, who showed me the value of being a teacher. You may be overworked and underappreciated, but I'm very thankful for all you've given me. Thanks also to my sister Nicole and my sister Susan and her husband, Tony, for all of their support. My aunts and uncles, Jack and Glenda Duclo, Carlos Molina, Teresa Molina, and Mariana Andridge, have guided me over the years. If not for my godparents, Rubén and Alicia Bilbao of Rosario, Argentina, this project would never have been conceived. My thanks to them for introducing me to their country and treating me as one of their own. I'd also like to thank their sons, Diego, Cristian, and Fernando, for their love and friendship and for being unafraid to give me a hard time when they thought I deserved it.

Last but not least, I want to thank Neela Nandyal for being by my side throughout the writing of this book. Her love, patience, and companionship have made this time easier. She has also been a careful reader—sometimes the only reader—of my work, and so she deserves credit for sharpening my prose as well. But the production of this book pales in comparison to our other creation, Nalini, who came into this world in 2009. Thanks to her for making each day a little brighter, for helping put things into perspective, and for sleeping through the night (at least most of the time).

Enemy in the Blood

Introduction

A Sickness in the Land

In 1937, Alfredo Palacios, one of Argentina's most recognizable politicians, went on a fact-finding mission to the country's impoverished northwestern provinces.[1] Although he represented the city of Buenos Aires in the national senate, Palacios specialized in exposing the conditions of the poorest of the poor, a mission that necessarily took him to the provinces. Through the windows of his touring car, at every turn Palacios witnessed astonishing "portraits of misery." Filthy, overcrowded shantytowns festered around provincial capitals. Families starved in spite of the gifts of a lush, fertile subtropical environment, often substituting bitter yerba maté tea for meals. Most poignantly, children toiled, barefoot and bent, in sugarcane fields. Stepping out of his car, the dandyish Palacios—with distinctive handlebar mustache, and dressed in a three-piece suit, bow tie, flowing scarf, and white hat—stood out among crowds of barefoot children. On the outskirts of Tucumán, Northwest Argentina's major city, he recorded the appalling living conditions in one of these miserable slums. He testified later on the floor of the national senate:

> Made of wattle-and-daub, straw, adobe, and canvas, these dilapidated dwellings measure, generally, three by four meters. The floor is made of dirt; inside, [there are] dirty, battered cots, or blankets thrown on the floor, and a bunch of crates instead of chairs. There, promiscuously, live men and women, of all ages. . . . That is where children grow up, crowded together, without knowing the most elementary notions of hygiene; malnourished, atrophied, the majority with physical defects, malarial, or with the degenerative stigmas of syphilis and alcohol. Many do not go to school, according to their own parents, because they are needed for work, especially in the time of the harvest or the preparations for the planting of sugar cane.[2]

Photographs accompanying his report, entitled *El dolor argentino* (Argentina's sorrow), reinforced his poignant accounts: one picture after another of disheveled families, standing in front of their decrepit shanties, humbly averting their eyes from the merciless gaze of the camera.

Building on decades of critique by public health doctors, social reformers, journalists, and politicians, Palacios viewed the Northwest as a land apart from the rest of Argentina, weighed down by manifold, mutually reinforcing problems. Distance from markets, primitive infrastructure, reliance on monoculture, and irrational exploitation of resources curtailed the region's economic growth. Wealth and income were spread unevenly, with paltry wages for agricultural workers and the persistence of latifundia that created virtual serfdoms in some areas. Agricultural migrants drifted from place to place, carrying their unstable and vice-ridden ways with them, undermining the moral roots of society. Illiteracy was rampant; children went hungry. The lower classes ended up devastated and abandoned. Everywhere, Palacios saw misery, immorality, indifference, and injustice.

Palacios also observed that sickness, disease, and degeneration had reduced the region's neediest to prisoners of their physical state. Aided by advice from prominent local public health doctors, such as Salvador Mazza and Carlos Alvarado, Palacios recited a litany of diseases and conditions—some familiar, some strange—that afflicted the region, such as malnutrition, tuberculosis, syphilis, and Chagas disease. But one disease in particular, seemingly inescapable and entrenched, controlled the prospects of the region: malaria. This parasitic, mosquito-borne illness was both cause and effect of the region's misery. Malaria thrived in the region's hot, humid, subtropical environment but also flourished opportunistically in bodies worn down by alcoholism, malnutrition, overwork, and material deprivation. Echoing many of his contemporaries, Palacios feared that malaria would "in a short time lead to a fatal degeneration of the race."[3] The sorry state of the Northwest was, to Palacios, an indictment of a nation on the wrong path: "We can never be a great, responsible, and progressive people if we lack citizens who are physically and morally sound, who are capable of exploiting our enormous riches and of governing and defending the patrimony of our cultural inheritance."[4]

As a socialist and muckraker, Palacios was often a dissident, or at least a thorn in the side of the powerful.[5] Yet, in his racial anxiety, nationalist fervor, and preoccupation with disease's ravaging effects on society, Palacios articulated a durable discourse that knew no political boundaries. Starting around the 1890s, solving the Northwest's malaria problem captured the imagination of generations of conservative aristocrats, progressive sanitarians, state public health agents, entomologists, epidemiologists, engineers, physicians, labor rights activists, educational reformers, newspaper editorialists, and political economists, irrespective of party affiliation or regional background. In Argentina, controlling malaria was more than a narrow public health question. For those involved in the campaign, it was a fight to reclaim the body and soul of a region and a nation.

Public Hygiene, Modernization, and Uneven Development

In this book, I examine the discovery, control, and eradication of malaria in Argentina from 1890 to 1950.[6] My central argument is that malaria control was driven by a larger project of constructing a modern identity for Argentina. Insofar as development meant building a more productive, rational, orderly, hygienic, and healthy society, the persistence of a "tropical" disease such as malaria prevented Argentina from joining the ranks of modern nations. Malaria came to symbolize the most "backward" part of the country, the Northwest, whose lethargic social and economic progress perplexed regional and national leaders. In malaria, advocates of modernization found a potent symbol of a malaise that was social, biological, and environmental in nature. Yet, a sometimes muddled understanding of the relationship among disease, society, and the environment would have a problematic influence on malaria control on the ground—with surprising consequences.

The narrative begins with malaria's emergence as a social problem in the late nineteenth century, which coincided with a growing recognition of Argentina's pronounced interregional disparities. By the late 1800s, Argentina was booming, developing into one of the most prosperous countries in the world. Steady economic growth, an influx of European immigrants, and urbanization transformed Argentine society. Denizens of Buenos Aires, known as "Porteños," self-consciously modeled their city on the great capitals of Europe, and the city bloomed with sophisticated shops and restaurants, wide boulevards, and large, elegant green spaces. In the capital, the national government invested in potable water systems, sewers, garbage collection, and disease control, with the aim of creating a sanitary urban environment. Simultaneously, a generation of influential scientists—the *higienistas,* or "hygienists"—campaigned against unhealthy habits and vices, with a mixture of didactic health education, progressive legal reforms, and aggressive social control. To national leaders, sanitation and hygiene were hallmarks of civilization, and public health scientists were key agents of modernity.[7]

Yet during this vibrant era of economic growth, demographic explosion, and cultural transformation, Argentina's subtropical Northwest lagged far behind, with large swaths of it seemingly frozen in the country's colonial past. Regional and national elites viewed northwestern society with a profound sense of anxiety. Under the sway of late nineteenth-century positivism, they sought to classify and diagnose the multiple problems of the region: grinding poverty, illiteracy, malnutrition, ill health, demographic decline, cultural backwardness, indolence. Malaria emerged as a symbol of this malaise and as a conceptual bridge between the social and environmental components of the Northwest's ills. In short, the disease became a useful marker of regional difference, those internal cleavages that undermined the continuous consolidation and development of the modern nation-state.

Meanwhile, Argentina's political and intellectual elites adapted European ideas of "scientific racism," which was manifested in eugenics, environmental determinism, and public hygiene campaigns.[8] Leaders of the malaria control effort worried that the disease diminished the vigor of the "national race" and sought to understand it in the terms of contemporary race science. Some believed that the searing and unforgiving environment of the Northwest itself produced an inferior race, with malaria acting as one of the most malicious tools in nature's arsenal. More optimistically, most hygienists argued that the particular environments that served as sources of malaria could be transformed and sanitized. In the process, improvements in public health would entice immigrants from Europe and thus gradually whiten the creole or mixed-blood Hispanic stock of the Northwest.

To these elites, combating malaria was part of a larger effort to control nature in order to transform the makeup of northwestern society. The presumption that controlling nature would transform society found support in the late nineteenth-century science of malaria. In this period, the miasmatic theory of disease causation prevailed, and geographic surveys were considered key epidemiological tools. It was widely accepted that malaria emanated from insalubrious and therefore unproductive landscapes, preferentially attacking those people who worked closest with the soil. Thus, fighting malaria was predicated on the physical transformation of unhealthy environments.

Taken together, concern over regional development, anxiety over the fate of the Argentine race, and the etiological framework of miasmatic theory and medical geography buttressed the claims of provincial elites and public health advocates who promoted malaria control as a pathway to social and economic progress. They developed a narrative of progress, arguing that malaria control would create a healthier working class and, via wetland drainage, transform unhealthy malarious environments into productive urban and agricultural landscapes. In turn, such development would make the Northwest more inviting to European immigrants and their "civilizing" influence. Thus malaria control would initiate a virtuous circle of improved health and accelerated economic growth, bringing this peripheral region into the orbit of national development.

Convinced of the urgency of the malaria threat, around 1900 the National

Department of Hygiene intervened to address the problem, first with a cycle of regional malaria studies, followed by legislative proposals. In 1907, the national congress approved Law 5195, creating the national Malaria Service, with authority in the afflicted provinces. Thus, Argentina became one of the first countries in Latin America to embark on a domestic malaria campaign.

Yet controlling malaria proved to be no simple matter, and complete eradication took several decades. Indeed, a major obstacle to the project's success was the overpowering concern with malaria's role in the larger process of social development. Malaria control advocates tended to support strategies that related to deeper transformations of nature and society, such as wetland drainage, channelization, tree plantations, and other hydraulic and agricultural controls. Even after miasmatic theory faded, superseded in scientific circles by the mosquito-and-parasite-based etiology, control efforts still revolved around *saneamiento,* or "environmental sanitation." The older notion of malaria as a disease *of place* proved to be surprisingly enduring.

Environmental sanitation had staying power in large part because of Argentina's fascination with foreign science. In particular, hygienists and politicians alike embraced a socially ambitious model of malaria control transplanted from Italy. The impressive reclamation of the Pontine Marshes and other malarious "wastelands" in the 1920s and 1930s seemed to demonstrate how comprehensive malaria control efforts could transform a region, its landscapes, and its people. However, advocates of an Italian-style environmental sanitation strategy overlooked its poor fit with the ecology of Northwest Argentina. Only when leaders of the campaign learned to tailor control measures to the reality of local conditions, particularly the habits of local mosquito vectors, was malaria brought under control. The vital piece of the puzzle was that *Anopheles pseudopunctipennis,* the principal vector of malaria in the region, does not usually breed in swamps or marshes and was thus unaffected by large-scale saneamiento efforts. This realization demanded that Argentina's malaria control experts meet the Northwest on its own terms, concentrate on more focused interventions, and shed the largely imaginary geography that had inspired ineffective strategies.

The Geographical Imaginary of Malaria

Fundamentally, this book explores the place of malaria in the *geographical imaginary* of northwestern Argentina. As I define it, a geographical imaginary is a constellation of meanings and values ascribed to a place, usually from afar, which enables a distanced and abstracted understanding of nature-society dynamics in that place.[9] Distilling the complexity of a place to its essential characteristics establishes a framework for political intervention to promote social development. Quite similar to the geographical imaginary, the "regional discursive formation," a concept developed by geographers Richard Peet and Michael Watts, is a master narrative that outside experts use to talk about a region and its problems, simplifying its history, its problems, and the heterogeneity of nature and culture it contains.[10] In Argentina, the geographical imaginary provided a shorthand for state planners, hygienists, physicians, and other scientists to label the Northwest region, classify its problems, and launch projects for its development. The danger, disgust, and disgrace of disease colored geographical knowledge. In the analyses of Alfredo Palacios and his colleagues, metaphors of contagion, torpor, hazard, and decay bled across whatever line exists between the medical and the social, as the Northwest itself became pathologized.[11]

Such pathologized geographical imaginaries may develop at virtually any spatial scale, from urban neighborhoods, to sub-national regions, to entire nation-states and even world regions. The geographer Susan Craddock has demonstrated how the white majority in San Francisco viewed the city's Chinatown as an incubator of diseases such as bubonic plague, reinforcing Anglo efforts to segregate Chinese immigrants to that tiny, overcrowded district in the early 1900s.[12] Around the same time, public health reformers stigmatized the American South, claiming that the region's cultural "backwardness" had its roots in widespread "diseases of laziness," such as hookworm, pellagra, and malaria.[13] Late in the twentieth century, Venezuelan public health officials responded to cholera outbreaks by making scapegoats of the Indians of the Delta Amacuro region, who were already perceived as unhygienic and culturally retrograde.[14] Today, fear of epidemic HIV/AIDS colors nearly all portrayals of Sub-Saharan Africa.[15] As may be evident, the diseases that figure prominently in such geographical imaginaries are not themselves imaginary. Far from it: sickness and death are quite real. A geographical imaginary is not woven out of thin air; it assembles partial and mediated understandings of place into a narrative that defines the identity of that place and explains its problems.

Indeed, the geographical imaginary is necessary and inevitable in comprehending and managing the reality of large, modern societies.[16] However, when disease becomes such a strong and palpable marker of identity for a place or region, it has a number of problematic effects. For one, as Craddock puts it, the "ascription" of disease onto "particular structures, districts, or regions," tends to *naturalize* problems that are socially constructed.[17] Attributing poverty or underdevelopment to a disease such as malaria, a common theme in portrayals of regions stricken by that disease, may shift the focus from social and political-economic disparities related to labor exploitation, inequitable land tenure, or racial discrimination. The elevation of scientific managers—technocrats—to positions of power tends to further the depoliticization of social development as progress becomes a question of "curing" this or that medical or social ill.[18]

At the same time, the geographical imaginary of disease may exercise undue influence on what I term *models of disease-and-environment:* lenses for understanding the interaction between people and disease within the social, built, and natural environment.[19] These models are necessary to distill complex reality to the components and dynamics that are *essential* for the instrumental purpose of disease control. However, I propose that the "models" constructed by scientist-bureaucrats in public health are unavoidably influenced by broader social concerns. Indeed, any independence between the scientific and social/political realms is now seen as highly problematic in studies of the history of medicine and public health. Yet the relationship between disease model and geographical imaginary, both fixed on a certain place or region, helps us understand why autonomy of the scientific from the social is difficult to achieve.

In the field of the history of medicine, there has been intense effort to frame disease within broader political, ideological, economic, social, and environmental contexts.[20] In particular, recent studies of malaria—in Italy, Palestine, the southern United States, Brazil, Peru, and Mexico, among other places—have gone beyond the narrow stories of progress and achievement in the biomedical realm to situate disease within relevant discursive formations, ideological struggles, social transformations, and geopolitical affairs.[21] Perhaps more than most diseases, historically, malaria has been difficult to reduce to a single cause or a discrete set of associated risk factors. Instead, to use Margaret Humphreys's phrase, malaria has often been conceived of as a "knot" of intertwined social, biological, and environmental factors, such as poverty, race, differential immunity, malnutrition, climate, topography, and so forth.[22] Thus, malaria is often approached as a system or a syndrome.

While Humphreys, in her study of malaria in the American South, carried out the somewhat heroic task of disentangling the knot—analytically separating and evaluating the relevance of causal or associated factors—my goal is different. To expand on her apt metaphor, I wish to situate the "malaria knot" within a larger tapestry of the geographical imaginary. As Craddock has said, "The purpose of conducting a regional study of disease lies in the value of illuminating those knowledge systems, ideologies, social structures, and economic patterns that are peculiar to a particular place in time and that determine the precise interpretations and utilizations of disease."[23] For that reason, this book analyzes what is going on *around* the malaria campaign—the ideological, political, and scientific context—as much as it does the inner workings of the campaign itself.

Yet, the choice of geographical scale for delimiting "context" is an important one. Conventionally, historical works related to malaria or other infectious diseases have tended to define scale uncritically, choosing the typical spatial containers for a historical study, principally the nation-state, a city, or, in many case studies related to tropical disease, a colony. Possibly, this historiographic practice reflects the power of widely accepted statistical categories. Charles Briggs and Clara Mantini-Briggs, in their study of the Venezuelan cholera epidemics of the early 1990s, underscore the taken-for-granted quality of geographical categories in official public health discourse: for example, the World Health Organization (WHO) portrays "geographic regions and nation-states as natural units of disease transmission, surveillance, and containment."[24] Even in works that trace international expert networks and the diffusion of public health knowledge and practice, the solidity of scalar categories is taken for granted; nation-states serve as bounded entities, providing a backdrop for the movement of actors and ideas.[25]

In this book, I take a distinct position. Building on the work of Briggs and Mantini-Briggs, I argue that spatial categories may appear natural, yet are actually constructed as part of larger official narratives about public health problems.[26] In the Argentine case, the malaria problem and spatial categories (specifically, region and nation) were co-constructed. Geography was not merely a backdrop to the malaria issue; nor can geographical entities and relationships be defined retroactively for historical actors. Rather, the construction of *geographical identities* was central to the discourse of malaria in Argentina. The political and scientific conversation about the disease—which went on for about sixty years—was really part of a larger conversation about modern regional and national identities. These identities were never fixed, but instead constructed relationally—in relation to one another and to other geographical identities.[27] In one direction, looking inward, elites saw geographical division and difference that undermined a coherent national identity and progress.[28] Looking outward, the nation's elites wondered how Argentina measured up to the "civilized" countries of the world.

This division and difference was eminently geographical—it revolved around historically distinct regions that still failed to coalesce. As Buenos Aires and the Pampas grew to a position of unquestionable dominance, the Northwest became the "other Argentina"—that is, the great "internal Other" that served as the mirror for examining the nation's flaws and shortcomings.[29] By the early 1900s, the identity of the Northwest began to coalesce around a concept of a *diseased region*. The gap between the Northwest and the more affluent, rapidly urbanizing, and politically dominant region around Buenos Aires seemed to grow ever wider over time. And malaria was the regional disease *par excellence*. Malaria, for the way it ravaged the body and shaped the attitude of its sufferers, became a powerful metaphor for the state of north-western society at large: frail, fatigued, anemic, apathetic, in dire need of modernization and reform. Although other diseases were greater killers, it was malaria's potency as a symbol of geographical *difference* that made it so threatening.

Just as importantly, the particular geographical framing of the malaria problem had a direct (and mostly counterproductive) influence on disease control "on the ground." In the prevailing geographical imaginary, the North-west was a diseased region, and malaria sprang from the interface between people and their environment: malaria was characteristically a disease *of place*. Scientific models, first based in miasmatic theory and medical geography, and later in the mosquito-parasite model of malaria transmission, sanctioned this perspective. In this context, sanitizing the landscape, primarily through wet-land drainage, seemed to be a key step in promoting development. Later, the positive experience of other countries employing wetland drainage for ma-laria control and rural development, particularly Italy, corroborated the de-velopmentalist model of malaria control. Yet, as we will see, this model was ill suited to the ecological reality of the Northwest. Thus, the problem lies not with a geographical imaginary in itself, but rather in those portrayals that substantially obscure or distort a region's problems when clarity is needed for effective social action.

Northwest Argentina: A Region and Its People

Since this book focuses on the power of geographical imaginaries, we will come to know the Northwest mainly through the eyes of historical actors involved in the malaria campaign. Their vision of the region, while always partial and often misguided, is a key part of this story. However, most read-ers require a more conventional initiation to this unfamiliar region. Today, Northwest Argentina officially includes six provinces, roughly from north to south: Jujuy, Salta, Catamarca, Tucumán, Santiago del Estero, and La Rioja (fig. I.1). This legal territorial designation originated in the 1940s with the regional planning initiatives of the first presidency of Juan D. Perón (many of which were tied directly to public health, as we will see in chapter 5). Until the mid-twentieth century, the region was usually called *el Norte* (the North), though it had fuzzier boundaries that sometimes embraced the federal terri-tories of Chaco and Formosa.[30] Although it is somewhat anachronistic, I will use the term *Northwest Argentina* throughout the book, for the sake of consis-tency. It is also worth noting that the vast majority of the malaria campaign's activity was concentrated in just three provinces, Tucumán, Salta, and Jujuy.

The Northwest's political divisions do not correspond at all to its physio-

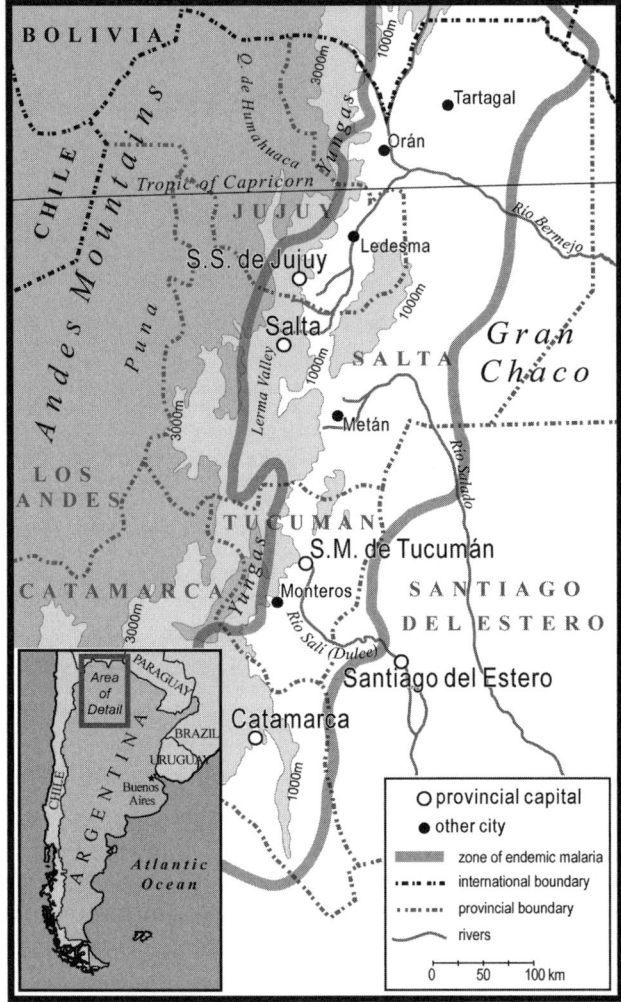

Figure I.1. Map of Northwest Argentina, ca. 1930, by author.

graphic zonation, which can be envisioned as three overlapping swaths that trend roughly from north to south. Moving across these swaths from east to west, elevation generally rises and the climate and landscape change accordingly. The Gran Chaco, a vast semi-arid scrubland, comprises the easternmost swath. As flat as Kansas, the Chaco features intermittent streams, seasonal marshlands, and thorny, scrubby vegetation. Though often called El Impenetrable, "the Impenetrable," opinions differ as to the origins of this label: some believe it derives from the hardpan soils that stymied the excavation of wells, while others credit the stands of thick vegetation that European settlers and armies found disorienting and nearly impassable. Due in part to its difficult geography and extreme climate, with temperatures of 40° Celsius typical in summer, the northern Chaco was one of the last areas of Argentina to be effectively integrated into the national state. Until the 1880s, indigenous tribes, such as the Mataco, Toba, and Wichi, lived peaceably and crossed unfettered over the barely controlled boundary between Argentina and Paraguay and Bolivia.[31] Similar to what happened in the Great Plains of the United States in the same period, railroads helped open the region to capitalist development. Cattle ranching and the exploitation of *quebracho colorado,* a hardwood used for tannins, railroad ties, and fuelwood, became major industries in the early 1900s. The Chaco ecological region dominates the eastern part of Salta Province, all of Santiago del Estero, and a portion of Tucumán.

Moving westward from the Chaco, as the Andes come into view, one gradually enters the subtropical foothills and valleys. Historically and today, most of the population of the Northwest has lived in this zone, which is also the center of agriculture, industry, and trade. The abrupt rise in elevation presents a major control on regional climate, especially the spatial distribution of rainfall. During the summer, moisture-laden winds traverse the Chaco and meet the Andean foothills; in turn, orographic lift produces rainfall, most of which falls on land below 2,500 meters. As these rising air masses lose their moisture, more arid conditions prevail at higher elevations. Precipitation patterns are highly seasonal, with marked wet and dry periods. San Miguel, the capital of Tucumán Province, receives on average over 100 millimeters of rainfall in each month from November through March, but only 20 millimeters monthly from June to September.[32] As a result of this seasonal pattern, stream flow is also highly variable: rivers draining the intermontane valleys tend to have wide, rocky beds that carry trickles of water in braided channels during the winter but turn to torrents in the summer. Heavy rainfall, warm temperatures, and rugged topography produce the typical vegetation type of middle elevations on the eastern front of the Andes, the Yungas. In Argentina, the Yungas biogeographic province, which extends well into Bolivia, is typified by subtropical hardwoods, including characteristic local trees such as *lapacho, cebil,* or *tipa;* microclimatic variability; and high species diversity in flora and fauna.[33]

Further westward, as elevation rises, the Yungas yield to more arid valleys, the Puna, and the highest peaks of the Andes. Moving upstream alongside the Río Grande in Jujuy, for example, one encounters the abrupt transition from humid subtropical lowland, through remnants of the Yungas forests, and into the arid, steep-walled valley known as the Quebrada de Humahuaca. Flanked by numerous alluvial fans, promontories of richly colored sedimentary rocks, and sparse vegetation, the *quebrada* has hosted a succession of agropastoralist civilizations for thousands of years, thanks in part to the virtues of irrigation.[34] Farther to the south, the Calchaquí Valleys offer similarly impressive canyon-land vistas, along with irrigated viticulture. At higher elevations, extremely dry conditions prevail, manifest in vast salt flats of the Puna, an extension of the Peruvian-Bolivian altiplano. This high plateau, not far from the Atacama Desert of Chile, is sparsely populated and has seen its fortunes rise and fall with dreams of exploiting mineral wealth, whether tin, copper, or, today, lithium.[35]

Mining, in fact, indirectly determined the region's settlement and control by the Spanish, starting in the mid-1500s. The colonial economy of the region was initially oriented not toward Buenos Aires, but north toward the mining district of Potosí, in present-day Bolivia. The precipitous growth of population and demand for food, animals, and other goods turned the present-day Northwest into a trade hinterland of Potosí. To service the mining center, the Spanish established a "line of settlements" linked on an overland trade route, starting with Santiago del Estero in 1553, followed by San Miguel de Tucumán, Salta, and San Salvador de Jujuy by the end of that century.[36] Politically, the region was integrated into the Viceroyalty of Peru, and Spanish armies subjugated the indigenous groups of the region, such as the Diaguita-Calchaquí. Yet even today, Quichua speakers remain in Santiago del Estero, while the Kolla of the Salta-Jujuy highlands maintain an indigenous identity.[37] The indigenous and Hispanic creole ethnic mixture of the region, combined with distinctive cultural landscapes, led one foreign traveler to remark in 1921, "It is within the district embracing Tucumán and Santiago del Estero that Argentine life begins to shade imperceptibly into the Bolivian or Andean."[38] While the roots, substance, and meaning of regional identity have always been hotly contested—as this book will show—contemporary scholars affirm the strong cultural affinities between Northwest Argentina and its Central Andean neighbors.[39]

Even before Argentina achieved its independence from Spain, the Northwest lost ground to Buenos Aires and the fertile Pampas that surrounded it. As the mining district of Potosí began its inexorable decline in the early 1700s, so went the fortunes of Tucumán, Salta, and Jujuy. Meanwhile, the Spanish crown's mercantilist policies eroded, and Buenos Aires emerged as the key port for the Río de la Plata basin. The creation of a viceroyalty with its capital in Buenos Aires in 1776 gave political validation to the emergent economic reality, and the Northwest eventually assumed the role of a remote hinterland to the port city. Although the Northwest played a key role in the Argentines' war against Spain, subsequent decades of political turmoil exacerbated the region's isolation and marginalization. In each of the provinces, caudillos and traditional oligarchies ruled, resisting economic change and efforts at political unification.[40] Complicating matters, the region was situated in a geopolitical cul-de-sac, sharing long borders over rough terrain with Chile and Bolivia, limiting somewhat the potential for international trade.

Remoteness, lack of good roads, and political strife put the Northwest at a disadvantage, and the region became largely disconnected from the process of capitalist expansion that connected Argentina to world markets. As the country as a whole experienced an economic boom in the late 1800s, the Northwest's prospects seemed to evaporate; as David Rock has remarked, Argentina's "growth enhanced rather than erased regional disparities."[41] Notably, from 1870 to 1910 the Northwest's population grew at a much slower pace than the rest of Argentina, which was buoyed by an influx of European immigrants (fig. I.2). Yet isolation also fostered the development of a largely self-sufficient internal market in the Northwest. Tucumán, particularly, had a "balanced and diversified economy that produced a variety of agropastoral goods and manufactures" by the middle of the nineteenth century.[42] But this province, with its dense population, high levels of capitalization, relatively egalitarian agrarian structure, and thriving bourgeoisie, proved exceptional in the Northwest. Technological innovation, investment, and political change came slowly to the other provinces, still dominated by conservative oligarchies, where semi-feudal conditions prevailed. The arrival of the railroad in Tucumán in 1876 initiated a new economic reorientation: while the region became the country's principal supplier of sugar, other regional industries deteriorated in the face of competition from cheaper foreign goods flowing through the port of Buenos Aires.

Thus by the early 1900s the seasonally hot and humid fringe where the Chaco plains graded into the Yungas foothills became the *zona azucarera,* the "sugar zone." The *ingenios* (sugar mills) of Tucumán set the technological and managerial standards for the region, and this tiny province produced over 80 percent of the nation's sugar by 1895.[43] Farther to the north and into the tropics, in the valleys of the Río Grande and Río San Francisco, the Jujuy-Salta sugar complex developed, somewhat later and on much larger, vertically integrated plantations.[44] Sugar wrought a dramatic environmental and social transformation throughout the Northwest. Previously unexploited land was put into sugarcane, most of the Yungas forests were lost, either to make way for fields or to provide fuel wood for the energy-intensive ingenios, and irrigation works expanded, especially on the large sugar estates. Meanwhile, the sugar zone became a magnet for migrants from other parts of the Northwest, as the rest of the regional economy reoriented toward the demands of the ingenios.[45]

This area of dynamic social and environmental change provided prime conditions for endemic malaria. Northwest Argentina was one of those sub-

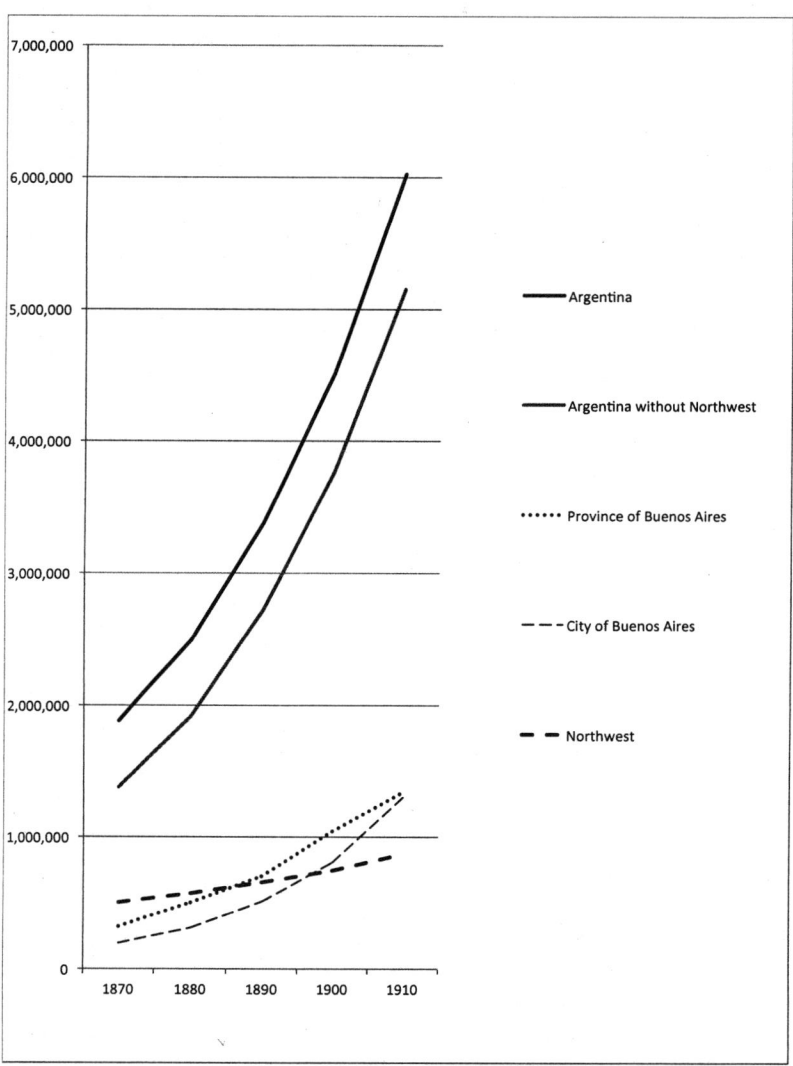

Figure I.2. Population change, 1870–1910. These are government estimates of decadal population change based on 1869, 1895, and 1914 national censuses. Northwest includes Tucumán, Salta, Santiago del Estero, Jujuy, Catamarca, and La Rioja. Argentina, Comisión Nacional del Censo, *Tercer censo nacional, levantado el 1 de junio de 1914* (Buenos Aires: Talleres gráficos de L. J. Rosso, 1916–1919), 2:xii.

tropical and warm-temperate areas of the world, along with the Mediterranean basin and the southern United States, where malaria thrived well into the twentieth century.[46] The Northwest, like these other regions, provided a climate that was broadly favorable for malaria transmission but, more importantly, featured environmental conditions appropriate for anopheline mosquitoes, particularly the *Anopheles pseudopunctipennis* mosquito, which lurks as an enigmatic protagonist of this book. This species is the highest-altitude malaria vector in the world, tolerating a broad elevational range, from about 500 to 2,500 meters above sea level.[47] At the same time, other often-invisible factors, such as grinding human poverty, unsanitary conditions, malnutrition, and internal migration, combined with natural conditions to make malaria endemic. Indeed, despite the virtual eradication of malaria, the Northwest, especially in remote outposts near the Bolivian border, continues to be something of a hotbed for vector-borne diseases, such as Chagas disease, dengue fever, and leishmaniasis, thanks to a combination of hazardous social and environmental conditions.[48]

Plan of the Book

While this book follows the long narrative arc of malaria control, from the recognition of malaria as a social problem to its effective eradication, each chapter brings a different theme into sharp focus. The first chapter centers on the primary issue of malaria and regional development. We will see how political and scientific elites of the Northwest linked malaria control to broader development goals and used the threat of disease to transform urban and rural landscapes of Tucumán and Salta. Chapter 2 explores the early years of the national Malaria Service, focusing on how state agents interpreted the nature-society dynamic of malaria through rational, bureaucratic practices of surveying, mapping, and administration. Their sometimes hasty appraisals of the disease ecology of the region suggested control strategies linked directly to wetland drainage, the perceived path to regional development.

With the malaria campaign floundering in the 1920s, political and ideological influences on the campaign multiplied and became more complicated. During this time, conflicting ideas of national "racial health" begin to affect the campaign, as explained in chapter 3. Argentina's malariologists looked admiringly to Fascist Italy for validation of large-scale environmental sanitation techniques, which were based on an organic or "socio-ecological" model of society. At the same time, however, regional scientists began to shape the ideology and scientific practice of the malaria campaign, sometimes in conjunction with American scientists from the Rockefeller Foundation, whose involvement in the malaria campaign was cut short by political intrigues. Chapter 4 analyzes an important shift in malaria control strategy that took place during the 1930s. Here, conflicting implications of the idea and practice of "ecology" are explored. Under the guidance of Carlos Alvarado, a revitalized Malaria Service shed a broad socio-ecological vision of progress, in exchange for narrowly focused control strategies that drew on insights from the budding science of ecology.

In chapter 5, I develop the theme of historical convergence to understand the rapid mobilization and success of the climactic battle against malaria in Northwest Argentina, which culminated in the effective eradication of the disease by 1950. This phase also represented the most overtly politicized use of malaria control, with populist leader Juan D. Perón using eradication as a platform to dramatically showcase his ambitious new public health policy. The conclusion offers lessons for understanding the relationship among development, environmental change, and malaria control today.

1

A Cure for Backwardness?

The Rationale for Malaria Control

The pulchritude of the streets, the regularity and frequency of street cleaning, also reminds me of German cities. Men armed with brooms and dustpans are always on the busiest arteries, cleaning and sweeping all day. . . . One must ponder the admirable effort of the municipality of Buenos Aires to sanitize and embellish the city, creating in this place of brick and iron a splendid mantle of vegetation and shade that nature had not provided.

—Jules Huret, *La Argentina de Buenos Aires al Gran Chaco,* 1913

Outside of the capital [Buenos Aires], all of the country can be written off as unhealthy. There are neither sewers nor running water, except in a few cities; there are no drainage or irrigation works, hospitals and sanitaria are practically unknown—in sum, all that the most elementary precepts of hygiene and health recommend, in order to make a region inhabitable, are missing.

—*Tribuna Popular,* Salta, 1905

At the end of the nineteenth century, there were, in a sense, two Argentinas.[1] In the thirty years or so since the end of a protracted cycle of political strife, Argentina had experienced a demographic and economic explosion. Primarily through the export of agricultural products, such as beef, wheat, and wool, the economy grew dramatically in the littoral region (in historical usage, Buenos Aires and the other provinces of the lower Río de la Plata basin). Networks of telegraph and railroad lines branched out through the fertile plains of the Pampas. Port cities such as Buenos Aires and Rosario grew upward and outward, fed by a steady stream of European immigrants. Buenos Aires was refashioned to reflect and rival the great European capitals of the day, with wide avenues, enormous parks, stately architecture, and trolley cars.[2] Prosperity enhanced the legitimacy and stability of the nation-state, as economic success and political consolidation were, in David Rock's words, "reciprocal and mutually reinforcing."[3] The nation's borders were established and secure, and the military subjugation of the country's native peoples had opened up the interior to be settled and reshaped by ranching, farming, and commerce.

This dynamic period transformed Argentine society. Yet intense interregional inequities marred Argentina's tide of prosperity. Far from the thriving ports and the fertile lands of the littoral, much of Argentina's interior found itself practically frozen in time. In economic and demographic terms, the country's most stagnant region was the Northwest, that corner of Argentina bordering Chile and Bolivia. This long-settled area, unlike the "empty" expanses and great cities of the Pampas, was mostly disconnected from Argentina's export-oriented boom. While the country as a whole experienced a demographic explosion, the Northwest experienced a net loss in population. Serious deficiencies in public health, including high infant mortality rates, rampant infectious diseases, and malnutrition, along with migration to other parts of Argentina, flattened population growth rates. Making matters worse, the region attracted just a small portion of the flow of immigrants from Europe to Argentina. Meanwhile, poorly developed transportation networks and distance from international markets diminished prospects for economic growth, and monetary and tariff policies killed local industry.[4]

In a land of apparently unending progress, the Northwest was largely static and inert. This intensifying polarization became a source of concern for elites of both regions. Leaders of the northern provinces saw great yet unfulfilled natural potential in their home region. For others, including many politicians, intellectuals, and scientists in Buenos Aires, the seemingly intractable problems of the region implied that national unification was still unfinished business. The persistence of such backwardness in a country making otherwise rapid progress challenged dearly held ideals of both liberal political economy and positivist science.

In this context of anxiety over sharpening regional disparities, malaria rose to become a problem of national importance, beginning in the last decade of the nineteenth century. While the disease was widespread in the Northwest at the time, it was not especially deadly, and other illnesses easily outranked malaria in the region's mortality ledger. Yet it was construed as such a threat to national well-being that by 1907 Argentina's congress had mobilized the resources of the federal government to undertake an intensive malaria control campaign. Why should this disease, above all other health and social problems in the Northwest, rise to such prominence? Why would containing malaria become an issue of national importance?

Malaria control emerged as a political issue because of the disease's role as a powerful symbol of the Northwest's malaise: malaria was a palpable marker of regional difference. Other diseases, such as tuberculosis or dysentery, may have been far greater killers, but malaria, unlike these illnesses, was basically isolated to the Northwest. Toward the end of the nineteenth century, social reformers, politicians, and scientific modernizers increasingly seized upon malaria as clear evidence of the region's underdevelopment.[5] Others proposed the stronger argument that malaria was the *root cause* of the Northwest's myriad shortcomings. Over time, elites developed a social narrative for malaria: the disease debilitated the working class, thus hindering economic development; it weakened the human organism, making it more vulnerable to the effects of physical and social ills, such as tuberculosis, alcoholism, and coca abuse; and it discouraged the influx of foreign immigrants and capital that were driving progress in Buenos Aires and the Pampas. Meanwhile, the failure to reclaim "waste" lands, particularly marshes and swamps, into productive and cultivated landscapes hindered the agricultural progress of the Northwest. Such lands were often synonymous with malaria hazards, so reclaiming them became seen as imperative to stimulating both good hygiene and agriculture. In short, elites proposed that the control of malaria would initiate a virtuous circle, leading eventually to idealized landscapes of health and wealth.

In constructing the political agenda for malaria control, elites sought to enact a certain type of development, one based on the rationality of modern science. When these men declaimed on the prospect of social progress, they did not advocate merely a brute form of capitalism; rather, they argued, often with great ardor, that science would lead the Northwest, and Argentina generally, away from "barbarism" and toward the ever-elusive goal of "civilization." Public hygiene was one of the great proving grounds for the role of science in this struggle between civilization and barbarism. The experience of Buenos Aires, itself in emulation of the great capitals of Europe, had demonstrated that investments in sanitary infrastructure could lead to social progress. Scientists played increasingly prestigious roles in the modern Argentine state. The Northwest's elite—many of them accomplished figures in medicine, engineering, and other sciences—wanted desperately to show their own region was on the same level of scientific excellence as the rest of the country, indeed, the world. Malaria control provided a key opportunity for such a demonstration.

This chapter focuses on the initial cycle of political action to control malaria as it developed into a problem of national interest. I begin with a more detailed examination of the role of science in Argentina's push toward modernization in the late 1800s, especially in the arena of public health. Underlying elites' diverse interests in public health was a constant preoccupation with Argentina's standing as a "civilized" country, in explicit comparison with Europe and North America. While this larger discourse of civilization and hygiene propelled efforts to control malaria, international science also played an influential role in how the disease was framed. Crucially, these initial framings of the malaria problem developed during a period of great flux in the scientific understanding of the disease. Malaria science in the 1890s mixed miasmatic and germ-based theories of the disease's etiology, justifying strong causal links between environment and disease. Although scientific consensus would eventually shift, the landscape-based ideas would become ingrained in strategies to fight the disease; these ideas were collectively known as *saneamiento,* or "environmental sanitation."

The remainder of the chapter traces the genesis of the "malaria problem" in the Northwest and the initial, tentative steps to control the disease. The key figure in publicizing the malaria problem was Eliseo Cantón, a scientist-politician of Tucumán. His work helped to inspire and legitimize early civic and provincial measures to control malaria. In Tucumán, the Northwest's most dynamic province, the governing class advocated malaria control for its potential benefits to agrarian development, but investment in sanitation actually ended up concentrated in the provincial capital. Meanwhile, in Salta, whose slow progress was more typical of the Northwest, malaria was construed mainly as an urban problem from the start. In both places, the transitional character of malaria science around the turn of the century legitimated the disease's connection to a broader set of sanitary and social problems.

Public Health and Development in the Two Argentinas

Improving public hygiene was central to Argentina's modernizing efforts in the late nineteenth century. The so-called Generation of 1880—a group of scientists, intellectuals, and political leaders—promoted a coherent program of national development derived, in large part, from European liberalism. This closely knit network of social elites presided over the consolidation of the Argentine state, the country's incorporation into the world economy as a provider of foodstuffs and raw materials, and the demographic explosion driven by European immigration. More broadly, the Generation of 1880 viewed national development as the product of a struggle between the forces of "civilization and barbarism," embraced Enlightenment rationalism and Positivist science, and celebrated all things European.[6]

These ideological tendencies converged perfectly in the public hygiene movement, a concrete and durable legacy of the Generation of 1880. As historian Diego Armus suggests, the "spirit" of scientific hygiene thoroughly permeated fin-de-siècle Argentina: it infiltrated an "infinity of spheres of social and individual life" and appealed to those across the political spectrum:

"liberal-conservative reformers, social Catholics, socialists, and even anarchists."[7] The value of hygiene was progressively internalized and reflected in such diverse social spaces as the hospital, the home, the workplace, and the streets, as well as in a transformation of individual behavior that eventually served as one pillar of a consumerist society.[8] The spirit of hygiene led also to tangible gains. The "pulchritude" of Buenos Aires observed by French journalist Jules Huret in this chapter's epigraph was the product of decades of investment in sewage, potable water, sanitation, and urban beautification. Yet, such advances made their way slowly to the interior provinces. This section explores the uneven growth of scientific hygiene in the late nineteenth century since this movement provided the main ideological and institutional framing for the beginnings of malaria control.

Advances in public hygiene and medicine play an important role in historical assessments of Argentina's "golden age" around the turn of the twentieth century. On the one hand, many historians celebrate the brilliance, foresight, and leadership of turn-of-the-century hygienists, mainly for their concrete contributions to the health and well-being of Argentine society.[9] While few doubt the benefits of improvements in basic sanitation and public health, in recent years scholars have offered more incisive critiques of the generation of progressive hygienists, underscoring their elitism, paternalistic attitude toward the working class, racial anxieties, perpetuation of male privilege, motives of social control, and inequities in implementation of public health reforms.[10] Whether critical or laudatory, few historians doubt the important role played by hygiene and allied sciences in shaping modern Argentina.

To the Generation of 1880, hygiene not only was the basis of improved health and well-being, but also served as a symbol of civilization. To them, nothing was quite so important as bringing Argentina into the ranks of the world's civilized nations. Their vision of progress entailed a conscious embrace and imitation of European (and, to a lesser extent, North American) cultural and economic institutions, along with a rebuke of Hispanic tradition.[11] Julia Rodriguez writes,

> Late nineteenth-century Argentine elites established a tradition of Eurocentrism that implied self-denigration and an idealization of all that was foreign. Intellectuals expressed an indiscriminate admiration for European art, music, architecture, food, and language. . . . They worshipped the values that they believed made Europeans and North Americans successful—hard work, thrift, and intelligence. These values, they believed, translated politically into democracy, secularization, and rational states and economically into a humming economy and profit. They envisioned an Argentina that, through emulation, would follow

the same path to development as western Europe and North America. They imagined themselves more European than South American.[12]

A key idea here is the "path to development." Argentina's liberal elites deplored most aspects of Hispanic culture, which they cast as retrograde. Only by emulating the most sophisticated nations could Argentina move along the path from barbarism to the glory of civilization and all it entailed.

This preoccupation with civilization and barbarism is worth examining more closely since it says so much about the way the Generation of 1880 framed issues of culture, race, nation, and health within a unified discourse. The political philosophers who preceded and inspired the Generation of 1880—most notably, Domingo F. Sarmiento and Juan B. Alberdi—laid the groundwork for liberal nation-making. Perceiving the poor moral, physical, and intellectual qualities of the country's creole, or *criollo,* stock, Sarmiento and Alberdi aggressively promoted European immigration as the solution to Argentina's longstanding cultural deficiencies.[13] Sarmiento memorably argued that "the principal ingredient towards order and ethics in the Argentine Republic is immigration from Europe."[14] Alberdi, political thinker and pioneering educator, expanded on this idea: "Each European who comes to our shores brings more civilization in his habits, which will later be passed on to our inhabitants, than many books of philosophy. We understand poorly what can't be seen and touched. A hard-working man is the most edifying catechism. . . . Do we want to sow and cultivate in America English liberty, French culture, and the diligence of men from Europe and the United States? Let us bring living pieces of these qualities . . . and let us plant them here."[15] Alberdi also formulated the famous dictum *Gobernar es poblar,* "To govern is to populate," establishing the promotion of European immigration as fundamental government policy. Under the direction of liberals such as Nicolás Avellaneda and Julio Argentino Roca, the Argentine government encouraged immigration through agricultural colonies, reimbursement of travel expenses to Argentina, and orientation and placement services for immigrants.[16] The racial ideas of Sarmiento and Alberdi became a standard part of the official government discourse; the introduction to the 1895 national census, for example, stated that the infusion of "Germanic, Anglo-Saxon, and Scandinavian races" would result in "a new and beautiful white race produced by the contact of all European nations fecundated on American soil."[17] In demographic terms, immigration transformed Argentina: by 1914, 30 percent of the country's population was foreign born; by comparison, immigrants made up only about 13 percent of the US population at the time.[18]

To be sure, the oligarchic Generation of 1880 did not view the effects of massive European immigration as completely salutary for the national character: by the turn of the century, the influx of Europeans of "lower quality," such as Italians, Spaniards, and Eastern Europeans, preoccupied elites; and many hygienists turned toward study and reform of the unruly urban milieu that immigrants had created in Buenos Aires.[19] Nevertheless, the Generation of 1880 continued to admire and attempted to emulate European ways, although elites tended to harbor fantastic and romanticized notions of the Old World: as Rodriguez argues, "It was not a real Europe that the Generation of 1880 emulated but rather an *idea* of Europe and what these Argentines considered Europe's most civilized and cultured nations, especially France and Britain. But Europe was, in fact, no paradise."[20]

In harmony with these generally Europeanizing tendencies, the Generation of 1880 also believed that a powerful modern state would be guided by the teachings of science; a more rational state could orchestrate society's energies toward constructive ends. According to historian José Luis Romero, the liberal oligarchy was determined to reform the state along these lines: "Instead of the ancient, semi-colonial state that endured until 1880, it seemed urgent to create a modern and vigorous state, endowed with the legal instruments that facilitated the full utilization of the flood of humanity that it now possessed for the realization of dreams of material wealth. All spiritual coercion, all of the forces that competed with the state, needed to be swept away; all of the instruments of government, on the other hand, had to be perfected and concentrated in the state."[21] While the government they created was far from perfect, the Generation of 1880 did manage to gradually consolidate power in the national state.

The alliance of state and science derived largely from the philosophy of European Positivism, which found favor in many other Latin American countries (Brazil, particularly) in the late nineteenth century. Most identified with the French philosopher Auguste Comte, Positivist thinking promoted empiricism and applied it to understanding and reforming the social arena. As Rodriguez says, "Comte's motto, 'Order and Progress,' appealed to members of the new Argentine ruling class. They saw it as a sure fix to the monumental 'backwardness' of their country."[22] As their confidence in science intensified, elites reframed problems such as malnutrition, poverty, overcrowding, and hazardous working conditions not as the outcome of social and economic processes, but rather as scientific conundrums whose causes, effects, and cures could be understood through rational means.[23] In Argentina, the role of science in identifying and correcting social problems extended not only to medicine and hygiene, but also into the fields of social pathology, psychology, criminology, and demography.[24]

Positivism, Europeanization, and the "civilization versus barbarism" discourse converged in the "science" of eugenics, which had many adherents among the leaders of Argentina's hygiene movement. As Nancy Leys Stepan argues, emphasis on hygiene and education distinguished the South American brand of eugenics that prevailed in the early twentieth century.[25] Contemporary European eugenicists, building on Darwin's evolutionary theory, Mendellian genetics, and the "Social Darwinism" of Herbert Spencer and others, increasingly adhered to the notion that biological characteristics were immutable. As a result, charity and social reform could never change the weakest members of society; the only way to prevent racial degeneration was to weed out those with undesirable traits, through specific immigration and marriage policies, or even forced sterilization. In contrast, a somewhat milder eugenics developed in South America, based more on Lamarckian concepts; in this formulation, learned or acquired characteristics could be passed on to future generations. Thus, progress in public hygiene or social welfare could lead to incremental improvements in individual organisms and the "race" as a whole.[26] As Eduardo Zimmermann points out, this premise underscored such diverse state projects as the control of infectious diseases, prevention of alcoholism and other vices, and the legislation of labor conditions for women and children.[27] "Racial poisons" or "social plagues" could be prevented, cured, or diminished through the rational application of modern science.[28] Thus, Argentinean eugenicists promoted public hygiene and education to forge and improve an Argentine "race," even as they advocated the "whitening" of this race through European immigration.

Promoters of eugenics and scientific hygiene interacted in well-connected, expert networks. Even as Argentina's population expanded and an urban mass society developed, into the early 1900s the world of national medical science was intimate and restricted. The medical school at the University of Buenos Aires was the nucleus of the "alliance of state and science for the advancement of hygiene."[29] By the late 1800s, the Facultad de Medicina eclipsed its peer institution at the University of Córdoba, becoming the premier site of medical research and training. The creation of other institutions solidified the country's scientific network. These included professional organizations such as the Argentine Medical Circle, Argentine Medical Association, and National Academy of Medicine; medical journals, such as *La Semana Médica;* and government agencies, most notably the National Department of Hygiene (Departamento Nacional de Higiene, known by its Spanish acronym, DNH), which figures prominently in the malaria story.[30] Hygienists were politically well connected, an integral element in the Generation of 1880. Formation in the medical sciences was a source of social prestige, and scientists were able to translate their scientific precepts into concrete political action. Pioneering hygienists such as Guillermo Rawson, José María Ramos Mejía, and Eduardo Wilde moved easily between the realms of science and politics, attaining high-level posts in liberal administrations, while other hygienists were active in electoral politics.

Notably, this network had a geographical structure, a detail that scholars have often overlooked. The core of this network was undoubtedly in Buenos Aires, and its influence spread inward toward the provinces. At the same time, the network extended outward, internationally, to some extent toward Uruguay and Brazil but, more pertinently, to Great Britain, France, and Germany. Just as in commerce, Buenos Aires served as the entrepôt for scientific innovations that tended to flow from abroad to the capital and from the capital out to the provinces. International medical conferences, sanitary organizations (such as the Pan American Sanitary Bureau, after 1900), exchange programs, the hiring of European faculty at the medical school, and the circulation of foreign medical journals were all elements that helped facilitate the incorporation of Argentineans into international scientific networks.[31]

The constant onslaught of epidemic diseases in Buenos Aires stimulated hygienists and gave urgency to their efforts. As in Europe, a general decline in health conditions accompanied early, explosive urban growth. At the same time that elites extolled urbanism as the apotheosis of civilized living, they were fully aware of the mortal dangers that it presented. An 1871 yellow fever epidemic in Buenos Aires, which killed about 8 percent of the city's population in four months, was a watershed event that launched the modern hygiene movement in Argentina.[32] With every succeeding epidemic, the state accrued power to promote and manage public hygiene. In the late 1800s, Buenos Aires faced epidemics of scarlet fever, cholera, bubonic plague, smallpox, measles, and diphtheria, even as the city's population skyrocketed.[33] With national development staked to international maritime commerce, the state invested in port sanitation to fend off global pandemics. A focus on the port led also to increased monitoring of immigrants' physical and mental health, to prevent the entry of degenerative or threatening elements. Established in 1880, the DNH became the central government institution for the promotion of hygiene, gradually accumulating responsibility for port sanitation, quarantines, infectious diseases, vaccination, hygiene education, venereal diseases, demography, food safety and inspection, medical exams and licensing, and the bacteriological institute.[34]

Somewhat at odds with the laissez-faire economic ideology of the Generation of 1880, the state became increasingly interventionist in matters of public health, especially where the urban poor were concerned. By the early 1900s, the government had a role in regulating cemeteries, slaughterhouses, bars, and brothels and controlling the width of streets and the height of buildings. Reporting of infectious diseases to the DNH and smallpox vaccination became obligatory. The government expanded its police powers to inspect and sanitize suspected "foci of infection" and to quarantine infected individuals in hospitals built expressly for that purpose.[35] Major epidemics became a rarity; infant and general mortality rates dropped dramatically. Hygienists could claim, legitimately, that health conditions and living standards in Buenos Aires were on par with those of the great European cities. Other major cities, such as Rosario and Córdoba, followed suit.

However, these innovations were much slower to reach the interior provinces and rural areas. In the first decade of the twentieth century, many hygienists would lament the geographical "disequilibrium" in health and sanitation that characterized the country, advocate the expansion of the power of the DNH into the provinces, and introduce measures for centralizing public health regulations under a national sanitary plan. Such radical changes in governance stalled due to the obstacles presented by constitutional federalism.[36] The national malaria campaign was an early attempt at centralization and expansion of state power over sanitation and hygiene.

The "Gospel of Hygiene" found favor in Argentina's Northwest, as well, among progressive politicians, scientists, and social reformers.[37] Many were repelled by what they perceived as the ignorance and backwardness (retraso) of their home region; just as Buenos Aires had successfully imitated the advances of Europe, so did many elites of northwestern cities hope to emulate the culture and values of the national capital. These elites realized, however, that significant projects to address the region's dire public health crisis were impossible, given the provinces' paltry financial resources. In malaria, these progressives would find a public health issue to galvanize attention at the regional and national levels.

Malaria Science in Transition

When did malaria become a problem in Northwest Argentina? Presumably, malaria had existed in the region since Spanish colonial times, perhaps even earlier.[38] In the local dialect, the illness was called *chucho,* a word derived from the Quechua *chúhchu,* meaning "shivers" or "chills."[39] This vernacular term indicates the longstanding relevance of the illness in popular thought, but it was the intellectual labor of scientists, politicians, and journalists beginning around 1890 that created the "malaria problem"—that is, malaria as the subject of sustained public attention and political debate.

Crucially, malaria became a social and political problem in Argentina during a time of great flux in scientific knowledge about the disease. In the latter half of the nineteenth century, advances in international malaria science redefined the disease and its relationship to the environment. For approximately twenty years, prior to acceptance of the mosquito's role in transmitting the disease-causing parasite, the scientific consensus mixed miasmatic and microbiological explanations of malaria etiology. Such an etiological framework reinforced the idea that malaria was a disease *of* the environment, generated by specific landscapes such as marshes and swamps. As a result, the analytical lens of medical geography typified early studies of malaria. Recent historical research has shown that bacteriology did not replace geographical and miasmatic explanations of disease abruptly and universally; rather, this transition was gradual, occurring at different times for different diseases.[40] In Argentina, a hybrid miasmatic-microbiological framework allowed malaria control to be linked to other sanitation efforts, such as the development of potable water and sewage systems. Moreover, this idea was "sticky": the broadly construed relationship between malaria and environment would continue to influence discourse and policy for decades, despite scientific innovations that might undermine this perspective.[41]

Well into the 1800s, the scientific understanding of malaria was based on miasmatic theory, which held that some illnesses emanated from corrupted environments.[42] Adherents of this theory accepted miasmas as invisible but real elements of nature and viewed certain landscape features and seasonal changes as sources of specific ills. Swamps and marshes were particularly fearsome: the heat of spring and summer led to the fermentation of stagnant water and the emanation of noxious vapors, which combined with other decomposing matter and were carried by the wind to produce a variety of human illnesses.[43] Other places of decay and decomposition in the rural and urban landscape were frequently singled out as hazards in need of cleansing or removal from human settlements: sewers, cemeteries, prisons, slaughterhouses, and so forth.[44]

Miasmatic theory was especially well suited to explaining the consistent recurrence of temperate-zone malaria in particular places at certain times of year. Though malaria in the nineteenth century was found through most of the world, in environments ranging from the Mississippi River basin to Italian cities to Andean valleys, in the popular and scientific imagination it was most identified with marshes or swamps. In such places, stagnant water combined with ambient heat to accelerate the processes of decomposition, fermentation, and emanation of malarial miasmas. There are linguistic cues to this landscape-based understanding of the cause of malaria. The English word "malaria" derives from the Italian *mal aria,* literally meaning "bad air." *Paludismo* and *paludisme,* terms for malaria in Spanish and French, respectively, come from the Latin word for swamp, *palus.*[45] Indeed, in Spanish-language documents of the late 1800s related to malaria, the meaning of such phrases as *terreno palustre* is ambiguous, since it could mean either "swampy terrain" or "malarious terrain" or both. Such vagueness cannot be completely resolved: rather, we should recognize that to the nineteenth-century mind, swampy and malarious landscapes were often one in the same. Yet we should also be aware that swamps and marshes were not viewed as the exclusive sources of disease-carrying miasmas.

Today, the notion of invisible, disease-causing emanations from the land may seem vague and imprecise, even outlandish. However, by the mid-nineteenth century a fairly sophisticated and internally logical body of miasmatic theory had developed. Physicians and other scientists did not necessarily make random, unsystematic appeals to the idea of miasma to explain illness. In the United States, for example, a government commission drafted an 1863 study, "Nature and Treatment of Miasmatic Fevers," that described the precise parameters of environmental conditions that produced malarial fevers. According to the report, miasmas rarely developed at temperatures below 60° Fahrenheit, and their development was halted completely at the freezing point; miasmas became more "abundant and virulent" as one approached the equator or the sea; dense vegetation was particularly hazardous because it trapped wind-blown vapors emanating from malarious locales; and previously healthy places could turn malarious because of a "turning of the soil," whether for agriculture or the construction of buildings, railroads, and canals.[46] Surveys such as this one relied on scientific tools of meteorology and topographical survey, not careless speculation. In addition, an abundant amount of empirical evidence supported miasmatic theory, and the drainage and sanitation of supposed malarial hazards often had the desired effect of diminishing the disease on a local scale.[47]

Toward the end of the nineteenth century, microbiological and miasmatic notions coexisted in scientific studies of malaria. In the 1870s, Italian scientists hypothesized the existence of a malaria bacillus, similar in form to the recently discovered tuberculosis bacillus. A few years later, in 1880, Alphonse Laverán, a French military doctor stationed in Africa, viewed the malaria germ under a microscope for the first time. Using blood samples taken from soldiers ill with the disease, Laverán saw protozoa in the shape of spheres and crescent moons, in rapid movement within and outside of red blood cells. This microorganism would come to be known as the plasmodium parasite, the infectious agent of malaria.[48] This discovery was soon confirmed by scientists in Italy, Germany, and Russia. Further laboratory studies revealed the microscopic evidence of the different parasitic agents of malaria, which corresponded to distinctive patterns of symptoms, mainly the periodicity and intensity of fevers and chills. Moreover, it could now be confirmed that quinine extract, whose curative powers over malaria had long been known, worked by destroying the parasite.

Yet one crucial question remained unresolved: how was the malaria parasite introduced into the human bloodstream? Scholars offered many hypotheses, falling into three broad camps: the parasite was waterborne, airborne, or insect-borne. Yet for almost twenty years after Laverán's discovery, no conclusive evidence was found to support any of these ideas. In the meantime, the concept of miasma was modified, with geography remaining central to comprehending malaria. The "malarious place" continued to be a salient category, but rather than emanating invisible vapors, many scientists believed that these fearsome places released, somehow, the newly identified infectious agent, the malaria parasite. Thus, prevailing medical notions of malaria mixed the old and the new.

Eliseo Cantón and the Construction of the Malaria Problem

During this transitional phase in malaria science, when miasmatic and microbiological explanations coexisted, malaria emerged as a subject of great scientific and political interest in Argentina, thanks largely to the work of Eliseo Cantón (fig. 1.1). A prominent figure in the world of medicine and public hygiene, Cantón had a lasting influence on malaria science and policy. His scientific studies—particularly *Malaria and Its Medical Geography in the Argentine Republic,* published in 1891—combined innovations in bacteriology and parasitology with detailed explorations of the physical environments of the Northwest, including descriptions of climate, hydrology, vegetation, soils, and geology. Cantón viewed malaria as a product of the environment: insalubrious landscapes generated malarial germs. In almost encyclopedic fashion, Cantón described the sanitary conditions of several northwestern places, illustrating the immense scope of, as well as local variation in, the malaria problem. He advocated malaria control not only for its health benefits, but also for the potential economic gains that would accrue to agriculture, industry, and local governments. Cantón, reflecting the ideology of the liberal oligarchy, also portrayed malaria as a racial poison and repellent to the civilizing force of European immigration. To him, the most efficient and long-lasting means of controlling malaria was to eliminate the sources of infection, which meant sanitizing insalubrious landscapes through drainage, cultivation, tree plantations, and other rational and productive land uses. In short, Cantón developed the fundamental bases for malaria control, which would prove surprisingly resilient despite major changes in understanding the disease's etiology.

Cantón crossed frequently and easily between the realms of science and politics. A native of Tucumán Province and a member of its ruling class, he studied at the prestigious Colegio Nacional in the provincial capital, which in the late 1800s matriculated most of the province's future leaders in medi-

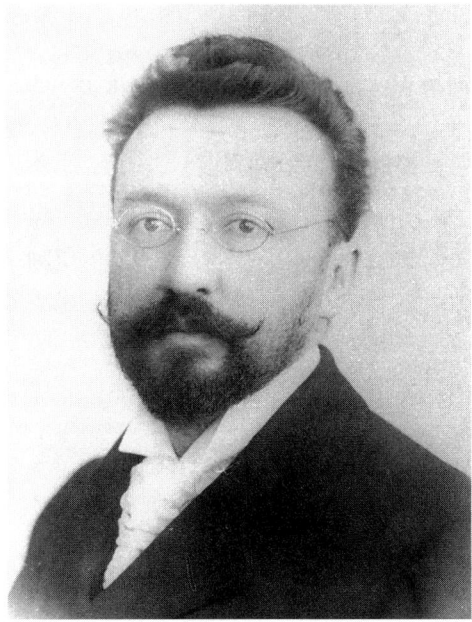

Figure 1.1. Eliseo Cantón. Photograph courtesy of the Archivo General de la Nación, Buenos Aires, Argentina.

cine, public health, education, and government, many of whom were close friends and colleagues of Cantón.[49] Subsequently, he studied medicine at the University of Buenos Aires, specializing in the pathologies of the Northwest. Soon after receiving his medical degree Cantón, along with Alberto L. de Soldati and Tiburcio Padilla Sr., organized the campaign against a cholera epidemic in Salta and Tucumán from 1886 through 1887. This leadership role fostered a political career for Cantón, which included terms as a provincial and national legislator from 1890 to 1912.[50] In this capacity he campaigned tirelessly for malaria control, civic beautification, construction of potable water infrastructure, and other sanitation measures. Later, he served for many years as dean of the medical school in Buenos Aires, the nexus of state and scientific interest in public health. Thus, Cantón was a politically well-connected member of an increasingly visible and influential class of elite intellectuals: "members of the Generation of 1880 and their students, the scientist-bureaucrats."[51] He directed his scholarly work, such as *Malaria and Its Medical Geography,* toward this audience; as a result, such works were a seamless hybrid of scientific treatise and political advocacy.

One influential aspect of Cantón's work was a methodology that relied on geographical surveys of areas afflicted by malaria. In this sense, Cantón was a product of his era, when medical geography was a standard lens for understanding health and disease. For example, medical geographies of every province of Spain had been published in the late 1800s, medical topographies were an instrument of British rule in colonial India, and many travel narratives of South America included descriptions of regional sanitary conditions.[52] Medical geography provided a framework for understanding the regional scale and the often-rural character of malaria in ways that hygiene, focused mainly on the city, could not.[53] Cantón was the first to survey malaria incidence throughout northern Argentina. *Malaria and Its Medical Geography* included detailed descriptions of nearly every department (i.e., county) of the northern provinces and territories, with details of topography, climate, soils, and hydrology; social and economic data; statistics on incidence of malaria and other diseases, when available; and identification and anecdotal accounts of several specific malaria hazards in the region. To give just one example, he described the province of Jujuy in these terms:

Its geographic situation, between 22°10′ and 24°20′ latitude, and bisected by the Tropic of Capricorn, places it within the environmental conditions most appropriate for the development of malarial fevers.

Fierce heat (referring to its plains), soils charged with organic elements, and rainfall nearly as abundant as that of the Chaco: nothing more is required for the *malaria bacillus* to develop with all of its energy, giving rise to the appearance of fevers as serious as those in the province of Salta.[54]

Within Jujuy, however, he found substantial geographic variation, with malarial conditions worsening, generally, as one moved east from high plateaus and valleys, through the humid foothills, to oppressively hot lowlands. Finer-scale distinctions in topography or climate helped explain the malaria situation for specific locales, such as the department of San Antonio, in the foothill region: "The department in general does not have large lagoons or swamps where malaria germs develop in such proportions as to occasion explosive epidemics, but there are low-lying, easily flooded areas and small marshes where malaria develops without any difficulty."[55]

Nearly everywhere he looked, by reading the landscape, Cantón found a local environmental source of malaria. In Rosario de la Frontera, near the Salta-Tucumán border, Cantón blamed irregular, rolling topography that allowed for the formation of marshes and lagoons. The "exuberant" vegetation of these wetlands, under the influence of summer's heat and humidity, produced an infamously malignant form of malaria, known as *chucho de la frontera*. In Yerba Buena and Tafí, just west of the capital city of Tucumán, malaria sprang not from wetlands, but from the "fierce and virgin earth" itself; the soil's intense fertility produced thick forests with abundant leaves and flowers, from which the "malaria germs developed prodigiously."[56] Wet rice farming was to blame for the persistence of malaria in some parts of southern Tucumán Province, while poorly constructed railroad embankments nearby produced miasma-generating pools of stagnant water. Meanwhile, in Catamarca malaria germs were ingested directly from a contaminated water supply. Though miasmas were usually invisible, they could be seen in the early-morning mists that formed over marshes and low-lying areas. In all, Cantón detailed the scope and cause of the malaria situation in about seventy different locales, throughout northern Argentina, even into the province of Corrientes and the territories of Chaco and Misiones.[57] Cantón synthesized his epidemiological findings in a large and exquisitely designed color map, offering the first cartographic portrayal of the disease in Argentina.

Using the empirical data from his malaria surveys, Cantón developed a general model of the environmental causes of malaria, which occupied the bulk of the book. Understanding the nature of the disease-causing agent—whether it was of "gaseous origin" or "miasmatic material" or a "microorganism"—was not the "primary objective" of the book. Rather, it was "sufficient for us to know that, whatever its nature, it occurs in places well known to us and evolves under specific conditions."[58] Thus, his primary concern was how environmental factors combined to give rise to malaria, and how these factors could be controlled or minimized. Cantón concluded that three elements were the "*sine qua non* of malaria: soil rich in organic matter, burning sun, and humidity."[59] Each was a necessary, but not sufficient factor in producing localized outbreaks of malaria. Fertile soils presented an organically charged medium for malaria to generate, whether as germ, gas, or vapor. The malignancy of malaria was roughly proportional to the intensity of ambient heat, explaining the generally favorable conditions of the subtropical north for the production of malaria, locally extreme conditions north of the Tropic of Capricorn, and the seasonal rhythm of malaria incidence. Humidity was broadly construed to include rainfall, water tables, damp soils, rivers, streams, canals, reservoirs, marshes, swamps, lagoons, puddles, and fogs. Where the three factors combined, a place became a source or focus of infection; absence of one of these factors would make an area malaria-free. In addition to the three major elements, Cantón also found other geographical factors influencing malaria. Proximity to a source of infection and direct contact with the land—as among farm laborers—increased the chances of acquiring the disease. By relocating to a slightly higher elevation, one could escape the influence of miasmatic clouds—Cantón estimated that a four-hundred-meter rise in elevation was sufficient. Prevailing winds, depending on their origin, could disperse miasmas.

Since malaria emanated from the landscape itself, Cantón deemed environmental sanitation (saneamiento) to be the key method of controlling malaria. He envisioned a future where the same key environmental forces that produced malaria (heat, abundant water, and fertile soils) could be managed and harnessed rationally, at once eliminating the harmful disease and providing for economic development. Nothing could be done to control the heating power of the sun, so sanitation efforts would focus on soils and water. Malaria hazards, according to Cantón's analysis, were found most often in "virgin" landscapes that had yet to be tamed and cultivated, where exuberant subtropical vegetation was allowed to flourish unchecked. The "vegetative potency" of these landscapes, including forests (bosques), scrublands (monte), or marshes and swamps (pantanos and ciénagas), had to be "diminished by way of repeated cultivation" in order to make malaria disappear.[60] He promoted every kind of agriculture (except wet rice farming) and scientific forestry as more rational, sanitary uses of the soil. Plantations of eucalyptus trees—which had been introduced to the Northwest from Australia in the 1870s—were especially beneficial. These trees dried out waterlogged soils, captured most of the nutrients available for other vegetation and malaria germs, and purified the air with their characteristic fragrance.[61] Of course, Cantón sought to eliminate sources of stagnant water, in cities and the country, yet counseled that wetland drainage had to be done in the winter months and followed by immediate cultivation of the area, or else risk unleashing malaria into the atmosphere.

With his emphasis on geographical survey and uncovering environmental causes, Cantón devoted relatively little space to the human element: how malaria was contracted, how it developed inside the human body, how it could be prevented or cured. Cantón presented a thoroughly anticontagionist perspective that precluded any transmission of germs from one person to another, directly or indirectly. At the same time, malaria had a deadly effect when combined with other illnesses, such as tuberculosis, gastrointestinal disorders, small pox, and cholera. In turn, these diseases, along with popular vices and habits such as alcoholism and sleeping outdoors, could make the human body vulnerable to attacks of malaria. Cantón wrote that malaria, "having become the lord and master of the soil in which it is propagated, . . . finds shelter and adapts well to all sorts of epidemics, but without permitting itself to be displaced by any of them, whatever their deadly power might be."[62] This stipulated relationship between malaria and other illnesses permitted Cantón, and others later on, to assert that malaria was one of the most dangerous and widespread diseases in Argentina, despite its apparently minor role as a direct cause of mortality. After Cantón, malaria was often treated rhetorically as a stand-in for other pathologies: that is, the consistent source of ill health that reigned between epidemics of more lethal diseases.

Cantón and his colleagues framed the malaria problem in the dualistic terms that prevailed among Argentina's Generation of 1880: that is, national development as a struggle between civilization and barbarism. In an 1897 speech at the medical school in Buenos Aires, he compared attitudes toward hygiene in "civilized nations" such as Great Britain, which had made large investments in sanitation, to those of Argentina: "What more eloquent example, what more suggestive fact could we find to prove the triumph of sanitary engineering and public hygiene, than the vigorous race of the English people in comparison with our own weak race, brought down by malarial fevers?"[63] The insidious character of malaria made it a racial poison; its continual presence in the air, soil, and water of the Northwest led to gradual racial degeneration. In an 1893 speech to the Círculo Médico Argentino, a leading organization of physicians in Buenos Aires, he made the case for increased investments in sanitation, particularly to improve malaria-infested water supplies. He argued that malaria "is an illness that eats away incessantly at the [human] organism, that destroys the physical body and enervates the moral being, that deprives man of his noblest initiatives, and even worse, degenerates the human species. Do you want proof? Travel through those populations [of the North] in the summer, drink the water that they consume; you don't have to look too carefully at the race to find certain indices of regression."[64]

The causes of racial degeneration could be found in the environment. Malarious landscapes were the epitome of untamed, unhealthy, and unproductive land, while agriculture and industry were civilizing, hygienic forces. Cantón stipulated an inverse relationship between a place's degree of civilization and the destructiveness of malaria: "Malaria does not belong to the class of diseases that are born and develop in human settlements, but rather comes alive in the solitude of the forests or in the uncultivated and deserted lands, fleeing as savages do from centers of population."[65] Such assessments vilified unused land as not only wasteful but downright dangerous. Thus, he repeatedly argued, investment in hygiene and sanitation was not merely an act of benevolence, but rather a shrewd economic strategy, moving the region and country along the path of development.

Malaria was an obstacle to one of the most important civilizing forces, European immigration. According to Cantón, the progress of the Northwest depended on an infusion of European immigrants who would educate through example and mix with the criollo population.[66] Gradually, the superiority and potency of the European race would overpower the inherent deficiencies of the criollo stock. Here, Cantón echoed the racial formulations of the Generation of 1880, inspired by such luminaries as Alberdi and Sarmiento, and anticipated the racialist ideas of Argentine eugenicists and hygienists such as José María Ramos Mejía, Emilio Coni, and Gregorio Aráoz Alfaro.[67] But he also transmitted the attitude of Tucumán's ruling class: sugar elites perceived criollo workers as "uncivilized and, above all, unreliable."[68]

To promote immigration, provincial governments had to commit to bringing malaria under control. Once malaria began to diminish, the curative and civilizing power of the immigrant would take hold. Cantón envisioned a future order where biological reality legitimated social hierarchy: European migrants, though superior in most respects, lacked experience of malaria and therefore needed to be protected from manual labor. Therefore, "the native sons" (criollos), who were more acclimated to the disease, would continue laboring in sugarcane, rice, and tobacco fields and, in general, "any occupations that put man in immediate contact with the soil," including, ironically, as laborers in sanitation works.[69] The precise social or occupational role for Europeans was left unstated, but Cantón was convinced that malaria prevented these superior beings from revitalizing the stagnant Northwest.[70]

The basic arguments of Cantón's *Medical Geography* would be largely accepted in the years that followed, both in scientific research and political action on malaria. Malaria was the most prevalent endemic disease of the Northwest; and though it caused little mortality on its own, it debilitated the working population, made it more vulnerable to other diseases and vices, and gradually degenerated the race. The fear of malaria kept foreign immigrants away from the Northwest, and since immigrants were the major force for civilization and economic development in Argentina, without the control of malaria the Northwest could not hope to make progress. Finally, malaria originated in unhealthy, unproductive landscapes; and the transformation of these environments, whether intended for development or sanitation, served both purposes. These ideas persisted despite the rapid changes in understanding of malaria, especially the incorporation of the role of the anopheles mosquito in the transmission of the disease. As the experiences of two northwestern provinces, Tucumán and Salta, demonstrate, fear of malaria could be marshaled to justify urban and rural development via the transformation of insalubrious landscapes.

Malaria and Development in Tucumán

Political efforts to address the malaria problem began at the local level: provincial elites of Tucumán and Salta built arguments for developing sanitation and directed local and national funds toward those efforts. Studying these cases more closely is important since they provide further insight into elites' preoccupations with sanitation as the foundation of progress and civilization, demonstrate how the work of Cantón and other scientists was used to build political arguments for malaria control, illustrate sanitary conditions in the provinces during the late 1800s, and show the impact of sanitation works on local landscapes and society. We will also see how the deficiencies of locally administered sanitation campaigns led to the increasing involvement of the national government in public health matters of the Northwest.

From early on, the political elite of Tucumán used the threat of malaria to rationalize the need for government planning and subsidies of agricultural development. The ruling class of Tucumán exemplified a provincial oligarchy, tied to one major industry, that enjoyed favorable relations with a strong national executive branch during the period of Argentina's intense economic expansion, from 1880 to 1914.[71] The Tucumán oligarchy, composed mainly of large landowners, agro-industrialists, and their scions, nurtured the sugar industry. As Donna Guy explains, the Tucumán oligarchy successfully maintained subsidies from the national government for the industry through direct stimuli such as railroad construction as well as protectionist measures such as tariffs, quotas, and internal taxes. The additional cost of subsidized sugar was usually passed on to urban consumers of the littoral.[72] This transfer of funds through the national government to Tucumán's government was the price of maintaining political order. Despite frequent global and domestic crises of overproduction, subsidies allowed the sugar monoculture of Tucumán to intensify, with the area planted to sugarcane in this small province increasing almost tenfold between 1888 and 1915.[73]

As a result, Tucumán's political-economic circumstances differed somewhat from those of the rest of the Northwest. There was a thriving real estate market, an expanding and dynamic bourgeoisie, and a relatively large contingent of small- and medium-sized farmers, independent from the sugar mills. Tucumán was also a magnet for farm laborers throughout the northwest region, especially during the *zafra* (sugar harvest) that took place during the winter dry season. Tucumán's population grew much faster than that of neighboring provinces, though much of that growth came at the expense of those same provinces, especially Santiago del Estero and Catamarca, rather than from European immigration.[74] Transportation and communication networks, along with protectionist policies, integrated Tucumán effectively into the structure of the national economy. Tucumán's elites were also well connected to the national ruling class, whose leading figure, Julio Argentino Roca, was a Tucumano by birth and generally supportive of provincial interests.

For all of these reasons, Tucumán was not nearly as "stagnant" or "backward" as neighboring provinces, although it is important to note that the province's own elites often applied such terms in severe self-criticism. Far from passive, and concerned about falling behind the rest of the country, the provincial oligarchy used government action to pursue an energetic developmentalist agenda. This program was based on the construction of public works, particularly roads, railroads, dams, and irrigation canals at state expense (frequently by channeling federal funds) to ensure the expansion of agricultural production. For example, during the 1890s Governor Lucas Córdoba led the effort to build a dam at La Aguadita on the Río Salí, to irrigate new lands to the east, in the department of Cruz Alta, which became a major zone of sugar production; and several more dam-building and irrigation initiatives followed.[75] At the same time, Tucumán's governing elites tended to direct provincial budgets and private funds toward the modernization and beautification of the provincial capital, San Miguel.[76] As we will see, improvements in hygiene, including malaria control, arrived in the city first and later spread to sugar mill towns and the countryside.

Initially, Tucumán's leadership linked malaria control to agricultural development, anticipating or echoing many of Cantón's concerns. Two major concerns united malaria control and agrarian development: drainage and labor. Drainage for sanitation purposes could be combined with the rationalization of agricultural water use. Tucumán's water supply and sanitation problems, in the formulation of some elites, stemmed not from an absolute moisture deficit—the province was well watered during the long summer—but rather from an imbalance in the distribution of water. The fertile lands nearest the foothills supported high yields of sugarcane and a dense human population, but they suffered from permanent or seasonal excesses of water that produced expanses of wetlands. Meanwhile, soils in the drier eastern half of the province could not be effectively exploited without channeling water through irrigation canals. Draining and filling swamps, the key sites of miasmatic emanations, and channeling their excess waters to parched terrain would thus serve a dual purpose by putting more land into production and reducing threats to human health.

Following this line of reasoning, in a January 1889 address to Tucumán's legislature, the progressive governor Lindero Quinteros highlighted the "intimate connection" between irrigation works and the sanitation of malarious landscapes.[77] It was not so much the disease itself as the category of "malarious lands," virtually synonymous with wastelands, that was the target of improvement. "Through the sanitation of malarious lands," wrote Quinteros, "will come the stimuli to the agricultural producer by way of foresighted laws. The causes that maintain our agricultural wealth stationary will also disappear, teaching the worker that his efforts will not be sterile when certain regions can count on easy and inexpensive irrigation, and that his lands will no longer be just one more dead asset on his hands."[78] For the next two decades, proposals to study or improve the province's irrigation systems nearly always carried a sanitation rationale.[79] These included proposals for building dams and associated irrigation networks at state expense and the prohibition of bodies of stagnant water on private or public lands. Few of these proposals turned into laws, and few of those laws were actually executed. Nevertheless, the persistence of the idea among political elites is noteworthy and indicates the larger development framework in which they imagined malaria. "Waste" lands, from the perspective of production, were synonymous with insalubrious lands.

Beyond the direct connection between environmental sanitation and rational use of water for agriculture, sanitizing "malarious lands" would also help solve the province's labor shortage by encouraging immigration from Europe. In 1898, a national commission investigating agricultural development confirmed that the province's population growth had not kept pace with the sugar industry's high demand for labor, making the province dependent on indigenous peoples and criollos from nearby provinces, especially for the labor-intensive zafra. Although the foreign-born population in Tucumán doubled between the censuses of 1895 and 1914, most European immigrants settled in San Miguel, not in the countryside. Only a small fraction of the massive number of immigrants arriving in littoral ports each year chose to cross the Pampas and settle in Tucumán. In 1914, according to the national census, Tucumán had only 32,618 of the 2,357,952 foreign-born residents in the country, or roughly 1 percent.[80]

With Tucumán's economy thriving, what was preventing immigrants from pouring into Tucumán in search of opportunity? Many speculated that the region's high disease burden and fierce climate—construed as the same problem—repelled Europeans, who found it more difficult to acclimate to such conditions. Thus the 1898 commission's report referred vaguely to "etiological considerations" and "very notorious causes" that inhibited immigration.[81] Cantón was more clear: "Make malaria disappear from the regions where it is endemic, or at least tend toward its decline, and we guarantee that agriculture will develop on its own. Workers go where fertile lands exist, as in the provinces of the North, but fear of malaria stops them in their tracks. To fight malaria, then, is to promote agriculture."[82] Governor Quinteros, for his part, hoped to transform Tucumán's agrarian sector through colonization schemes similar to those enacted in the provinces of Santa Fe, Córdoba, and Entre Ríos: "The drainage and sanitation of malarious lands is . . . a necessity that commands us, if we wish to bring to our land the civilizing labor of the immigrant," said Quinteros.[83] Such planned colonization efforts never came to fruition, but such statements reflect the elites' preoccupation with attracting European immigrants to improve land and life in the Northwest. Revealing their social priorities, elites seldom noted the impact that malaria had on the well-being of the laborers already employed in agriculture, local criollos and indigenous groups, instead placing emphasis on guaranteeing the health of Europeans not yet arrived. Strangely though, no one seems to have pointed out that a sizable portion of immigrants were coming from parts of Spain and Italy where malaria was as commonplace as it was in the Northwest.

Although they focused mainly on agricultural development, provincial elites also used the threat of malaria to campaign for sanitary improvements in the city. In August 1895, Eliseo Cantón, by then a member of the national congress, proposed a bill to authorize a loan of one million pesos from the federal government to the province of Tucumán for the construction of a potable water supply in its capital and largest city. On the floor of the Congress in Buenos Aires, Cantón offered a long and grandiloquent speech in defense of his proposal that echoed many of the sentiments and findings of his well-regarded works on malaria and public hygiene. As if speaking of two different countries, Cantón compared the fortunes of Tucumán with those of the city of Buenos Aires. In the nation's capital, ordinary citizens enjoyed a temperate climate, fresh sea breezes, and clean and abundant water; meanwhile, in Tucumán, people lived as if "under a Biblical curse," forced to endure fierce heat, foul and heavy air, and impure water.[84] In Tucumán's capital, Cantón observed, the general mortality rate was approximately forty-four per one thousand, a rate unknown in any "civilized country," while in Buenos Aires it was much lower, on par with European capitals.[85] Fully one-third of Tucumán's deaths could be attributed to malaria, argued Cantón, either ordinary malaria, "pneumonia of a malarious origin," or "gastroenteritis due to malaria."[86] Cantón's arguments were persuasive: Tucumán obtained its loan, and by 1898 the first potable water was delivered to the city. Years later, one local historian reflected that this event marked "a victory of civilization" for the citizens of Tucumán.[87]

Civic beautification complemented the development of sanitary infrastructure in the elites' quest for civilization. They used the threat of malaria to build support for the creation of public parks. In San Miguel, malaria played a key role in the long campaign to build Parque 9 de Julio, the city's major public commons. At the time of San Miguel's relocation to its present site in the seventeenth century, the central plaza was situated about five blocks from the western bank of the Río Salí. Over the next two hundred years, the main channel of the river migrated about two kilometers east of the city center, leaving behind a low-lying area dotted with marshes and prone to seasonal floods. This area, covering about four hundred square blocks, was often cited as the source, first, of malarial miasmas and, later, as a breeding ground for malaria-carrying mosquitoes. Thanks mainly to the efforts of Alberto L. de Soldati, a national senator from Tucumán, the federal government contributed over 100,000 pesos to the drainage and filling of the area to create the city's main park, Parque 9 de Julio, which served, as one newspaper remarked, both "hygienic and aesthetic purposes." One of the era's best-known landscape architects, the French immigrant Carlos Thays, designed the park, which still features drainage channels and eucalyptus groves that testify to saneamiento's role in civic beautification. The major parks in Salta (Parque San Martín) and Santiago del Estero (Parque Francisco de Aguirre), also constructed in the first decade of the twentieth century, were similarly inspired by elites' concern for simultaneously fighting malaria and creating well-ordered and verdant public spaces.[88]

The Tucumán oligarchy often assumed a paternalistic attitude toward the "subaltern" classes, seeking to "civilize" and "moralize" them through cultural events, labor regulations, public education, and public health legislation.[89] In their treatment of public health issues, elites' paternalism is transparent; and in this respect, they shared the outlook of hygienists in the national capital. Sometimes the sugar mills themselves provided services (such as free medical care) toward this end, but usually the provincial government (often channeling funds from the national state) provided hospitals or sponsored public health campaigns. Elites' interest in public hygiene was driven by boosterism and civic pride, and possibly by the common tendency of scions of industrial elites to attempt to distinguish themselves in the arenas of arts, science, and medicine. Many of the "native sons" of Tucumán's close-knit oligarchy from the late nineteenth and early twentieth centuries, such as Eliseo Cantón, Gregorio Aráoz Alfaro, and Alberto L. de Soldati, were models of the hybrid scientist-politician, going on to play key roles in legislating malaria control and other aspects of public hygiene. These elites were a vanguard of a progressive class, which did not necessarily dominate Tucumán politics, but did make important contributions in public health, education, and the arts.

This constant striving for the hallmarks of "civilization" and "progress" had a negative counterpart, which could be described as a regional inferiority complex. Tucumán's oligarchy was extremely self-conscious of the region's shortcomings, constantly comparing the sluggish Northwest to the rapidly advancing Buenos Aires.[90] Elites' concerns went beyond objective evaluations—say, comparisons of population growth or mortality rates—and into debates over the validity of perceptions. Malaria was of paramount concern not necessarily because it was truly dangerous, but rather because the *perception* of such a risk abroad had the effect of denigrating the region as a whole. One Tucumán newspaper encapsulated malaria's perceived "geography of danger" in this way: " 'The malarious lands,' they say with terror in the littoral and in foreign lands when talking about this region of the country. And before this phantasm, immigration holds back, capital does not take risks, labor does not dare to come here, to challenge the dangers of the endemic. Such dangers are exaggerated—we know that—but we must do everything we can to make the endemic disappear, precisely for that reason: because at a distance, the phantasm exhibits enormous contours."[91] In such statements, Tucumanos acknowledged that external perceptions shaped the geographical imaginary of the Northwest. These perceptions were slow to change and threatened the region's economic well-being. The "phantasm" of malaria even undermined Tucumán's efforts to become a tourist destination, particularly during its characteristically sunny and mild winters.[92] The Tucumán elites viewed themselves as a progressive, civilizing force, yet found it necessary to constantly prove that they "belonged" in the modern age and that provincial culture was "at the same level as Europe"—or at least Buenos Aires.[93] This competition with Buenos Aires, along with the usual veneration of cities in Spanish America, may explain why the benefits of malaria control, hygienic modernization, and beautification accrued to San Miguel before the rest of the province. Yet at other times regional elites took advantage of the perception of backwardness, in an almost strategic fashion, when advocating for national government funding for sanitation and development.

Hazards of the Urban Environment in Salta

North of Tucumán, the provincial capital of Salta was another notorious hotbed of malaria. Today, the city nicknamed Salta la Linda (Salta the Pretty One) is a major tourist destination, a garden spot known for its benign climate, picturesque streets, colonial architecture, and cleanliness. Salta's situation at the turn of the twentieth century, on the other hand, could hardly have been worse. In 1901, a commission organized by the National Department of Hygiene warned, "The index of general mortality in Salta is the highest known in the country and the depopulation of the city is accelerating."[94] The president of Salta's own Board of Hygiene wrote, "It would not be an exaggeration to compare Salta to a floating asylum of colossal dimensions, such is the number of the sick, and the quantity of the water that wells to the surface."[95] Epidemics of every type assailed the people of the city, who lived also with the constant burden of malaria.[96] Even as late as 1916, an article in the US-based *Geographical Review* reported that Salta maintained "its reputation for paludinal fever."[97] Compounding Salta's miserable sanitary state was a moribund economy, provincial fiscal crisis, and a tradition-bound ruling class. Compared with the dynamism of Tucumán, Salta seemed like a sleepy, ailing vestige of the colonial era.

What accounts for Salta's tremendous change from a "veritable pesthole" at the end of the nineteenth century to a clean, healthy tourist attraction a hundred years later?[98] In many ways, the story of how Salta confronted its demographic crisis and transformed its alarmingly substandard hygienic conditions is a classic tale of urbanization and modernization: a maturing city overcomes the misfortunes of geographical circumstance through a constant, purposeful reshaping and domestication of the natural environment. The story of Salta also shows that associations between the health of a place and the health of its people are always strong and persist despite changes in popular understandings of medicine, biology, and environment. Miasmatic theory framed early assessments of Salta's unsanitary conditions and recommendations for how to improve the city's public health at the end of the nineteenth century. Concrete advances included a detailed public health census, mapping of sanitary hazards, construction of a potable water infrastructure, drainage of wetlands and saturated soils, installation of a sanitary sewer system, and civic beautification through tree planting and the creation of a major city park. Older ideas that associated disease and landscape would continue to influence sanitation efforts, reshaping the urban landscape for years to follow.

Without fail, nineteenth-century political elites, journalists, and hygienists indicted Salta's sixteenth-century founders as the culprits in the city's dire sanitary situation. At the northern end of the valley that would bear his name, the Spanish army officer Hernando de Lerma selected a marshy area, surrounded by rivers and streams, for a new settlement.[99] Unfortunately, according to Cantón, Lerma "did not have the opportunity to study the geology of the terrain, letting himself be guided only by the attractions of a magnificent and beautiful landscape."[100] This boggy plain had a slight incline roughly from northwest to southeast, and at the time of Spanish settlement it was crisscrossed by numerous creeks and dotted with marshes and lagoons.[101] While the Spanish may have chosen this site for the natural protection it afforded from indigenous tribes, promoters of civic hygiene in the late 1800s lamented "the laziness and selfishness" of the city's founders, who had "condemned succeeding generations to suffer the inclemency" of the site they chose.[102] The combination of summer's heat, humidity, and flooding produced unhygienic conditions, which at the end of the nineteenth century were framed in a mostly miasmatic discourse. Nevertheless, despite the shortcomings of its site, Salta became an important colonial trading center since it lay on a key supply route between Tucumán and the mining district of Potosí, in modern-day southern Bolivia.[103] As the economic center of gravity in Argentina shifted decisively toward the littoral in the late colonial and early republican period, however, Salta faded in importance and fell into a state of steady decline.

Since the early colonial era, the city and private landowners had constructed various canals in an effort to rectify streams, reduce the saturation of the soil, drain lagoons and marshes, and carry away storm water. By 1900, a rudimentary drainage network was in place. The Canal del Sud or Tagarete drained the downtown area: it was an open canal, roughly ten feet wide, running from west to east in the middle of a major thoroughfare, three blocks south of the central plaza. Six blocks north of the plaza, roughly parallel to the Tagarete, was the Zanja del Estado. Both discharged into the Zanja Blanca or Tincunaco, which ran from north to south along the foot of Cerro San Bernardo; this large canal carried water into the Río Arias. This system, however, was far from perfect. Its capacity was limited: summer rains tended to overwhelm this network of drainage canals, and water took its natural course, flowing across the city from northwest to southeast, through the streets. As the soil underlying the city became saturated, springs developed in streets and even inside houses. With the water table so near the surface, human waste in pit latrines or street gutters frequently contaminated drinking water from wells. In 1895, a sanitary commissioner reported that thousands of tiny springs were "invading" the city, many of the city streets were completely flooded, and the ground beneath the houses was practically an "immense swamp" that seriously threatened the lives of the city's inhabitants.[104] With its high water table, wrote Cantón, the city practically "floated on an immense subterranean lake."[105] Moreover, the city was "surrounded on all sides"—particularly toward the southwest and southeast—by marshes, swamps, and lagoons, the "principal foci of infection."[106] A survey undertaken by the National Department of Hygiene in 1901 identified 62,876 square meters (about 6.3 hectares) of marshes in the city and its immediate vicinity.[107] The largest of these, the Laguna de Chartas, would merit mention in nearly every report on Salta's sanitary conditions, into the 1930s.

According to all contemporary observers, this unhygienic environment not only offended the senses—comments often focused on the nauseating sights and smells of city streets—but also gave rise to diseases of every kind. Building on a hybrid microbiological-miasmatic etiology, public health reformers focused on the relationship among soils, waters, and air. To them, the soil was in essence a semi-permeable membrane, which in healthy cities offered a discrete barrier between subterranean water and the atmosphere. The problem in Salta was that the soil, water, and air mixed promiscuously, creating miasmas charged with contaminated organic matter and dangerous microorganisms.[108] These miasmas were almost synonymous with malaria. Echoing Cantón, a local physician wrote that in Salta "the conditions for the development of malaria are always found together: soil charged with abundant organic matter, permanent humidity, and the heat necessary for fermentations, conditions which are joined with generally poor domestic and individual hygiene."[109] A few years later, the National Department of Hygiene reported that contaminated soils of the city were "appropriate for the development of every kind of micro-organism, and constitute breeding grounds for specific pathogens and poisons, and their decomposition gives rise to the formation of great quantities of unhealthy and poisonous gases."[110] Malaria germs and other microorganisms contaminated the rustic water supply, dependent on wells. Thus, the air people breathed, the water they drank, and the food that they ate were little better than poison.

Sanitarians and journalists worried that the city's appalling sanitary conditions would lead to demographic stagnation, perhaps even an outright population collapse. Local newspapers took a consistently alarmist tone in their reporting of epidemics, mortality, births, and deaths. In some years, deaths outnumbered births in Salta, and with minimal immigration from abroad or other provinces, Salta's population growth had stagnated.[111] Sanitary surveys corroborated Salta's status as the deadliest city in Argentina: the general mortality rate in the city from 1894 to 1900 was, on average, an astounding 44.2 per 1,000. By comparison, in 1899 the death rate in Buenos Aires was 17.0 per 1,000; in London, 19.2 per 1,000; and in Madrid, 30.1 per 1,000.[112] From 1869 to 1895, no city in Argentina had grown as slowly as Salta; in that period, as Salta grew by about 21 percent, Buenos Aires expanded by 254 percent, and Rosario by 290 percent.[113]

Of the specific diseases that assaulted the city, malaria was viewed as the principal cause of death and misery. As the disease most closely associated with the city's pernicious physical environment—its contaminated soil, water, and air—malaria was seen as the "soil" in which the "seeds" of other diseases might find purchase. Malaria, which was seldom treated properly, created a state of general malaise and illness, affecting almost every person at some time in his or her life. In Salta, malaria was commonplace: a census of sanitary conditions taken in 1897 found that 1,288 of the city's 15,000 residents reported a bout of malaria in the preceding year; malaria outranked the next leading cause of illness by a ratio of about nine to one.[114] Malaria was assumed to be everywhere: breathing the air or drinking the water could be sources of infection. In this situation, the frail populace was made more vulnerable to other illnesses. Salta suffered regularly from typhoid fever, dysentery, pneumonia, typhus, and tuberculosis. It faced frequent epidemics, including cholera (1886–1887), smallpox (1890, 1901–1902), diphtheria (1892), influenza (1894), pertussis (1896), measles (1896–1897), and bubonic plague (1899–1900).[115] Salta's population was deficient in other ways; the province had the second-highest rate of "idiocy" (after Jujuy) and extremely high incidence of deafness and goiter.[116] In sum, health conditions in Salta were pitiful and ripe for reform.

Upper-class Salteños viewed the city's public health woes and unhygienic environment as poignant evidence of Salta's lack of a civilized culture. They condemned the filthiness, ignorance, laziness, and fatalism of local people. Such archaic traits held back progress and led to neglect of the urban environment, which in turn conditioned cultural norms. A self-styled progressive segment of the upper class predictably assailed the culture of the lower classes. Dr. Ricardo Aráoz, president of the local board of hygiene, disparaged the "the poor nutrition of the working class, their disorderly habits, the fact that they sleep on the floor," along with their chaotic backyards, "where all matter of filth accumulates, [including] excrement, garbage of every type, horse droppings, waste water, etc."[117] A local newspaper condemned popular vices, such as the consumption of yerba maté tea, which "predisposed the organism to easy access by malarial microbes."[118]

Yet, perhaps surprisingly, newspapers and public health advocates reserved the most ferocious critiques for Salta's tradition-bound oligarchy.[119] Imbued with a spirit of *noblesse oblige,* progressive critics held the working class blameless for their conditions: they did not know any better. The government, however, had abdicated its responsibility for promoting the well-being of the citizenry, teaching them the ways of civilization, and maintaining them in hygienic living conditions. With the city once again under the threat of bubonic plague, one newspaper wrote: "We have achieved a certain level of culture and civilization, which the moral education of the lower class contradicts entirely. The distinguished society of Salta is similar to a dress made of luxurious silk that hides the underwear of a filthy person, and the municipality should take care of such incongruities, since it is charged with safeguarding public health."[120] Local newspapers consistently lambasted the municipal board of hygiene as corrupt, inert, and indifferent in the face of epidemics and unable or unwilling to enforce sanitary regulations.[121] Assessments of municipal hospitals and clinics were equally pessimistic: these were places where poor people went to die, not to be cured.[122] In short, the growing clamor for improving public health was backed by a potent moral critique: paternalistic, yes, but thoroughly critical of Salta's civic culture, from top to bottom.

Given the limitations of local leadership and resources, Salta turned to the federal government for help. In an 1897 letter to the president of the National Department of Hygiene, the head of the local board of hygiene pleaded for federal intervention to address Salta's sanitary problems. Without such help, "the population will continue to be decimated, immigration will keep its distance, and our fertile soils will serve only to produce diseases of every kind."[123] Almost immediately, the DNH responded favorably, budgeting 100,000 pesos for a preliminary study.[124] This study, building on the work of Aráoz, entailed a detailed survey of the city's topography and geology, a house-by-house survey of the built environment and available sanitary infrastructure, and comprehensive epidemiological statistics.[125] The resulting report by the DNH recommended comprehensive transformation of the city's infrastructure. The first priority was to drain the soil and reduce the number of marshes in and around the city. Existing canals would be deepened, straightened, and lined with rocks or concrete, but the most significant change to the civic landscape was the construction of a major new drainage canal, running from north to south, about six blocks to the west of the central plaza. This rock-lined canal was intended to capture part of the load of the Zanja del Estado and to drain the western marshes, in particular the massive Laguna de Chartas, via smaller ditches. This channel, today's Canal de la Esteco, would empty into the Río Arias, ten blocks due south of the plaza. As another measure for draining the soil, the sanitary commission proposed the planting of eucalyptus and pine trees southeast of the city center, near the marshy confluence of the Canal de Tincunaco and the Tagarete. The next step was to improve the system of rainwater drainage. Streets in the city center would be paved, and a system of gutters and storm drains, leading to the city's various drainage canals, would be constructed.

The DNH also projected a separate system for provision of clean, running water. The source of the city's water supply would be the *quebrada* (narrow canyon) above the town of San Lorenzo, about ten kilometers northwest of the city. The water from this fresh stream would be delivered by the force of gravity to the city in a main pipe running beneath Caceros Street, which bisects the city from west to east. The final element in the sanitary plan was to construct a system of sewers and a filtration plant, even though flush toilets were practically unknown in the city. The entire project was budgeted at 1,176,373 pesos, a rather high amount for an impoverished city of fifteen thousand people. The Department of Hygiene took pains to justify this amount, performing an elaborate calculation of the monetary benefits of the plan: if the mortality rate could be cut in half, with each human life valued at 1,215 pesos, the project would pay for itself after five years.[126]

More important were the effects that sanitation would have on investment, development, and immigration. Following Cantón's line of argument, the sanitary commission argued, "The day that Salta can give guarantees of health and recovers the commercial activity it had in another era, . . . surely its sons will not emigrate because the immense lode of a prodigious nature and a beautiful climate will forcefully attract not only the native sons, but also immigrants arriving in the country in search of new regions, where they can carry the contingent of their reproductive force."[127] The "crossing of the races" or racial mixing that would follow from increased immigration would lead to a decline in inbreeding, viewed as another cause of poor health, and contribute to the "physical, moral, and intellectual development of new generations."[128]

This plan was quickly executed. In 1902 the national congress approved the plan and disbursed the funds necessary to carry it through; the following year, Salta's provincial legislature began to make the necessary acquisitions of land and water rights.[129] By 1905, construction had begun, first on the widening, deepening, and lining of the Zanja Blanca.[130] With the assistance of other federal funds, the area designated for special tree plantations was developed into the city's major park, known today as Parque San Martín. This lovely green space, designed by the legendary French landscape architect Carlos Thays, is today forested with trees originally planted as part of sanitation efforts; and the park's centerpiece is a magnificent fountain in an artificial lagoon.[131] Thus began the long transformation of Salta from a city of filth and disease to "Salta la Linda."

Conclusion

This chapter has traced the "discovery" of malaria as a social and public health problem in Northwest Argentina. Although the disease, known vernacularly as *chucho,* had been endemic in the Northwest for centuries, it was only in the 1890s that politicians, hygienists, and social reformers began to pay close attention to it. The recognition of this disease threat stemmed from a nexus of broader developments in political ideology and scientific knowledge. First, during this period malaria became an important marker of regional difference. The political elites of the Northwest, especially the sugar oligarchy of Tucumán, seized upon the debilitating presence of malaria to explain the region's characteristic "backwardness." Building on this idea of disease as a marker of regional difference, many provincial and national elites put forth the argument that malaria control could be a tool for regional development. Eliseo Cantón and other members of the ruling class believed that controlling malaria through agricultural and urban sanitation measures, particularly by reclaiming of wetlands, would initiate a virtuous circle of health and progress. Sanitation of malarious lands would open up new areas for agricultural development, improve the health and productivity of the rural proletariat, and, perhaps most importantly, attract the "civilizing labor" of European immigrants.

Finally, many of the basic assumptions about malaria, and its relationship to the natural and social environments of the Northwest, developed during a period of great flux in scientific understanding of the disease. Scientists mixed elements of germ theory (or bacteriology) with older, landscape-based miasmatic concepts. Even laypeople saw the world this way: a 1908 article in a Tucumán newspaper made reference to both "malaria-carrying mosquitoes" and "poisonous miasmas" emanating from marshes.[132] Within such a hybrid framework, scientists and political figures could find cause of the disease in certain landscapes, particularly marshes, swamps, and other wetlands. With this understanding, they could also link malaria to other modernization efforts. The ideas and experiences of this formative period would also have a decisive impact on the ways that malaria scientists constructed models of malaria and the environment and formulated control strategies based on these models. Specifically, the Malaria Service would hold fast to landscape-based models that dictated, preferentially, drainage and reclamation of rural and urban wetlands. The directors of the national malaria campaign, into the 1930s, would continue to associate agricultural development and malaria sanitation, without strong consideration of mosquito dynamics. The late nineteenth-century construction of the malaria problem would prove to be surprisingly persistent.

2

Launching the Campaign

Suffice it to say that we cannot aspire to a place among the cultured
peoples of the world as long as we have not put into practice the means
of combating illnesses and reducing the death toll, up to the limits that
science permits, and in that way assure the general welfare, which is the
essential purpose of government!
> —Alberto de Soldati, *Diario-Senadores,*
> September 23, 1905

In 1900, malaria "invaded" the city of Santiago del Estero. Even in a region accustomed to epidemics, the virulence of this outbreak was alarming. Although only some 150 kilometers southeast of Tucumán's capital, the
city had until that time been considered beyond malaria's endemic zone.[1] In
fact, Cantón had not even bothered to mention Santiago, Argentina's oldest city, in his medical geography. Lying at the edge of the vast Chaco plain,
the somnolent, colonial-style city enjoyed a semi-arid climate and absence
of marshlands, qualities that had once made it a refuge for malaria sufferers
from Tucumán.[2] Yet, by the time malaria reached its peak in the city in 1902,
approximately 72 percent of its 11,409 residents had been infected, a rate far
higher than any previously recorded in Argentina.[3]

As in Salta and Tucumán, Santiago del Estero's government was ill equipped
to handle the epidemic. A hastily assembled board of hygiene, led by Dr.
Antenor Alvarez, conducted comprehensive epidemiological and topographic
surveys to determine the source of the problem, not unlike the legendary
actions of John Snow during the 1854 cholera outbreak in London. Alvarez used epidemiological maps to pinpoint the principal breeding ground for
malaria-carrying mosquitoes near the city's center.[4] This body of stagnant
water adjacent to the Río Dulce was the unintended outcome of a badly
planned levee, which had blocked an outlet for flood water. Alvarez arranged
for the site to be drained, filled, planted to eucalyptus and other trees, and
converted into a large city park. The sanitation of this site appeared to conclude the epidemic almost as dramatically as it had begun, with new malaria
cases declining steeply after 1902. For years afterward, this incident would
be cited in Argentina as the classic success story of malaria control through
environmental sanitation.[5] Alvarez himself, in future publications and con-

ference papers, would reflect on this apparent triumph and reinforce the association between wetland reclamation and malaria control.[6] He would also parlay this public health success story into a political career, eventually representing Santiago del Estero as governor and national senator.

The Santiago del Estero epidemic proved pivotal in the history of malaria control in Argentina. Integrating important advances in international malaria science, Alvarez recognized the mosquito's role in malaria transmission and applied that knowledge to control efforts for the first time in Argentina. Discovering and scrutinizing the mosquito's routines would become the fixation of malariologists worldwide for the next fifty years. Yet in Argentina, at least, recognition of the mosquito's role did not represent a clean break with past conceptions of the malaria problem. Just as miasmatic and microbiological frameworks coexisted through the 1890s, the role of the mosquito was rapidly accepted without completely displacing older concepts of malaria etiology.[7] The mosquito connection simply offered a clarification of earlier views: that is, a more precise explanation of why certain landscapes, such as marshes, swamps, and other areas of standing water, became malaria hazards. More importantly, Alvarez's sanitation efforts in Santiago confirmed that drainage of infectious foci could rapidly reduce malaria incidence. Thus, the emergence of the mosquito hardly altered conventional and commonsense notions of malaria's place in the landscape and how to attack the disease at its source. The basic logic behind *saneamiento* was not questioned.

The epidemic in Santiago del Estero was crucial for another reason: to many prominent hygienists and politicians, it suggested that malaria was spreading from its source in the Northwest to other parts of the country. Cantón's medical geography, legislative studies of malaria in Tucumán, and reports on Salta's sanitary situation, discussed in the previous chapter, generally portrayed malaria as endemic and entrenched, not a traveling epidemic. Malaria had been seen as a constant presence in the areas where it was found, although its intensity could vary seasonally and from year to year. It was the product of the particular conditions *of a place* and characteristic of that place, not a contagion that spread from place to place. In this sense, malaria was distinct from diseases such as cholera or bubonic plague, which indeed traveled, often over large distances, as newspapers of the Northwest reported, nervously and expectantly.[8] Quite suddenly, after the Santiago del Estero epidemic, the nature of malaria had changed: it seemed poised to spill beyond its traditional boundaries, threatening the rest of the nation.

Although Buenos Aires was a long way from Santiago del Estero, the spreading threat of malaria made it a national problem, not one of purely regional scope. Perceptions of a peripatetic menace, however irrational in retrospect, provoked concern among hygienists and politicians in Buenos Aires.

The problem now seemed much closer to home. Argentina's hygienists had always been obsessed with threats from abroad, but now danger appeared to be spreading from the interior toward the capital. Advocates of federal intervention to address the malaria problem, whether from the affected provinces or not, embraced this new geographical imaginary. In the aftermath of the Santiago epidemic, the national government, mainly through the action of the DNH, took an increasingly active role in addressing malaria.

In this chapter, I focus on the formation and early action of the national Malaria Service and its reception in the Northwest from roughly 1900 to 1920.[9] During this time, the social power of hygienists in Argentina reached its zenith. They were supremely confident in their own knowledge and ability and in the capacity of rational science to solve social problems. The creation of the Malaria Service extended the national "alliance between state and science" into the provinces to promote national development.[10] The Argentine state played a key role in constructing the malaria problem by enframing it in particular ways. As many scholars have noted, modern states operate according to bureaucratic logics that grant them a particular "way of seeing." States use tools of "scientific" statecraft—including surveying, mapping, and statistical compilation—to enable more rational and orderly visions of the societies under their control and to deepen the reach of the state into social life.[11] Throughout the world, not least in early twentieth-century Argentina, public hygiene was a key avenue for increasing the state's control over social life while naturalizing and depoliticizing its acts through a verbal and visual rhetoric of rationality. The malaria campaign in Argentina fits this modern concept of the state's role. Yet scientific statecraft did not pay immediate dividends, in large part because the self-assured ideology of progress through science and technical mastery of nature concealed state agents' muddled understanding of the human ecology of malaria in the Northwest.

This chapter begins with an exploration of the bureaucratic and political genesis of the national Malaria Service. The deliberations of scientific advisory committees of the DNH and the national congress over malaria control policy reveal the diverse rationales behind the malaria campaign and how these translated into campaign strategy. Next we examine the initial action of the Malaria Service, with a primary focus on a series of surveys conducted by DNH bureaucrats in the Northwest in 1911. Here, the theme is the particular "ways of seeing" employed by state agents, typified by the use of new technologies that offered rapid appraisal of the afflicted region. These surveys, representing a continuation of medical geographic methods, offered a hazy understanding of the epidemiology of malaria, mainly confirming the landscape-based notions of saneamiento. The remainder of the chapter examines the practice of malaria control into the 1920s, moralistic and unrealistic attempts at hygiene education, and the setbacks and frustration that the Malaria Service encountered due to fiscal crisis and popular resistance.

Toward a National Malaria Campaign

The epidemic in Santiago del Estero triggered a new cycle of study, debate, and legislation on malaria, this time at the national level. Complying with directives from the president and national congress, and under the auspices of leading hygienists, the DNH took control of the malaria problem, becoming the exclusive government agency for all matters related to the disease. In 1900, the DNH published its first pamphlet on malaria prevention, which explained the newly discovered role of the mosquito in malaria transmission, and distributed gratis fifty thousand copies of it throughout the malarious zone.[12] Around the same time, the DNH conducted investigations on the malaria situation in each of the affected provinces.[13] The first national commission on malaria convened in Buenos Aires in May of 1902 to synthesize the results of these provincial surveys, discuss the latest scientific advances from abroad, and develop a national policy to control the disease. This commission was led by Dr. Carlos Malbrán, one of Argentina's leading bacteriologists, a native of Catamarca, and president of the DNH, and included leading hygienists and politicians from the Northwest.[14] Eventually, after some legislative fits and starts, the prescriptions of this commission evolved into Law 5195, which established the legal, administrative, and technical bases for malaria control in 1907. Most importantly, it created the Malaria Service, under the direction of the DNH, with authority in the afflicted provinces, making Argentina one of the first Latin American countries to create an agency expressly for the purpose of malaria control.[15]

The creation of this new institutional framework required compelling political arguments, especially to overcome a key structural obstacle to creating a national malaria control program: constitutional federalism. The respective roles of the provincial and national governments had been the focus of decades of conflict in Argentina, a debate not completely settled with the constitution of 1857 and the federalization of Buenos Aires in 1880. Though the national state became ever more powerful in the late 1800s, the principle of provincial autonomy was still cherished in many quarters. Thus, proponents of malaria control developed a case that transcended parochial concerns. Malaria control advocates, still influenced by a medical geography framework, characterized malaria as entrenched in the peculiar social and environmental conditions of the subtropical Northwest, yet they also portrayed the disease as a national threat. Provincial governments, hygienists claimed, were incapable of addressing the problem while the DNH had the necessary resources and technical know-how. Ultimately, the support of local politicians and media in the Northwest made the national malaria campaign possible. Regional elites relinquished provincial autonomy to procure what was essentially a federal subsidy for local development.

Hygienists affiliated with the DNH amplified the basic arguments for malaria control that had emerged before 1900. Malaria was the main obstacle to progress in the regions where it was endemic, predisposing the population to other diseases, debilitating labor, and leading to high mortality and gradual depopulation while discouraging the civilizing force of European immigration. Malaria, Malbrán asserted, was the "principal" factor of the Northwest's elevated morbidity and mortality; though it was not necessarily lethal on its own, it eroded the resistance of the human organism to attack by other illnesses. Despite the recognition of the mosquito-and-parasite etiology of malaria, it was still widely construed as a product of hazardous or insalubrious environments that urgently required sanitation. In relaying the planning activities of the DNH and congressional debates on malaria control, the media of Tucumán and Salta approvingly reproduced this development-centered case for the campaign.[16]

Although the impact of malaria on the Northwest was clear, how could it be considered a national problem? First, malaria seemed poised to spread from the endemic zone to other regions of the country. Hygienists seized upon the epidemic in Santiago del Estero as the foremost exemplar of this phenomenon, but also made the dubious argument that the provinces of Córdoba, La Rioja, and Catamarca had only recently begun to experience malaria, following the development of improved transportation routes that connected these peripheral areas to the core of the malarious region in Salta, Jujuy, and Tucumán.[17] The 1902 commission concluded that "either in sporadic or epidemic form, it can be said that malaria has been observed in all of the Republic." They even cited the speculative claim of Guillermo Rawson, a patriarch of Argentina's hygiene movement, that malaria epidemics had occasionally occurred in the city of Buenos Aires, in marshes around the Palermo district.[18] In congressional debate on the malaria bill, Antonio F. Piñero, representing the national capital, emphasized the spatial trajectory of the disease: it was a mobile threat that had to be stopped, or else it would destroy the "vitality of the nation" in a way that "no other country on earth" had experienced.[19] Thus, Piñero reasoned, the necessity of federalizing the malaria campaign superseded questions of provincial autonomy.

Here, Piñero gestured at a more subtle argument for malaria control, which conceived of the nation as an *organism* whose integrity was undermined by any threat from within or without. Malbrán argued that a national law for malaria control was necessary because "trying to defend the vital and productive elements of extensive and important regions, and the sanitary and economic solidarity of the country, demands safeguarding its weak points, so that the *national organism* does not suffer."[20] In 1900, Soldati wrote to Piñero that malaria "not only debilitates the body, but also drains the energy of the soul, making the populace passive and indifferent, apt to endure tyranny, and incapable of reaction."[21] Unafraid of superlatives, on the floor of the lower house of congress Piñero argued that malaria threatened to produce "the degeneration of our race." In turn, Soldati appealed to the powerful obsession of Argentina's liberal elites, the struggle between civilization and barbarism: passage of the malaria bill, and public health legislation generally, was indispensable if Argentina wished to join the ranks of "civilized nations."[22] Piñero and Soldati referred to the "shame" (*vergüenza*) of malaria's continued existence and the injustice of regional inequalities it reflected in such a rapidly advancing country.[23] This rhetoric of this incipient organic nationalism, connecting race, nation, health, and environment, would only intensify over time.

Probably the decisive and most practical argument for the intervention of the national government was that the provinces lacked the financial capacity and scientific expertise to manage malaria control. The alliance between science and the state for the promotion of national development had its own geographical imaginary, in which Buenos Aires was clearly the metropole, and the provinces and territories, its satellites. To Malbrán and most of his fellow hygienists, the DNH was the only agency with the expertise, resources, and knowledge to carry out government action in matters of public health. The fatalism and inertia of the malarious Northwest stood in stark contrast with the optimism and progress of the scientific hygiene movement in the capital. Malbrán proclaimed the new avenues opened by a microbiological understanding of the disease: thanks to the "conquests of science," malaria no longer had "absolute dominion" over the regions where it was endemic.[24] With scientific tools in hand, fighting malaria was mainly a question of government taking wise action based on the "counsels of science."[25] In this respect, malaria control advocates shared the vision of Julio A. Roca and the Generation of 1880: a powerful central state, organized on rationalist principles, should orchestrate national development.[26]

Surprisingly, perhaps, provincial media readily accepted the superior capability and natural authority of the national government in matters of public health. Newspapers in Tucumán and Salta concurred that their local governments were not up to the challenge of malaria control, or any other action in favor of public health. The papers complained incessantly about local and provincial boards of hygiene that were charged with a broad set of duties, such as the maintenance of sewers, drains, and canals; responding to epidemic outbreaks; managing medical clinics for the poor; and guaranteeing the safety of food and medicines. These boards, according to local media, were idle, incompetent, and corrupt, habitually abandoning their public duties in the face of public health emergencies.[27] In Salta, the condition of the major hospital, El Milagro, became the basis of dark satire that featured smug and inept doctors ushering their patients toward untimely deaths.[28] Medical assistance in the countryside was practically nonexistent, except in some sugar mills; without competent and scientific care, citizens turned to *curanderos* (folk healers) and patent medicines. Moreover, local media wrote approvingly of politicians who could obtain federal subsidies for provincial development. Tucumán's delegates to the national congress, such as Soldati and Cantón, were especially adept at procuring federal funds not only for disease control, but also for hospitals, parks, and irrigation and drainage canals.

Thus, in the Northwest the birth of the federal malaria campaign was celebrated: as one Salta newspaper put it, "All of you people with faces pallid and lips dry from fever, listen: at last, your suffering is going to end."[29] After the passage of Law 5195 in 1907, provincial legislatures quickly ratified DNH authority over malaria control. The governor of Tucumán remarked that "the action of the national government, with the powers that it has available, simplifies this problem enormously, offering us the definitive sanitation of the malarious regions in a relatively short lapse of time."[30] To hygienists of the DNH, this was an early though tentative victory for the centralization of public health authority in the national government. Probably few at the time would have wagered that it would take another forty years before the disease would be effectively eradicated in the Northwest.

Surveying the Malarious Lands

Despite the existence of previous medical geographies and the knowledge of local experts, the Malaria Service did not yet know the territory under its jurisdiction. Large-scale topographic maps were nonexistent or incomplete, administrative boundaries were vaguely defined and subject to change, and essential demographic, social, and economic data were also hard to obtain. More central to the issue of malaria control, the directors of the DNH lacked a vision, literally, of the Northwest. What were housing conditions like? Where were medical services available? Which communities would be best served by Malaria Service clinics? Most importantly, where were malaria hazards located; what was their extent; how could they be sanitized; how much would it cost? To answer such questions, the newly installed directorate of the Malaria Service confronted the unfamiliar territory of the Northwest through the classic explorers' tools of surveying and mapping. Maps were accompanied by other essential technologies of the modern state, photography and statistical compilation. All together, they comprised a new "way of seeing" particular to the state, a bureaucratic spatial conquest.

In 1911, José Penna, president of the DNH, commissioned a special survey of the malarious lands, headed by Germán Anschütz, a physician, and Antonio Restagnio, a sanitary engineer. In effect, this was the third major appraisal of the geography of malaria in the region, following Cantón in 1891 and the DNH commission in 1902. In May and June of 1911, this expedition surveyed parts of the provinces of Catamarca, Tucumán, Salta, and Jujuy by railroad, on horseback, by car, and on foot. The *Annals* of the DNH published the results of this survey in 1911 and 1912.[31] At over one hundred pages, with dozens of photographs, maps, and diagrams, the survey provided detailed descriptions of the geography of the malarious zone, locale by locale. Anschütz and Restagnio also synthesized the survey results into a general sanitation plan or model. The apparent precision, technical proficiency, and comprehensive scope of the surveys demonstrated the "distanced sense of vision" with which the state held and exercised its power.[32]

Malaria Service maps had at least three intertwined objectives, some more apparent than others. First, they served as general and specific descriptions of northwestern locales, which served to increase the state's storehouse of geographic data. However, since there is no "pure" description or one-to-one correspondence between the map and the object being mapped, a process of simplification and generalization immediately took place.[33] This process was implicated in a second objective: the Malaria Service analyzed data from its surveys to characterize schematic or generic spaces where malaria was likely to be found. Thus these maps served as a rubric for interpreting landscapes and planning control efforts throughout the region. The least apparent, but still fundamental, purpose of these mapping projects was to deepen and extend the presence of the national state in the Northwest and to establish effective control over social space.[34]

All three of these objectives—description, abstraction, and extending state power—were interwoven in the presentation of the survey. Restagnio and Anschütz presented critical data in three key modes: the itinerary, the map, and the photograph. Discoveries from each mode of presentation—each "way of seeing"—were cross-referenced to one another. The bulk of the report consisted of a detailed itinerary of the expedition, presented mostly as journey segments from one railroad station to another. By 1911, several railroad lines crisscrossed the Northwest, mainly to link the region's *ingenios* (sugar mills) to national markets. The density of this rail network was highest in the principal sugar-growing province, Tucumán, where most lines ran roughly north-south, perpendicular to the general drainage pattern. For most of the expedition, the surveyors identified potential malaria hazards as they moved along the rails, probably at full speed and with few stops.

Anschütz and Restagnio located the hazards precisely, with reference to towns, landmarks, or railroad kilometer markers. For example, traveling south along a 115-kilometer stretch of the Provincial line in Tucumán Province (Ferrocarril Noroeste Argentino), the surveyors identified over ninety distinct hazards, including "excavations with water" 300 meters outside of Lules, "excavations for embankments, with water and very swampy, and full of aquatic vegetation" between 103.0 and 101.7 kilometers, near Famaillá; and numerous "irregularities" and "depressions" in the terrain where water could collect.[35] As the Provincial line cut directly across the general drainage pattern, railroad embankments slowed the flow of water from the foothills to the west, borrow pits for excavations filled with water, and poorly designed bridges and culverts created bottlenecks. Thus Restagnio and Anschütz recognized, at a glance, that natural features alone could not explain the abundance of standing water, and instead they blamed anthropogenic features resulting from railroad engineering. Their report is filled with several such itineraries (displayed as tables) along all of the major rail lines of the region, and usually only around major population centers did they get a closer look, on horseback, on foot, or by car.

The detailed itineraries were cross-referenced to sketch maps (*croquis*). These very large-scale maps (about 1:1,000 scale) depicted malaria hazards such as marshes, swamps, excavations, ponds, streambeds, and other areas of standing or sluggish water, along with a limited number of other features (such as railroads and buildings) for context. Though simple, these maps follow many of the conventions of modern cartography, including a plan view, standardized symbols (e.g., for railroads and roads), text labels, and consistent scale. The real-world coordinates of each *croquis* are established only by reference to the accompanying itinerary. The report culminates in a set of strategic maps, which graphically display a generic, recommended plan for sanitary engineering in the region.

The DNH surveyors also represented the northwestern landscape in photographs. Forty photographs accompanied just one report of the 1911 expedition, published in the *Annals* of the DNH, and these were reproduced in other reports. Most of these photos depicted malaria hazards in the landscape, organized not by location along the itinerary, but instead by type. One type of malaria hazard, "marshes located in the irregularities and depressions of the terrain, located within the urban or suburban area of malarious communities," was exemplified in photos of marshy areas of towns in Salta, Catamarca, and Tucumán. Generally, the images depict landscapes improbably devoid of people, although buildings, fences, houses, and railroad tracks indicate a human presence. Even in a series of photos of "model" residences—in the sense of "typical," not "ideal"—of the vulnerable poor, the only human figures are presumably men affiliated with the DNH expedition, dressed as they are in coat, tie, and hats. Overall, the photographs served to illustrate the specific malaria hazards discussed in the text and displayed on the maps, but they also played the role of model—what DNH engineers should look for in the field. Finally, the photos served a prospective function. These were the "before" pictures—the disorganized, unattractive, unsanitary present—that would one day be compared to photos of the same sites after sanitation works had been implemented. Subsequent DNH publications, as well as the work of the Rockefeller Foundation, which is explored in the next chapter, made frequent use of these before-and-after series to show the progress of malaria control work.

Synthesizing their field surveys, Anschütz and Restagnio developed a general typology of malaria hazards in the Northwest and a strategy to eliminate them. Almost invariably, these hazards were areas of standing water, whether natural or anthropogenic, seasonal or permanent. Restagnio, the chief engineer, envisioned a network of canals throughout the region to permit "continuous movement of water," similar to contemporary plans for the development of irrigation in Tucumán.[36] This ambitious canal network would capture springs at their source, preventing them from turning depressions into marshes; allow them to pass unimpeded beneath railroads; drain irrigation waters from the fields; and deliver all of this water to the many rivers and streams crossing the area.[37]

The comprehensive and authoritative presentation of the DNH survey concealed the surveyors' selective, partial, and distant perspective on the malaria problem. Crucially, Anschütz and Restagnio accentuated those aspects of the malaria problem that could be viewed from a moving train: not people, parasites, and mosquitoes, but rather threatening or degraded *landscape features.* Just as importantly, only certain transportation corridors were surveyed, but this "view from the road" was extrapolated to characterize vast, unseen landscapes.[38] For the purposes of malaria control, these railroad corridors were hardly representative of regional landscapes: surveying mainly along railroad lines took them through a narrow corridor of abundant areas of standing water that resulted directly from the fact of the *railroad itself:* its numerous embankments, low bridges, undersized culverts, and borrow pits facilitated the pooling of water on the upstream side of the tracks. Extrapolating these conditions to the Northwest as a whole was unwarranted.[39] Just as crucially, the surveyors conflated visual evidence of a hazardous landscape with malaria risk. Just as in the deliberations of the 1902 conference, the mosquito plays a perfunctory, or implicit, role: no entomological surveys were conducted. Nor was there any attempt to link geographical survey to epidemiological data for particular locales, in order to ascertain if there was at least a spatial concordance between local hazards and malaria incidence.

Thus, despite the sheen of accuracy, objectivity, synoptic perspective, and detailed, technically competent draftsmanship, the Anschütz-Restagnio survey did not improve much on Cantón's medical geography of twenty years before. In fact, despite trying to distance themselves from Cantón, Anschütz and Restagnio reproduced his basic understanding of malaria as a disease *of* the landscape and his argument that malaria control served larger economic development needs through, for example, the rationalization of irrigation. The veneer of science imparted by surveying and mapping helped embed this model of malaria control, despite the lack of critical science that went into it.[40]

Malaria Control in Practice: The First Decade

Even as the team led by Anschütz and Restagnio surveyed the Northwest, the Malaria Service was getting organized. The early phase of the campaign was filled with optimism, ambition, and energy. Its agenda was the product of almost twenty years of geographic survey, scientific study, and political debate, and so the path to take seemed clear. The powerful rhetoric of the legislators in the national congress suggested that malaria control was imperative to the welfare of the region and the country as a whole, and the directors of the Malaria Service shared this belief. This confident attitude would make the early failures of malaria control especially disheartening.

As its creators intended, the malaria campaign extended the presence of the national state into the provinces. The Malaria Service had a centralized and vertically oriented administration within the DNH, headquartered in Buenos Aires, some one thousand kilometers away from the legally designated malaria zone.[41] Underneath the central authority were four regional directors with offices in the capitals of Tucumán, Salta, Jujuy, and Catamarca Provinces. Each province was divided into districts (*circunscripciones*), with clinics (*dispensarios*) in various cities and towns. A medical doctor, employed only part-time, supervised each district; his staff included nurses, orderlies, sanitary engineers, and squadrons of laborers (*peones*) dedicated to saneamiento tasks.[42] From the beginning, the service's districts covered almost the entire malarious region; opting for broad regional coverage rather than focusing effort in a few locales would prove to be a consequential choice.

The chief (*jefe*) of the service from its inception until the mid–1930s was Antonio Barbieri, an ophthalmologist. As its long-time director, Barbieri must have had considerable influence on the agency, but he remains an enigma since only the barest biographical details are available.[43] Although an eye doctor may seem like an odd choice for director of the Malaria Service, Barbieri had expertise in trachoma, a bacterial eye infection that was also endemic to the Northwest, and simultaneously led efforts against it. Other than in official reports published every few years, his pronouncements on malaria control were a rarity, and his contributions to basic research on the disease, practically nonexistent. Certainly, he was overshadowed by the directors (presidents) of the DNH, who also played a crucial role in crafting the policy and public image of the Malaria Service. The presidents of the department were some of the most important figures in the history of public health in Argentina, including Malbrán (1900–1910) and Penna (1910–1916), both key figures at the 1902 DNH conference on malaria, and Gregorio Aráoz Alfaro 1918, (1923–1928, 1930), one of Tucumán's "native sons."[44] All of them, unlike Barbieri, were active in politics, played the role of public scientist, and seemed to have more influence than Barbieri on the strategy of the campaign.

The Malaria Service strove, mostly unsuccessfully, to quantify the scope of malaria in the Northwest. Establishing baseline levels of malaria incidence was crucial for guiding local control efforts, evaluating their effectiveness, and ensuring the proper distribution of the agency's technical and human resources.[45] Penna had launched an initiative to increase the statistical capacity of the DNH, reflecting a general trend toward bureaucratic quantification.[46] From the beginning, the Malaria Service's reports were full of numbers—directors clearly fetishized statistical compilations, displayed in massive tables—but their utility was dubious. The Malaria Service generally inferred malaria incidence crudely, from the number of people seeking assistance at their clinics.[47] Such inferences led to equivocal conclusions: Did a rise in the number of malaria positives represent an actual increase in incidence of the disease? Or, did it simply reflect an increase in the availability, efficiency, or attractiveness of the Malaria Service's clinics? The malaria campaign was especially vulnerable to this confusion in its early years as its services became more intensely used throughout the region.[48]

Inconsistent diagnostic terminology of the era also confounded efforts to quantify the malaria problem. By 1910, experts worldwide recognized the existence of three different strains of malaria, each caused by distinct plasmodium parasites and producing characteristic clinical symptoms: *P. vivax, P. malariae,* and *P. falciparum*.[49] In addition to these three varieties, all of which were found in Northwest Argentina, the Malaria Service recognized dozens of other types of malaria, some of which might not be recognized today. These types included mixed infections of more than one parasite; fevers caused by malaria compounded by other diseases, such as typhoid; and malaria infections that were not mixed with other diseases but exhibited symptoms of those diseases. The Malaria Service's doctors diagnosed thousands of such cases and grouped them together under the heading "anomalous forms." The extremely high proportion of anomalous cases—ranging from about 10 percent of malaria cases in La Rioja to nearly 50 percent in Catamarca—casts doubt upon most of the service's malaria incidence data until the 1930s.

However, it is possible to make some telling generalizations about the scope of the malaria campaign's services and, to a lesser degree, the epidemiology of malaria in the region. Within just a few years of being established, the Malaria Service's clinics were an important element of the region's public health infrastructure. Its clinics were widespread and popular. From 1912 to 1915, the Malaria Service's clinics attended at least a half million people, if we count only those diagnosed with malaria, and untold numbers not diagnosed with the disease (see table 2.1). In 1915, over 84,000 malaria sufferers attended Malaria Service dispensaries in Tucumán alone; to put this in perspective, in the same year only about 7,500 people showed up at all of the province's public hospitals, combined.[50] The clinics attended patients year-round, though typically the yearly epidemic peak occurred from March through May (late summer to early fall).[51] The limited evidence from Aráoz's careful survey of Tucumán in 1914 shows that malaria incidence was generally quite high but also highly variable geographically. Most locales in the province had a malaria index of between 5 and 20 percent.[52] But in Tucumán's capital city, about 3 percent of the population suffered from malaria, while on the outskirts of the city, rates were much higher, as high as 37 percent.[53]

From its inception, the Malaria Service based its control plan on a dual strategy that entailed treatment and prevention of malaria through the use of quinine ("internal" prophylaxis) and an attack on mosquitoes (saneamiento or "external" prophylaxis). This two-pronged strategy had its origins in the meeting of the DNH malaria commission in 1902. Hygienists based mostly in Buenos Aires (such as Penna and Malbrán) saw internal prophylaxis as an extension of the revolutionary bacteriological research of Europeans such as Robert Koch. They viewed biomedical and pharmaceutical interventions, especially attacking the malaria parasite with quinine, as the key to success. In conjunction with using quinine as the main line of defense, hygienists advocated quarantine for malaria sufferers and general improvements in hygiene for the lower classes, including moderation in behavior, diet, and dress; elimination of vices, such as alcohol and excessive sexuality; and disinfection, improvement, or even condemnation of unhygienic domiciles. In short, proponents of internal prophylaxis prescribed hygienic measures that differed little from strategies used to fight contemporary urban maladies, such as tuberculosis.[54]

Table 2.1.
Patients diagnosed with malaria at Malaria Service clinics, 1912–1915

	Tucumán	Salta	Jujuy	Catamarca	La Rioja	All provinces
1912	19,909	19,790	8,833	5,420	1,372	55,324
1913	62,145	39,410	13,505	10,475	3,052	128,587
1914	96,170	44,977	14,914	14,598	3,966	174,625
1915	84,209	43,119	18,615	13,154	3,728	162,825
Total, 1912–15	262,433	147,296	55,867	43,647	12,118	521,361
Yearly average	65,608	36,824	13,967	10,912	3,030	130,340

Source: José Penna and Antonio Barbieri, *El paludismo y su profilaxis en la Argentina* (Buenos Aires: D.N.H., 1916), 68–69.

Note: Averages are rounded to nearest whole number; totals for Santiago del Estero are not included in the table because data were available for 1914 and 1915 only.

Meanwhile, advocates of saneamiento continued to focus on malaria as a product of the natural environment, taking the medical-geographic view essentially corroborated by the incorporation of the mosquito link. Proponents of saneamiento saw the strategy as an extension of the improvements in sanitation infrastructure in Buenos Aires, broadly construed to include potable water, sewers, proper drainage, street paving, garbage collection, and civic beautification through parks and boulevards. More specific environmental sanitation tactics were adapted from foreign experiences with malaria control, both in national and colonial settings, particularly Italy but also the Suez Canal, Panama Canal, Cuba, and the United States.[55] They also emphasized, as early provincial supporters of malaria control had, all of the side benefits that environmental sanitation could produce, such as opening up land for agriculture or improving efficiency of irrigation systems.

Internal prophylaxis depended on quinine, the only medicine universally acknowledged to prevent and treat malaria, until synthetic versions of it became available in the mid-1920s.[56] The Malaria Service generally prescribed quinine as a curative rather than a prophylactic, although treating malaria sufferers would also have the incidental effect of preventing the spread of the disease to uninfected persons. According to the directors of the Malaria Service, the reluctance of patients themselves precluded the preventive administration of quinine. Penna and Barbieri remarked that the "indolent" natives of the Northwest did not take malaria seriously and were apt to suffer through it, seeking treatment only when the symptoms became absolutely intolerable.[57] (Others, especially later on, would view this trait more favorably, as evidence of criollo stoicism, not passivity.) The drug was usually administered as chloralhydrate of quinine, via powder, pill, or intravenously. Patients of all ages complained of the extremely bitter taste of quinine, so the quinine pills were coated with sugar, while children often received chocolate candies containing tannate of quinine. The bitterness of the quinine was only its commonest and mildest side effect—in many patients, quinine led to upset stomach, vomiting, dizziness, and a characteristic ringing in the ears.[58] In 1929, a Salta newspaper reported three cases of lethal overdoses of quinine, including two children, in the city.[59] Due to the negative popular perception of quinine, many people eschewed this free medication and instead bought patent medicines. Salta and Tucumán newspapers advertised these medications, sold under such brand names as Esanofele Bisleri (apparently, a pun on "anopheles") and Antimalárico Cantani at least into the 1920s. The continued presence of these ads suggests both a demand for quinine alternatives and the persistence of malaria in these cities.[60]

While quinine may have played a role in preventing the spread of malaria, "external" strategies made significant changes to the landscape and offered the best proof of the campaign's strong attempts at social and environmental control. One favored strategy, at least initially, was to fumigate residences of those stricken by malaria. This tactic was among the most invasive utilized by the Malaria Service: after notifying the owner of the house, a team of laborers would remove the inhabitants, furniture, clothes, and other objects, close all doors and windows, and seal all cracks and vents as best as possible, using wads of paper or rags. In the *ranchos* (shanties) or other buildings that were difficult to seal hermetically, a large canvas or tent was used to cover the entire location. The workers would then burn sulfur or other fumigation agents for about an hour. After allowing the house to air out for a while, the dead mosquitoes would be swept up, and the walls bleached, then whitewashed, to prevent further infestation and make indoor mosquitoes easier to spot.[61] From 1911 to 1914, the Malaria Service fumigated sixty-four thousand residences in Tucumán, Salta, Jujuy, and Catamarca, using eighty-one thousand kilos of sulfur.[62]

Fumigation efforts directly targeted adult mosquitoes. More elaborate still were methods to eliminate mosquitoes in their egg, larval, or nymph stages. In the early years of the federal malaria campaign, the most effective chemical for this end was petroleum: a thin film of the liquid on the surface of water in ponds, open barrels, cisterns, and troughs would kill any larvae and prevent adult female mosquitoes from laying eggs. However, petroleum had many disadvantages, in that it led to accidental fires, poisoned water intended for consumption by people or livestock, and evaporated quickly.[63] Alternative substances for creating a mosquito-inhibiting film on water surfaces included olive oil, lime, and tar (which was abundant in Jujuy). The DNH recommended a wide array of other chemicals as insecticides, although some were clearly safer than others: sulfur, potash, hydrochloric acid, ammonia, calcium chloride, iron sulfate, tobacco leaves, and pyrethrum, an extract of chrysanthemum flowers.[64] Other control methods included stocking water deposits with small fish or crustaceans that would feed on mosquito larvae; the cultivation of certain algae; mechanically disturbing water surfaces with fans or paddle wheels; and the placement of metallic screens over barrels of water.[65] Despite having alternatives, in 1912 and 1913 the DNH utilized approximately twenty-seven thousand liters of crude oil, plus an unknown amount of refined petroleum, to destroy mosquito habitat.

The most important element of *profilaxis externa* was saneamiento—drainage and hydraulic engineering works for the sake of sanitation and broader development goals. A legacy of the framework developed by Cantón, the lessons of Santiago del Estero, and the recommendations of the 1911 DNH survey, such works consisted primarily of reclaiming wetlands (marshes, swamps, lagoons), clearing obstructions in irrigation canals and ditches, closing sewers, filling puddles and other small pools of standing water, leveling and resurfacing streets, and planting trees, such as eucalyptus and willow, that desiccated the soil. From the perspective of the Malaria Service, agrarian sanitation (*saneamiento agrario*) would, by ordering landscapes and clearing them of the threat of malaria, bring formerly unproductive areas into the sphere of national development. In fact, most foresaw a positive feedback effect from saneamiento: once the malaria threat was diminished in uncultivated areas, agricultural settlers themselves could become a force for controlling malaria because they, too, would clear overgrown vegetation, drain and fill swamps, and level fields.[66] Law 5195 obliged landowners, sugar mills, and railroads to exercise care during earth-moving projects that might create openings that could fill with water and thus become breeding grounds for mosquitoes; however, the DNH lacked resources and effective authority to force private enterprises to aid in sanitation efforts and received little assistance from provincial and municipal governments. Because of this lack of cooperation, along with a limited budget and the high cost of reclamation projects, the DNH focused its engineering efforts on small-scale undertakings in the most populated regions of the endemic area.[67]

Science, Hygiene, and the Masses

The directors of the malaria campaign, immersed in the pervasive ideology of scientific hygiene, aimed to make an even deeper imprint on society than quinine, fumigation, and drainage would allow. They hoped to transform what they perceived as the "backward" culture of the Northwest by instilling a "hygienic consciousness" among the masses in support of control efforts. The rural poor were the main targets of such efforts. Hygienists, all members of the upper class, severely criticized the poor, viewing their ignorance, indolence, and traditional ways as obstacles to progress. While acknowledging the role of poverty as a catalyst for malaria, the Malaria Service seldom framed the disease within a broader political-economic context of social inequality and miserable labor conditions. Instead, they targeted habits, vices, and attitudes that fostered unsanitary environments, facilitated the spread of infectious diseases, and weakened bodily constitutions. Corrective messages were conveyed in top-down fashion, from the enlightened scientific experts to the masses, via various media, including posters, pamphlets, lectures, and school lessons. Soon, however, the DNH grew weary of trying to change popular habits and came to favor control tactics that minimized the need for collaboration from the public.

As we saw in the last chapter, the state's scientific elite led a national effort to develop and instill a broad "hygienic consciousness" among the masses. Renowned hygienists such as Emilio R. Coni, Nicolás Lozano, and Gregorio Aráoz Alfaro hoped that the lower classes would internalize lessons in hygiene after incessant repetition, leading to changes in habits and lifestyle and concomitant improvements in health conditions.[68] These hygienists fused scientific concepts (mainly from bacteriology and medicine) with a paternalistic and conservative moralism, lamenting ignorance, laziness, and the persistence of immoral and degrading habits—especially alcoholism, excessive sexuality, poor nutrition, and a lack of hygiene.[69] The hygienic way of life was not only the key to health, but also a sign of modernity and sophistication.[70] Thus, scientific hygiene was an extension of the dominant framework of social progress of the time, the unceasing battle between civilization and barbarism.

Numerous private organizations for the promotion of hygiene were founded in the first decade of the twentieth century, nationally and in the Northwest. Coni helped found several of these groups, such as the Argentine Antituberculosis League, the Anti-alcohol League, the Argentine Society of Sanitary and Moral Prophylaxis (which targeted tuberculosis and venereal disease), and the Gota de Leche (Drop of Milk) league, concerned with care of infants.[71] The DNH collaborated in the formation and advancement of these organizations, and it also made hygiene education a more visible part of its own policy.[72] The political and cultural elite of the Northwest soon emulated these efforts generated in Buenos Aires. In 1909, the first two Gota de Leche centers opened in San Miguel to provide milk, vaccines, and free medical care for infants. Over the next decade, other locations opened in Tucumán, and this effort may have made a dent in the province's alarmingly high infant mortality rates.[73] In 1919, a group of progressive elites formed the Liga Sanitaria del Norte (Sanitary League of the North), whose goal was to "propagate the fundamentals of hygiene" throughout the region. In its charter, the Sanitary League stipulated, the "lack of cleanliness is the stamp of barbarism. The health of the race is a precious good that the nation needs urgently."[74] In affirmation of the league's objectives, the newspaper *El Orden* of Tucumán editorialized, "As long as we do not achieve the inculcation in the popular spirit of the most elemental notions of hygiene, which are now lacking, the malaria campaign and any other emergency campaign which is attempted will be a waste of time and money."[75]

During this period, there was considerable debate in Argentina about the social causes of health and sanitary problems. One dimension of this debate—to put it in today's terms—revolved around the issue of structure versus agency: To what degree were specific health problems, such as tuberculosis or malaria, embedded in larger political-economic structures? How much did environment determine individual behaviors and attitudes about health and hygiene? What degree of autonomy did individuals have to make the "correct"—hygienic—choices? Generally, hygienists of the Generation of 1880 took the view that the poor were ignorant, indolent, and prone to immorality, and as a result their poverty was a reflection of moral failures. However, by embracing the wisdom of modern science, reform was possible. On the other hand, a faction of reformers, of diverse political stripes including socialists, anarchists, progressive Catholics, and members of the emergent Radical Party, argued that sanitary problems were more deeply embedded in political-economic structures. Public hygiene could not be segregated from the social into the scientific realm, and efforts to change individual habits and attitudes were dubious and limited. As a result, many social reformers focused on advancing legislation to ameliorate widespread, miserable working conditions.[76] Others argued that diseases such as tuberculosis originated in the injustices of the "capitalist system" and that the scientific indications of hygienists were simply a distraction from the systemic faults of an unjust, autocratic, and oppressive society.[77]

For the most part, during its first decade the malaria campaign took the more scientific, reductionist, and moralistic view of the malaria problem, seldom situating the disease within a larger political-economic framework. For example, the exploitative, hazardous, and shockingly unhealthful working conditions of the sugar mills of the Northwest, especially those of the *zafreros* (seasonal harvest laborers) scarcely rated mention in the Malaria Service's discourse on the causes of malaria. The increasingly boisterous politics of Tucumán, where sugar workers agitated for better working and living conditions with some success, was similarly outside of the purview of the Malaria Service.[78] In this way, Argentina's malaria campaign reflected an international trend identified by Randall Packard: malaria control increasingly concentrated "on eliminating the proximate causes of the diseases—parasites and mosquitoes" with a proportional disregard for "the broader social and economic conditions that played a role in the epidemiology of the disease."[79]

But the messages conveyed through educational efforts were not *completely* reductionist or drained of broader social content. The Malaria Service viewed the disease as the root cause of a host of social and economic ills and believed that controlling it would usher in progress and civilization. The alternative view, that economic development would improve living conditions across the board, leading incidentally to a decline in malaria, did not coincide with the ideology of Argentina's hygienists, nor did it flow from the political mandate for the malaria campaign. Malaria Service leaders positioned themselves as disease control experts whose scientific outlook and status as state agents placed them outside of everyday political matters.[80]

The DNH adopted a wide array of methods to promote the malaria campaign, mainly producing pamphlets, posters, and handbills for distribution and display in public places. Stylistically, early malaria campaign propaganda was staid, informative, even wordy, with the occasional use of photorealistic graphics depicting mosquitoes, malaria symptoms, or areas of standing water. Mostly they contained straightforward messages. The title of one widely disseminated pamphlet expressed its simple intentions: *What Is Malaria? How Is It Transmitted? How Is It Combated?* Using the regional vernacular terms for malaria (*chucho*) and mosquito (*zancudo*) throughout, the pamphlet explained the contemporary understanding of malaria in direct but not simplistic terms. It included photographs and drawings of the distinctive postures of *culex* and *anopheles* mosquitoes in their adult and larval stages, to allow the reader to differentiate between harmless insects and dangerous carriers of malaria.[81] Such pamphlets were widely disseminated, especially to doctors and teachers, while posters with similar illustrations could be found in many public buildings, including schools, hospitals, railroad stations, and factories, as well as the Malaria Service's own clinics.[82]

In some places, the DNH helped to integrate malaria control and hygiene into the curriculum of public schools.[83] For example, a year after the passage of Law 5195, Salta's provincial Ministry of Education decreed the addition of several malaria-related topics into the school curriculum, such as parasitology, entomology, and climatology.[84] The DNH sponsored at least one scholastic essay contest on the malaria problem.[85] The newly formed University of Tucumán also produced its own malaria education pamphlet, possibly aimed at the province's schoolteachers.[86] Malaria Service officials gave public lectures, collaborated with local clergy, and conducted informal hygiene education as part of their clinical consultations. The DNH even produced short films and screened them at movie theaters, bars, public meetings, and schools.[87] Finally, local newspapers collaborated in elevating awareness of hygiene through their editorials and the publication of DNH press releases, official documents, and speeches.

Although most malaria education materials contained straightforward information about the disease, they were also laced with general pronouncements about hygiene. The DNH condemned habits and behaviors, often cast as vices, that either "predisposed" the body to infection or exposed people to mosquito bites. The DNH advised that alcoholism, late nights out, and excessive sexual activity were all behaviors that put people at risk for contracting malaria and other harmful diseases.[88] Such "notions of hygiene," however essential to their promoters, were often ill suited to the lived experience of everyday people in the Northwest. For example, during a trip to Tucumán soon after the passage of Law 5195, Carlos Malbrán advised such measures as "using mosquito nets over beds; metal screens in doorways and windows; portable mosquito-proof chambers for travelers; special clothing that consists of a darkly-colored fabric with a high collar and tight sleeve openings, kid gloves, and veils like those used by beekeepers."[89] Along the same lines, the DNH repeatedly advised against the practice of sleeping outdoors and discouraged men from going shirtless.[90] Theoretically, this was all good advice to avoid mosquito bites, but probably quite alien to farm laborers who withstood hours of intense work in a searing, humid environment and who struggled to provide themselves with ordinary clothing, let alone kid gloves.

Indeed, government hygienists were quite aware that the poor of the Northwest had little inclination or capacity for change, and they sometimes grew despondent over their indifference to, and ignorance of, all manner of threats to their health. Campaign directors and local newspapers lamented that the lower classes, as well as many local physicians, who presumably should have known better, did not view malaria with sufficient alarm.[91] The Malaria Service had little faith in the common rural folk. One official, commissioned to write hygiene education materials, remarked: "One must descend a little to see closely the psychological characteristics of the people of the country and the small towns and villages. . . . The man of the country limits his views and his actions to the soil that he cultivates and the livestock he tends; he has neither the time, nor the capacity—in general—to consider other matters. . . . [I]f his body is taken prisoner by physical ills, nearby is the *curandera* [quack or folk healer] in whose hands, by preference, he deposits his faith."[92]

Unsurprisingly, the hygienists had low expectations of the poor. Yet in the scourge of malaria they found a biological explanation of such inveterate ignorance and indifference. Malaria, according to one pamphlet, defamed the character of rural people: many who suffered the label of "lazy" or "obtuse" were not intrinsically that way, but probably just exhibited the symptoms of apathy associated with a perfectly curable disease.[93] A DNH poster announced that malaria, "in a chronic state, leads gradually to prostration and the ruination of the body and the spirit."[94] "Wherever [malaria] exists," said one pamphlet, "it diminishes effective labor and in some places, paralyzes industry."[95] Wherever malaria spreads, "poverty substitutes for independence, and the social burden increases, whether by way of sustaining invalids, or encumbering productivity."[96] Malaria, said the teenager María Bussolatti in a prize-winning essay, "profoundly affects the health, prosperity, and dignity" of the people, "diminishes their energy," and "destroys ideals, ambitions, and progress."[97] In such rhetoric, sympathy blurs into paternalism, with elites confident in their ability to dictate measures necessary for improving public health.

This paternalism had a basis not only in distinctions of class and expertise, but also in geographical difference. Hygienists reflected on the great chasm that separated the enlightened, progressive capital and the benighted interior provinces, articulating complicated and conflicted ideas about the nation's geography of health. On the one hand, hygienists believed that the production of scientific knowledge was essentially placeless and its values and concepts, universal. Nicolás Lozano, for example, argued that scientific discoveries and innovations should be judged by their scientific merits, regardless of place of origin, and that any positive and beneficial idea should be diffused widely.[98] He viewed the malaria campaign as a good example of this principle, in that it adapted control methods demonstrably effective in other countries; and, conversely, Argentina's methods could work equally well in other countries with similar conditions.[99]

At the same time, however, universal scientific knowledge flowed along specific urban to rural pathways.[100] Bussolatti, the adolescent advocate of malaria control, under the tutelage of Lozano, argued that scientific ideas of hygiene and disease control "should pass from the cities to the towns, from the towns to the countryside, and the echo of their resounding voice should overcome the distance that separates us [in Buenos Aires] from the provinces of the North, where the focus of this endemic [malaria] appears on the map of the Republic like a black stain, and which the national sanitary authority, with marked determination, tries to erase."[101] Here, Bussolatti takes the cartographic code of dark shading, as depicted on the DNH's maps of the malaria, and transforms it into a metaphor for moral failure. Even a so-called regional illness, such as malaria, reflected poorly on the entire nation; thus it was logical and necessary that the central government should "intervene to combat a state of things prejudicial to the name and progress of Argentina."[102] Under these circumstances, the outsider status of the DNH, indicated both by the distance that separated Buenos Aires from the endemic zone and by hygienists' social detachment, was a source of the agency's strength. Guided by the universal, disinterested principles of science, government hygienists could stay above the fray of politics, provincialism, and corruption.[103]

Extending this line of reasoning, some hygienists argued that inculcating the principles of scientific hygiene could create more perfect national citizens. Hygiene was the science that best served democracy since it encouraged the development of a popular class that was healthy, dignified, educated, and responsible, guided by logic rather than superstition, and inspired by nationalist ideals and appreciation for the state. Defining and cultivating citizenship had long been a concern of the hygienists of the Generation of 1880, even as exclusionary, elitist politics often made a mockery of liberal principles.[104] During the first years of the malaria campaign, hygienists came to terms with major changes in the political landscape of Argentina. The passage of the milestone Sáenz Peña Law in 1912 extended full voting rights and fuller citizenship to all adult males, initiating the demise of the liberal oligarchy that had dominated Argentina for fifty years. Some hygienists welcomed this broadening of the franchise and the potential for political equality that it presented, believing that it might bring helpful changes to the way public health was governed. Pedro J. García, the director of Tucumán's bacteriological laboratory, argued that increasing democracy also required a change in public health strategy, from coercive measures—such as the quarantine and *cordon sanitaire*—to collaborative, educational, and scientifically informed strategies.[105] Thus at least some hygienists were quite vocal in linking hygiene education to broader goals of democracy.

After a few years, however, the malaria campaign diminished efforts to educate the public about the principles of hygiene. For one, it was never clear if the message was getting across: considering that illiteracy was high—around 50 percent in Tucumán at the time—it is unlikely that wordy pamphlets and posters would have made much of an impact. Beyond the issue of effectiveness of educational materials, the DNH frequently adopted an aloof attitude toward the people of the Northwest. Despite their occasional insistence to the contrary, the DNH searched for ways to circumvent the lack of a "hygienic consciousness" in the region, rather than confront and reform it. This was another advantage of the saneamiento strategy: drainage, filling, tree planting, and other landscape-oriented measures could be done, in theory, with little confrontation, cajoling, or consent. If the public could not be trusted to change their attitudes and behavior, said Penna in 1911, then the Malaria Service would have to change the environment they lived in.[106]

Setbacks and Frustration

The malaria control campaign began with great fanfare, quickly establishing offices and clinics throughout the Northwest, transforming landscapes through environmental sanitation works, and curing the sick with free quinine treatments. Many progressive elites saw the malaria campaign as a harbinger of an even more important transformation of social habits and values, toward the inculcation of a hygienic consciousness, with social and economic progress to follow. Before long, however, the DNH curtailed the ambitions of the malaria campaign in the face of a number of setbacks. Financial limits proved crucial, as the service's budget shrank radically during a time of national economic contraction. The apathy of local governments, ordinary citizens, and the business community exacerbated the Malaria Service's fiscal woes.

The malaria campaign had begun during what most historians characterize as Argentina's *belle époque,* the apogee of the country's economic prosperity.[107] The rhetoric and design of the malaria campaign reflected the self-confidence of a nation on the rise. A confluence of events soon broke this confidence, however, as Argentina fell into economic depression from 1913 to 1917, a period when national output declined by an estimated 20 percent.[108] The government was thrown into fiscal crisis, and the Malaria Service was affected immediately. By 1917, the yearly budget of the agency was less than one-fifth of what it had been at its peak in 1912, one million pesos (approximately US $425,532 at the time).[109] These financial problems severely limited the scope of the malaria campaign. In March 1914, part of the staff was laid off and saneamiento works were suspended.[110]

For the next few years the Malaria Service elected to devote its entire limited budget to the maintenance of the free quinine distribution program at its clinics. Antonio Barbieri, the director of the service, believed that financial realities left him with no other choice, but he also made a virtue of necessity, arguing that quininization offered immediate care to those suffering from malaria, while the benefits of saneamiento were harder to gauge in the short term. While the financial situation of the malaria campaign worsened, the number of people attending the clinics did not drop off significantly. Meanwhile, at Tucumán's main provincial hospital, malaria cases rose steadily from 1915 to 1919, both in absolute terms and as a proportion of all admissions (fig. 2.1).[111] Whether this apparent increase in malaria incidence

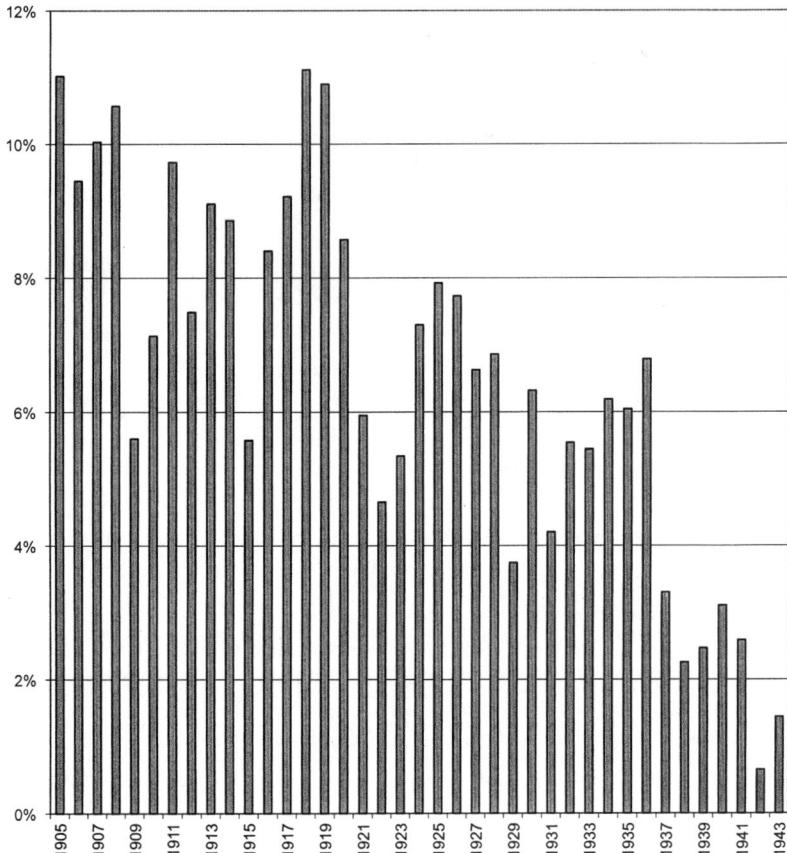

Figure 2.1. Percentage of malaria cases with respect to all admissions, Hospital Mixto, San Miguel de Tucumán, 1905–1943. From 1905 to 1927, original data were kept for Hospital Mixto (men's and women's hospitals); from 1928 to 1943, data were kept separately for Hospital Padilla (men's hospital) and Hospital Santillán (women's hospital). Note the steady rhythm of malaria incidence, starting with 1909: "low" years (troughs) separated by about five to seven years, and "high" years (peaks) also separated by about the same interval. *Anuario estadístico de la provincia de Tucumán,* 1905–1943.

arose from DNH cutbacks is difficult to say. Still, budgetary troubles surely compounded the problem of a campaign spread too thin, given that the Malaria Service's clinics, offices, and personnel were distributed across fifty different localities in six northwestern provinces.[112]

Provincial governments and local enterprises did little to collaborate with the cash-strapped Malaria Service. Adhering to the provisions of Law 5195, all of the Northwest's provincial governments had formally requested the action of the Malaria Service. Yet the law did not require the financial or even moral support of the provinces for the malaria campaign, and the provinces' minimal contributions to the malaria campaign were a source of constant irritation to the Malaria Service. Penna and Barbieri admonished the provinces for their ingratitude, arguing that malaria control was a "benevolent" campaign, "not only for the health of individuals and a great mass of population, but for the economic welfare of the provinces themselves."[113] In the Northwest, the provincial governments were worse off financially than even the national government. So, while provincial politicians frequently proclaimed the importance of public health and passed legislation to protect it, these efforts were mostly dead on arrival, since the provinces lacked the funds and infrastructure to implement such programs, an issue recognized in the original rationale for malaria control.[114]

Without the cooperation of local government, it was also difficult to procure the cooperation of local citizens and the business community.[115] Ordinary citizens in the Northwest may have embraced the Malaria Service for offering quinine treatment free of charge, and, indeed, well over one hundred thousand people showed up at the clinics each year from 1913 to 1915. Yet the Malaria Service grew frustrated with its recalcitrant clientele, who often failed to take the full course of quinine therapy, or else resorted to the ministrations of folk healers. The inculcation of a "hygienic consciousness" had failed to make even the most practical impact: as DNH president Gregorio Aráoz Alfaro said in 1918, quinine therapy alone would never bring malaria under control, "as long as we lack a populace with a level of culture sufficient for understanding the benefits of a continuous and methodical consumption of the medication."[116] While the Malaria Service attempted to enforce proper quinine therapy, its saneamiento work sometimes generated resistance, as in the case of a property owner in Jujuy who brought suit against the DNH for damages caused by sanitary reclamation works.[117] Such legal challenges were rare, but the DNH found it almost impossible to enforce certain provisions of the law, such as landowners' obligations to sanitize malaria hazards or the requirement that railroads place mosquito-proof screens on their passenger car windows. When coercion and threats of fines failed, efforts to collaborate with railroads, sugar mills, and other private interests were met mostly with indifference.

Conclusion

Thus by 1920 the campaign faced a serious dilemma. Since the 1902 malaria conference, and through the passage of Law 5195 and the organization of the

Malaria Service, the dual strategy of internal prophylaxis and saneamiento had been considered fundamental to success. Yet campaign resources were only sufficient to pursue one strategy or the other. Distributing quinine was more cost-effective in the short run, but it depended on the cooperation of people who lacked the knowledge, patience, and will to do so. Saneamiento techniques did not depend as much on cooperation or collaboration, and potentially produced longer-lasting benefits, but these were labor-intensive, expensive, and not exempt from conflicts. As we will see in the following chapters, the Malaria Service continued to focus on drainage and sanitary engineering works as the ideal solution. Too much was invested ideologically to do otherwise, given the strong link between saneamiento and broader development goals. In practice, though, the Malaria Service continued with a quinine-based program, though most agreed that this was a stopgap solution.

More broadly, the scientist-bureaucrats of the DNH framed the problems of the Northwest within their own particular geographical imaginary. The Northwest was a diseased region, where unhealthy people and insalubrious landscapes formed a vicious circle that prevented development of the region. As a result, the Northwest appeared as a "stain" on the mental map of the country, a shameful relic of an era where superstition and fatalism, rather than science and progress, ruled. Hygienists saw themselves as "missionaries of science" from the enlightened capital to the benighted Northwest; and they imposed a distanced, technocratic, and moralistic vision, practically devoid of critical analysis of the political-economic roots of public health crisis, onto the region and its people.[118] This somewhat patronizing perspective was largely internalized by social elites and media of the Northwest. Yet the first decade of malaria control proved that the DNH did not comprehend the society and environment under its jurisdiction. As we will see in the next chapter, the malaria campaign was often more interested in following the latest advances from abroad than in truly trying to understand the realities of the Northwest.

3

Foreign, National, and Local
Influences on Malaria Control

Malaria is the worm that rots away the foundations of the Argentine nation.
—Dr. José Tobías, "Contribución al estudio," 1923

In 1923, hygienists from across Argentina convened at the National Sanitary Conference in Buenos Aires. Contemplating nothing less than a complete overhaul of national public health administration, the delegates expounded on a multitude of sanitary problems and the grave threat they posed for the prospects of the nation. Though it had successfully sequestered itself from notorious international epidemics, such as cholera, plague, and yellow fever, Argentina still faced diverse and interconnected menaces, including infectious and venereal diseases, along with the social vices that amplified their damaging effects. The delegates widely agreed that unsanitary conditions not only tore apart the fabric of society, but also undermined the strength and vigor of the Argentine race and the basic biological foundations of the nation itself. Only a reorganization of the National Department of Hygiene (DNH), based on centralizing authority over public health in the national state, could provide the coordination, efficiency, and expertise necessary to prevent the deterioration of the race.

The proposed restructuring of the DNH went nowhere until the populist government of Juan D. Perón brought these reforms to fruition in the 1940s. Yet the proceedings of the 1923 conference offer a window into the ideology of the country's leading hygienists: their paternalism, their prioritizing of public health above almost all other concerns, their unabashed nationalism, and their fascination with racial improvement. Their ideology also colored the campaign against malaria, which was a principal concern for the hygienists at the 1923 conference, no matter their regional background. Representatives from the northwestern provinces, such as the Salteño José Tobías, author of this chapter's epigraph, argued that malaria "threaten[ed] to destroy the physical and intellectual vigor of an enormous mass of Argentines." Jerónimo del Barco, former governor of Córdoba, contended that the "gradual degeneration of the race" caused by malaria undermined the nation's military strength. Antonio Barbieri, the Porteño who headed the national malaria campaign, believed that he was leading more than just a public health effort: it was nothing less than a campaign to "invigorate the race."[1]

This ominous rhetoric accompanied a flurry of activity in malaria control. In the 1920s the players involved in the program multiplied, introducing diverse visions, strategies, and techniques, with uneven degrees of coordination. While the National Department of Hygiene continued its leading role, other international, national, and local actors increasingly influenced the course of the campaign. To take just one eventful year, in 1925 a group of Malaria Service officers returned from five months abroad studying malariology in Italy; the DNH entered into a cooperative agreement with the US Rockefeller Foundation; and the department published the results of an epidemiological and entomological study of the Northwest led the previous year by Peter Mühlens, a German scientist. That same year, Charles Nicolle, a French expert in tropical medicine, aided an Argentine researcher, Salvador Mazza, in the foundation of an institute of regional pathology in the Northwest. All the while, politicians debated the merits of investing in malaria control and other public health projects, while bureaucrats and officials jockeyed for position to protect their administrative turf.

This chapter examines the complex local, national, and international influences on Argentina's malaria campaign during the 1920s. We cannot understand the motives behind malaria control and the choice of specific control policies without reference to the broader political, ideological, and institutional context of Argentina in that era. To this end, this chapter focuses more on how this context shaped malaria control policy and less on whether and how policies impacted malaria control in action, which is a problem I return to in chapter 4. The 1920s saw a gradual change in the ideological hegemony of the hygienists inspired by the Generation of 1880. First and foremost, discussions of malaria policy took place in a public health discourse that was increasingly nationalistic, racialized, and organicist, as the rhetoric of the 1923 National Sanitary Conference demonstrates. At the same time, other varieties of nationalist thought influenced public health policy, generally, and malaria control, specifically. A resurgent regionalism challenged the purportedly elitist attitude and cosmopolitan outlook of Buenos Aires, offering an alternative vision of where the "true" heart of Argentine nationhood could be found: in the "creole" or Hispanic interior provinces. Reflecting this trend, elites of the Northwest increasingly asserted the region's autonomy and moral authority by creating regional institutions for education, scientific research, and the promotion of public hygiene. Finally, there was an increasingly prominent strain of anti-interventionism or anti-imperialism in national politics, with a concomitant suspicion of some foreign institutions, that debilitated productive innovation in malaria control.

During the 1920s and 1930s, such ideological currents shaped public health politics and swayed the mission of malaria control. Three interrelated episodes demonstrate the complicated relationship between the action of the malaria campaign and the political realm. First, Argentina's hygiene establishment, dedicated to improving an organic society, pushed the malaria control program toward an emulation of the Italian Fascist government's campaign of *bonifica integrale,* or "integrated agrarian sanitation." By the 1920s, the success of malaria control in Italy was well publicized, and its ambitious melding of agricultural development and vector control through marshland reclamation validated the concept of *saneamiento* that so many Argentine malariologists endorsed. Second, the chapter explores the rise of a school of regional medicine in the Northwest in the 1920s, led by Salvador Mazza, a pathologist originally from Buenos Aires, who adopted the northwestern province of Jujuy as his home. This organized interest in the unique disease ecology of the subtropical Northwest grew out of a broad-based development of regional institutions, such as universities. The regional pathologists also established close and productive research ties with scientists from the Rockefeller Foundation, whose brief but noteworthy affiliation with malaria control in Argentina is the third episode considered here.

Race and Health, Region and Nation

Although malaria was strongly identified with the Northwest, gaining infamy as the archetypal disease of the region, it was often construed as a national problem. As we saw in previous chapters, framing the disease in national terms might have been a strategic political maneuver: such a re-scaling of the problem amplified fears and legitimized the transfer of authority over malaria from inept provincial governments to the federal public health administration. As hygienists and social reformers continued to debate malaria control policy, the rhetorical appeal to national well-being only intensified, but with the fate of the Argentine "race" now taking center stage. During the interwar period, eugenics was part of the "cultural climate," and concerns over the quality and quantity of the *raza argentina* permeated discourse related to national development, across the political spectrum and beyond the narrow limits of self-identified eugenicists.[2] Public health advocates connected malaria to all of the major tropes in the racial-national discourse, such as concerns over population growth and immigration from abroad, preoccupation with racial degeneration, environmental determinism, the conception of the nation as an organism, regionalism, and the role of scientists in managing the population. The framing of malaria in racial and national terms served to perpetuate the longstanding model connecting malaria control with the problem of regional development.

Before proceeding, some clarification is needed on the subject of nationalism. I define nationalism broadly, as a constellation of ideas that construct the nation as a social fact. This definition derives from the notion that a national identity must be actively and continuously constructed, as opposed to conventional views that reify the nation as a self-evident category.[3] From this perspective, "nationalism" is a discourse that serves as an ideological support for political projects, not only in the obvious realm of national security, but also for such initiatives as economic development and the promotion of public health. This broadly construed nationalism should be differentiated from the political movement called "nationalism" or "conservative nationalism" that is central to Argentina's early twentieth-century history. This reactionary nationalist movement, bringing together traditional elites, the military, the Catholic Church, and other sectors, came to prominence at the end of the 1910s, gathered strength in the 1920s, and finally gained official power with a coup d'état in 1930 that initiated a decades-long line of authoritarian governments. While conservative nationalist thought does encroach on the public health discourse, the people, events, and ideas discussed in this chapter had little direct influence on nationalism as a discrete political movement. Yet, this analysis reveals continuities and commonalities between conservative nationalism and liberal positivism—the latter, the general basis for hygienists' social and political philosophy—rather than seeing them as diametrically opposed worldviews.[4]

Demographic stagnation continued to be a major preoccupation for hygienists, but by the 1920s this concern was coupled with growing ambivalence over the role of immigration from abroad. Despite explosive population growth in the previous decades, most hygienists continued to argue that Argentina was underpopulated relative to its great expanses, and they lamented the untapped potential of its land and other natural resources.[5] It also seemed that the demographic imbalance between the littoral and the interior (and between urban and rural) was only intensifying, an argument supported by an influential cohort of Argentine political economists, especially Alejandro Bunge, founder of the journal *Revista de Economía Argentina*.[6] To address this maldistribution, Barbieri and others pushed for government land colonization programs, even for the breakup of large landholdings, to make smaller, single-family farms available, in conscious emulation of the yeoman agrarianism identified with the United States at the time.[7]

In reality, however, the population of the Northwest was not declining but

Table 3.1. Average annual population growth rates, 1910–1925

Province	Total population growth rate (%)	Natural growth rate (%)	Migration growth rate (%)
Mendoza	3.32	2.05	1.28
Buenos Aires	3.20	2.21	0.99
Santa Fe	2.96	2.16	0.80
Capital Federal	2.75	1.36	1.38
Córdoba	2.65	1.90	0.75
Santiago del Estero	*2.41*	*2.28*	*0.13*
San Juan	2.32	1.87	0.45
San Luis	2.23	1.91	0.32
Entre Ríos	2.18	2.08	0.10
Tucumán	*1.75*	*1.43*	*0.32*
Corrientes	1.46	1.43	0.04
Jujuy	*1.41*	*0.60*	*0.80*
Catamarca	*1.41*	*1.34*	*0.06*
La Rioja	*1.30*	*1.25*	*0.05*
Salta	*1.24*	*0.99*	*0.25*

Source: Dirección General de Estadística, *La población y el movimiento demográfico de la República Argentina en el periodo 1910–1925,* Demografia Serie D. No. 1 (Buenos Aires: Gmo. Kraft Ltda., 1926).

Note: Provinces of Northwest in italics. In this period, there were only fourteen provinces plus the federal district (Capital Federal). National territories (e.g., Misiones, Chaco) were not included in original report.

growing (table 3.1). The region still faced severe public health problems and generally lagged behind the rest of the country in demographic and health measures. Nevertheless, population increased thanks to sustained high fertility rates and lower mortality deriving from progressive improvements in public health and nutrition, even while the region lacked a sizable contribution of immigrants from outside Argentina (table 3.2). Eventually, this prodigious fertility would underscore claims that the criollo of the interior was a source of national strength. However, due to problems of statistical compilation and reporting, as well as the strength of dominant discourses on the nation, hygienists were slow to internalize this demographic fact.[8]

Nevertheless, the status of the criollo, the poor "native stock" of Argentina that had been denigrated by an earlier generation of elites, improved, while the relative standing of immigrants declined. By the 1920s, a general consensus had emerged among social elites of diverse political associations: immigration from abroad was still necessary for national progress, but poli-

Table 3.2. Average annual mortality and birth rates, 1910–1925

Province	Infant mortality rate (0–1 yrs.)[a]	General mortality rate	Birth rate
Capital Federal	88.61	14.89	28.53
Buenos Aires	97.47	12.83	34.91
Santiago del Estero	*108.15*[b]	*13.52*[c]	*36.29*[c]
Corrientes	113.56	14.07	28.33
Santa Fe	116.48[b]	15.91	37.51
Entre Ríos	125.16	15.90	36.74
La Rioja	*127.49*[b]	*12.66*	*25.21*
Catamarca	*128.24*	*13.49*	*26.92*
San Luis	146.80[b]	17.26[c]	36.32[c]
Córdoba	152.37	19.52	38.47
Mendoza	188.05	23.35	43.82
Tucumán	*189.98*	*27.26*	*41.56*
San Juan	200.06[b]	26.36[c]	45.04[c]
Salta	*202.47*[c]	*26.37*[c]	*36.25*[c]
Jujuy	*230.11*	*30.01*	*36.06*

Source: Dirección General de Estadística, *La población y el movimiento demográfico de la República Argentina en el periodo 1910–1925,* Demografía Serie D. No. 1. (Buenos Aires: Gmo. Kraft Ltda., 1926).

Note: Rates expressed per 1,000 population, except infant mortality rate, which is expressed per 1,000 live births. Provinces of the Northwest are in italics. In this period, there were only fourteen provinces plus the federal district (Capital Federal). National territories (e.g., Misiones, Chaco) were not included in original report.

[a] 1914–1925 only.
[b] 1924 and 1925 data not available.
[c] 1925 data not available.

cies promoting "selective" immigration were required. In 1924, Gregorio Aráoz Alfaro, Tucumano and president of the DNH, reluctantly accepted that Argentina had failed to capture Europe's "best"—the Anglo-Saxon and Scandinavian "races"—and that Argentina would be a New World outpost of a "Latin" race composed mainly of Italian and Spanish blood. However, he cautioned that Argentina must admit only the most "healthy and able peoples, with a capacity for work and fit to bestow us strong generations."[9] Deficient immigrants brought not only physical ills transmissible to others (e.g., trachoma, tuberculosis), but also inherent defects that could contaminate the national gene pool and poison the morals of the social body.[10] At the same time, however, Aráoz Alfaro hoped for a future adapted to Argentina's cultural identity (reflecting, as he often put it, "our needs" and "our progress") rather than a wholesale transplant of European ways.[11] Immigrants had to be acculturated to a coherent and morally correct national identity.

This quest for a great and powerful nation, however, was constantly threatened by the specter of racial degeneration. Most elites involved with hygiene, social psychology, and other "sciences" viewed Argentines as components of a not quite amalgamated race that was damaged by social, biological, and environmental "poisons." In this formulation, social problems arose because of a compounding and concentration of these poisons, for example, in the slums of Buenos Aires, where sexual promiscuity, venereal disease, tuberculosis, filth, and overcrowding combined to produce a panorama of poverty and decay. In the Northwest, social reformers had long targeted malaria as the principal cause of racial degeneration. Depictions of the malarious criollo, however, grew progressively sensationalist in correspondence with the hegemony of racialist ideas. Leopoldo Bard, a national legislator from Buenos Aires, described the typical criollo laborer in these terms: "emaciated, thin, underfed, destroyed by the endemic disease [malaria], of a sallow or coppery color, poorly developed, haggard, shabbily dressed, and above all, with those peculiar features, with the expression of sadness, dejection, and indifference that constitute the most characteristic aspect of the malaria sufferer."[12] Tobías concurred: malaria, over generations, had shaped the "skeptical, indifferent, fatalistic character" of the criollos and damaged their genetic heritage as well.[13] In effect, the much-feared "degeneration of the race" was inscribed on the very bodies of poor criollos, and malaria was the foremost culprit.

Elites also believed that the natural environment played an important role in shaping culture, health conditions, and the quality of the race. Such "environmental determinism" was integral to social Darwinist and imperialist theories of racial classification in many countries.[14] In Argentina, the idea was also widespread and cut across ideological lines. Hygienists saw the searing, moist, and verdant conditions of the subtropical Northwest, via the medium of malaria, shaping the character and physical appearance of its people. More broadly, in keeping with the Darwinist spirit of the age, they believed that differences in the races of the world derived from long-term exposure to distinct climatic circumstances. Meanwhile, environmental determinist reasoning supported a line of political thought that was, generally, quite different from the hygienists' liberal positivism: namely, conservative nationalism, with its idea that national character sprang from the "synthesis between environment and history."[15] Thus, determinism was broad enough—some might say, incoherent enough—to support contradictory political projects, whether the liberals' aggressive pro-immigration stance or the conservatives' resurrection of the gaucho and criollo as authentic representatives of national identity. These mostly unresolved contradictions carried over into environmental determinism's role in Latin American eugenics. As Nancy Leys

Stepan has argued, the "soft" eugenics of many Latin American countries saw national racial "germplasm" as more malleable through changes to the social milieu (such as sanitation, hygiene, and education), not only through "hard" measures such as sterilization or regulation of marriage.[16] In this context, transformation of the environment through hygienic modernization was, in effect, a form of social engineering.

Immersed in such nationalist, racialist, and environmental determinist ideologies, many hygienists portrayed the nation as a super-organism of intertwined biological, environmental, economic, and social character, a portrayal that was also infused with a dose of patriotic mysticism. As Jeane DeLaney argues, both positivists, such as the leadership of the DNH, and cultural nationalists believed "that societies were natural organisms rather than creations of autonomous, free-thinking individuals," that is, "as the product of history, race and environment."[17] Aráoz Alfaro consistently held that the power of the national organism depended absolutely on the well-being of its people. Under the leadership of intelligent and progressive government, the promotion of a broad social hygiene would produce a "robust, energetic, virile, intelligent, and hardworking *Argentine race*" capable of producing a "great and strong" nation.[18] The case for malaria control fit well within this framework: could the nation be healthy, if its constituent parts—its regions—were not?[19]

That the interior provinces, and particularly the Northwest, were a drag on national progress was not a new idea. However, the 1920s saw a subtle shift in the portrayal of the region and the criollos who constituted it. Some, like Aráoz Alfaro—himself a northwesterner—did not see much hope in the region's native stock: European immigrants, "with all of their defects, have always been far superior to the criollo, generally indolent, capricious, and spendthrift," he reported in 1924.[20] But others elevated the criollo of the interior to the role of protagonist in the national project. As many scholars have noted, conservative nationalists such as Ricardo Rojas or Manuel Gálvez embraced Hispanic cultural tradition in a search for the "core" of national identity, very similar to German folk nationalism.[21] Conservatives in the provinces, such as Benjamin Villafañe of Jujuy, celebrated the Northwest as a "reservoir" of the "national spirit" while launching an extensive critique of Buenos Aires for its cosmopolitanism, corruption, and domination of the rest of the nation. National ethnic identity, as Oscar Chamosa puts it, became gradually "creolized"; the criollo served as a cultural type—much like the mestizo in other Latin American countries—that provided the discursive possibility of the erasure of cultural difference under the rubric of national integration.[22] Racial theorists gradually moved away from the Europeanizing bent of the Generation of 1880 and toward the consensus that national identity should be based on a shared Hispanic or Latin cultural heritage.[23]

During the 1920s and 1930s, the Northwest became the most "creole" of the national regions. In retrospect, this "creolization" was a discursive construction, but intellectual elites of the time saw it as a concrete reality: the region's long Hispanic roots and the subsequent lack of European immigration had sheltered it from the social and racial transformation experienced in the littoral. Gradually, controlling malaria and other endemic regional diseases became urgent not so much to open the door for immigrants, but to protect the criollo "brothers" or "native sons" in the Argentine heartland. For their part, elites in the Northwest stoked a regionalist-creole resurgence to spawn and nurture local institutions, such as those especially dedicated to public health, a phenomenon explored in more detail below.

This highly nationalistic, racialized, and organicist discourse on public health dovetailed perfectly with the prevailing focus on malaria control as a platform for regional development. As discussed in previous chapters, the regional development narrative placed malaria at the nexus of a host of economic, social, sanitary, and environmental ills. This expansive and holistic discourse on the disease invited large-scale and socially transformational control strategies. With development, racial improvement, and environmental sanitation so strongly intertwined in the worldview of hygienists, they looked to the Italian "bonifica" strategy, based on a similar socio-ecological perspective on national destiny, as a model for Argentina's malaria control program into the 1930s. Even after the Malaria Service moved control strategy in a different direction, the nationalistic, racialized, and organicist discourse continued to prevail in political debates on malaria control and public health, more broadly. For example, the social reformer Alfredo Palacios fixated on the unjust suffering of the poor criollo of the interior, an affront to the national conscience. As chapter 5 explains, the Peronists would take up this argument and, with their unprecedented use of state power, bring to fruition some of the grand vision of hygienists and social reformers.

The Italian Model and Master Narratives of Development

The socio-ecological vision of malaria control developed as new ideological elements grafted onto earlier developmentalist discourses. Tying more and more social problems together into "malaria's knot" raised the stakes for controlling the disease. Despite the professed urgency and scope of the malaria problem, however, the DNH seemed to make little headway against the disease. During the interwar period, Argentina's hygienists looked to Italy for the keys to success in fighting malaria. Since the late nineteenth century, Italy had been not only a leading center of scientific malariology, but also a major proving ground for malaria control policy. Then, starting in the 1920s, the

Fascist government of Benito Mussolini joined malaria control to a millenarian vision of landscape reclamation and agrarian development. Notable successes in large-scale environmental sanitation, especially the drainage of wetlands, served as a visible inspiration for the technocrats of Argentina's Malaria Service. Italy's experience confirmed the driving narrative of malaria control already in place in Argentina: a strong state, capable of sanitizing and reshaping dangerous, unproductive landscapes, could drive out disease, reorganize society, and unleash the potential of backward regions.

The defining characteristic of the Italian government's approach to malaria control in the 1920s and 1930s was its strong socio-ecological perspective, whereby land reclamation, rural development, and improved health were seen as linked results of malaria control. The umbrella term for this control philosophy was *bonifica,* which had roughly the same multivalent meanings as saneamiento did in Spanish, ranging from "reclamation or drainage" to "sanitation" or "rationalization." Depending on context or intent, bonifica could mean any one of these things or all of these things at once. For malaria control planning, bonifica was usually broken down into three parts, which corresponded roughly to a change of scale from the human body to the landscape to the region. *Bonifica umana* referred to treating or preventing malaria infections through the timely prescription of quinine. *Piccola bonifica* encompassed a suite of small-scale environmental strategies aimed at mosquitoes in their adult and larval stages. These strategies included drainage and filling of small areas of standing water; application of larvicides, such as petroleum or Paris green, to water surfaces; cultivation of aquatic plants and animals known to inhibit anopheline larvae production; recycling of water in ponds or fields by use of pumps or siphons; and fumigation of houses and other buildings.[24] *Grande bonifica,* which translated into Spanish as *gran saneamiento, saneamiento agrario,* or *saneamiento hidráulico,* consisted of massive drainage and land reclamation projects at the landscape scale: river valleys, marshlands, and so forth. The most ambitious grande bonifica projects operated on even larger scales, attempting to harness the hydraulic power of entire drainage basins and regions and distribute waters evenly and in a rational manner to prevent malaria and enhance agricultural productivity.[25]

In the 1920s, Mussolini co-opted the bonifica idea, using land reclamation as a base for the restructuring of rural Italian society and environment. The Fascists called this program *bonifica integrale* (integrated agrarian sanitation). They approached bonifica with millenarian fervor, using it as a major symbol of their hoped-for restoration of the golden age of the Roman Empire, captured in the slogan, "*Bonificare la terra per bonificare l'uomo, bonificare l'uomo per bonificare la razza*" (To reclaim the land, and with the land the men, and with the men the race).[26] The "bonification" of the Pontine Marshes was perhaps nothing less than a war to replace unruly and dangerous "first nature" with a planned, orderly, Fascist "second nature."[27] At its base, wrote Cesare Longobardi, a Fascist propagandist, bonifica integrale depended on a holistic, organic vision of nature and society working in harmony:

> It is no longer a question of carrying out this or that work, by itself and for itself—be it drainage, or irrigation, or protection against malaria, or reafforestation, etc.—but of considering organically, and in their technical, agrarian, and economic aspects, the aggregate of all the works and measures required in the several sectors, be they land settlement, social measures, the reconditioning of mountain-land, the control of watercourses, drainage, irrigation, aqueducts, the breaking up of new lands, the reconditioning and improvement of the soil, experimental work, roadmaking, the erection of villages, buildings, power-stations, the laying of electric lines, etc.[28]

Connected with other Fascist programs of rural colonization, intensification of wheat production, and promotion of population growth, bonifica integrale also involved rural electrification and the construction of "New Towns," Fascist model settlements.[29] In Italy, the draining of the Pontine Marshes through bonifica integrale was nothing less than "the most important domestic policy initiative that Mussolini's dictatorship pursued in the 1930s," according to Frank Snowden.[30] As the British malariologist Malcolm Watson argued in 1942, "For over two thousand years malaria defied all man's efforts to reclaim and cultivate the Pontine Marshes. But within the past decade, Mussolini, by destroying the anopheles, has colonized the area."[31]

In Argentina, nothing of the magnitude of bonifica integrale would actually be attempted, yet many in the Malaria Service, including its directorate, longed to transplant this transformative agenda to the Northwest. Barbieri, in particular, was impressed by the grand scale and vision of bonifica. Anticipating the words of Longobardi, Barbieri told the delegates of the 1926 National Medical Conference in Buenos Aires:

> We believe, and I am convinced, that the true sanitation of northern Argentina, not only with regard to malaria, but also to other subtropical endemic illnesses, such as hookworm, typhus, leishmaniasis, etc., can only be achieved with the agricultural transformation of the environment, and this by way of stable works of sanitary engineering, the "*gran bonifica and bonifica integrale*," as the Italians say, which considers, in addition to the hygienic sanitation of the soil, the problem of agriculture, irrigation, transformation of the squalid dwelling, etc.[32]

On the surface, there were many parallels between the malaria situations of the two countries. In both Italy and Argentina, malaria was restricted to peripheral regions that epitomized underdevelopment.[33] On some DNH maps, the Pontine Marshes and Northwest Argentina were juxtaposed at the same scale, a cartographic representation not only of their resemblance, but also of the much greater extent of malaria prevalence in the Northwest.[34] Malaria control in both countries depended on similar discourses of population decline and racial degeneration. The focus on reclamation of large areas of stagnant water was another common denominator. In this respect, Argentina had its own success story in the annals of malaria control, the bonification of Santiago del Estero in 1902. The Italian malariologist Giuseppe Sanarelli called it the "the most illustrative and perfect [work] known in contemporary anti-malaria literature."[35] Barbieri and others also perceived identical social causes of malaria in the two countries, particularly the persistence of a practically premodern peasantry, latifundia that monopolized the best agricultural land, and an absence of sanitation and education in the countryside. The Fascist "integral" approach had the advantage of tackling all of these problems at once.

The transformational potential of the Italian model served to entrench the methods already in place in Argentina. As shown in the previous chapter, from the very start the Malaria Service prioritized the reclamation of wetlands as a strategy with positive effects in multiple realms. When a lack of resources put such strategies on hold, alternative methods such as quininization were viewed as necessary but always second rate—quininization was mostly a palliative that failed to address the root causes of the endemic disease. Aráoz Alfaro, at the Third National Medical Conference in 1926 (whose keynote theme was malariology), declared that works of agrarian sanitation were the "most powerful and most radical" tools in the fight against malaria; and he advocated massive, landscape-changing techniques. Delegates to the conference ratified a new reform of malaria campaign strategy, which still featured the "dual strategy" of internal and external prophylaxis, but with stronger emphasis still on saneamiento, connected to a broader rationalization of the hydraulic landscape through effective irrigation policies.[36]

Ultimately, the national congress did not adopt these reforms to the existing malaria law. Still, with Aráoz Alfaro leading the DNH and restoring its budget to reasonable levels, the Malaria Service renewed its focus on saneamiento, mainly in works of *piccola bonifica* (small- and medium-scale reclamation). In the mid-1920s, throughout the Northwest the Malaria Service drained marshes, lagoons, and spring-fed pools; cleaned irrigation ditches; straightened river channels; and filled low-lying depressions. In many locales, the Malaria Service enacted the comprehensive irrigation and drainage net-

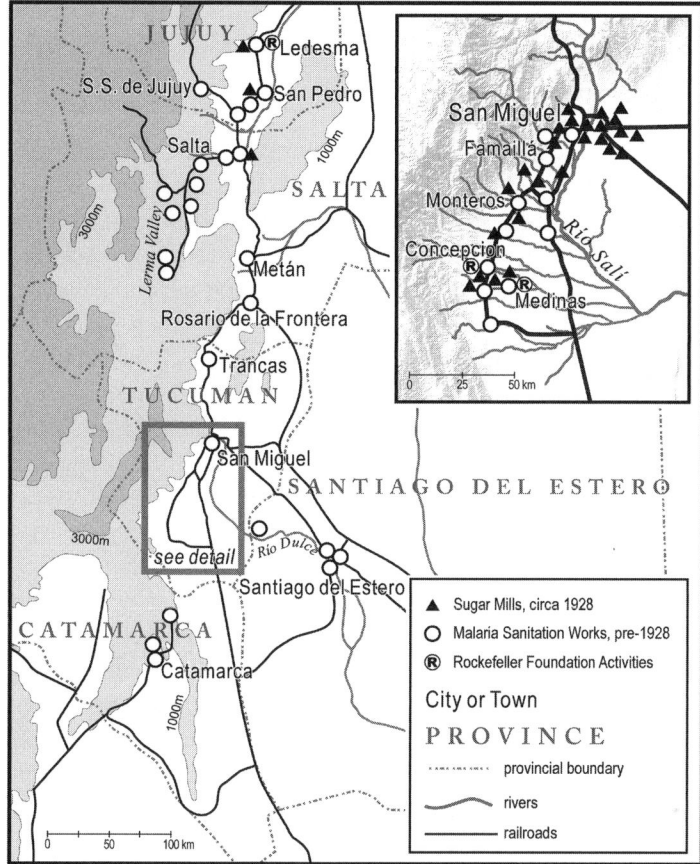

Figure 3.1. Map of Northwest Argentina, highlighting Malaria Service sanitation works, Rockefeller Foundation activity, 1925–1929, and sugar mills, by author. On Malaria Service works, see chapter 3, note 37; for Rockefeller Foundation activity, see chapter 3; for location of sugar mills, see Julio Bosonetto, "Distribución de los ingenios azucareros tucumanos," in *Geographia una et varia* (Tucumán: Universidad Nacional de Tucumán, 1951), 50.

works envisioned in Germán Anschütz and Antonio Restagnio's strategy maps of 1911, enabling the "continuous movement of running water." Overall, by the end of the 1920s the Malaria Service had carried out saneamiento works in at least thirty locales in the Northwest (see fig. 3.1).[37]

Traces of these works are still visible on the landscapes of the Northwest. From 1924 to 1926, in and around the intensely malarious town of Monteros in Tucumán, the DNH built 13,824 meters of canals and ditches, mostly alongside roads.[38] The troublesome El Tejar arroyo was deepened and straightened, and adjacent areas were filled and planted with eucalyptus trees to suction moisture from the soil. These eucalyptus trees, planted in the 1920s, are still visible on the banks of El Tejar today, as is an athletic field constructed on a filled marsh.[39] In 1927, the DNH drained and filled dozens of marshes and lagoons around Salta. Even the notorious Laguna de Chartas—a "frightful portrait of pain and misery," due to its reputation as a malaria hazard since the days of miasma—was finally drained, and its dry bed plowed for agriculture.[40] Today, a residential neighborhood, centered on Plaza Gurruchaga, sits on the reclaimed land. A slight topographical depression, rustic drainage ditches, and waterlogged soils in the plaza are subtle cues to the area's "insalubrious" past.[41] While the DNH bonifica work did not match the magnitude of draining the Pontine Marshes, such projects nonetheless showed their renewed commitment to reshaping the landscapes of the Northwest.

Strong Italo-Argentine institutional relationships in malariology helped transmit and sustain the Italian model in Argentina. These transoceanic linkages may help explain why the model became embedded despite its defects in practice. This binational expert network was established early and developed with renewed strength after the interruption of World War I. Exchange programs, for example, sent malaria control personnel from Argentina to study in Italy.[42] Likewise, Italian malaria experts came to Argentina to attend medical and public health conferences, such as the 1923 National Sanitary Conference, featuring Alejandro Lustig, an Italian biologist, physician, and senator, or the 1926 National Medical Conference, where Giulio Alessandrini and Gustavo Pittaluga presented papers and even a short motion picture on the successes of the Italian malaria campaign.[43] Since the Italian–Argentine relationship in malariology was well developed before the heaviest Fascist infiltration of malaria control began around 1928, the Argentines tended to ignore or diminish the Fascist ideology behind bonifica integrale. Mussolini's name was rarely, if ever, invoked, despite the obvious ways that bonifica integrale was used to enhance his cult of personality in Italy. Instead, hygienists tended to see bonification as a worthy expansion of state technocratic power, backed by a "scientific" analysis of social problems.

It is important to emphasize that Italian malariologists themselves were not intent on transplanting bonification, whole cloth, into Argentina. In fact, they usually emphasized the concept of mixed strategies, rather than one monolithic approach, as appropriate for malaria campaigns. Moreover, no one could claim to represent the "Italian School" as such, since it was dynamic and internally heterogeneous, with many strong disagreements about the nature of malaria and how best to control it. Pittaluga, for example, warned of the high financial costs of bonifica integrale.[44] In addition, unsettled scientific questions produced creeping doubts about malaria control methods among the Italians, including the perplexing phenomenon of "anophelism without malaria"; the strength of malaria in southern Italy, relatively free of the great swamps; and the findings of the 1927 League of Nations malaria commission. Cautious optimism, not overconfidence, pervaded the Italian school of malariology—if not the Fascist government of Italy—in the 1920s and 1930s.[45]

Yet, the more the malaria campaign in Argentina seemed to struggle, the more intensely bonifica-inspired efforts were praised and demanded. Malaria Service officials began using Italian terms, especially "piccola bonifica," interchangeably with their Spanish counterparts. In 1934, at the Fifth National Medical Conference, Nicolás Lozano and Domingo Selva proposed a "new orientation in the malaria campaign," composed of a costly escalation of saneamiento works and a concomitant reduction in emphasis on quinine dispensaries. But this "new orientation" actually reflected the long-standing preference for large-scale environmental sanitation works.[46] Into the 1940s, many reform-minded politicians, such as Alfredo Palacios, attempted to modify Law 5195 to codify the saneamiento orientation and grant the malaria campaign the power and resources that it had in Italy. Even after Carlos Alberto Alvarado had taken malaria control strategy in a completely different and more effective direction, as we will see in the next chapter, legislative proposals to reform the Malaria Service continued to promote an explicit imitation of the Italian school and attributed whatever success Argentina's malaria campaign had had to the partial replication of Italy's example.[47]

In summary, Italy's example validated two main aspects of Argentina's malaria campaign: landscape-based (saneamiento) strategies and the developmentalist orientation that portrayed malaria as the nexus of a whole suite of social ills. Transformation of the landscape was often conflated with mosquito control: the bigger and more visible the alteration of the environment, the better. Public health leaders in the two countries shared an organicist view of society, in which the nation was seen as a functioning organism composed of natural and human elements. While unable to execute control strategies at the same scale as in Italy—partially for want of landscapes truly analogous to Italy's Pontine Marshes—Argentina's malaria campaign forged ahead with its fight against nature. Public health leaders in Argentina, particularly Barbieri and Aráoz Alfaro, drew erroneous lessons from the Italian school: rather than redoubling efforts in malaria research, they assumed the solution was already available for import. The spuriousness of those geographical analogies would soon be exposed, however, in part through the productive scientific research of a new school of regional pathology in the Northwest.

The School of Regional Pathology

The development of "regional pathology" in the Northwest, spearheaded by Salvador Mazza, represents an interesting hybrid of scientific positivism (in epistemologies and methods), on the one hand, and regionalism and traditionalism (in foundational mission and public image), on the other. At the same time, retracing the connections of the scientists associated with this school to their peers in other countries indicates that regional science, far from being isolationist or parochial, depended on international scientific networks that largely bypassed national state institutions. Indeed, the regional pathologists constructed their professional identities in opposition to the national medical establishment, based in Buenos Aires, which they disdained for choosing urban comfort over fieldwork in remote places and ignoring the fate of Argentina's poorest, disenfranchised rural dwellers. These "abandoned peoples," to use Palacios's descriptor, suffered from malaria, Chagas disease, hookworm, goiter, leishmaniasis—vector-borne diseases or nutritional deficiencies that were characteristic conditions of poverty. Mazza and his cohort exemplify Marcos Cueto's "scientific excellence in the periphery," working in a backwater region within an internationally peripheral state.[48] Yet they were also a sometimes dissident group in the domestic scientific community, and as a result the impact of their research on malaria control was delayed.

The school of regional pathology developed in a context of resurgent regionalism. Assertions of regional identity in the Northwest appealed to collective memory of a glorious past of indigenous civilizations, Spanish conquistadors, bloody battles for independence, and gaucho patriarchs. While often striking the chord of traditionalism, northwestern regionalism did not simply reject positivism or rationalism. In Tucumán, the so-called Generation of the Centennial, a group of progressive but locally minded intellectuals and politicians, promoted a new, modern vision of the Northwest. They saw economic potential in the area's natural resources, strength in a cohesive though somewhat conservative culture, and beauty and order in the region's landscapes. Although a host of problems plagued the Northwest, regional political unity and a concomitant resistance to the hegemony of the littoral offered the opportunity for revival and growth.

One of the less-studied products of Northwest regionalism was the building of new educational, scientific, and public health institutions with a proudly local focus. A tightly knit network of progressive elites drove the building of these institutions. One of the foremost and influential members of this cohort was Juan B. Terán. Similar to his friend and fellow Tucumano Gregorio Aráoz Alfaro, Terán embodied the contradictory tendencies of a national intellectual elite in transition from the hegemony of positivist science and outward-looking, liberal political-economic theory to a conservative turn toward a search for the moral center of national identity.[49] Terán was the prime mover in founding the University of Tucumán in 1914, which proposed a new model of higher education focused on serving local needs.[50] In his inaugural address as first president of the university, he drew a sharp distinction between the new university and its predecessors in Buenos Aires and Córdoba.[51] The old schools were devoted to fine arts and philosophical abstractions, sufficient for producing a languid and self-centered elite; but, in contrast, Tucumán's university "aspire[d] to study the concrete truths of an unknown land."[52] Terán viewed Tucumán itself as a place where indigenous and Hispanic elements fused together, in fact creating the criollo roots of Argentina's national identity.[53] At the inauguration ceremony, Ricardo Rojas, a native Tucumano and one of the most influential of the conservative nationalist thinkers, laid out a radical vision of the objectives of the university.[54] Whether in science, humanities, or applied fields, everything would revolve around local questions and necessities.[55]

True to the ambitions of its founder and supporters, the university quickly became the nucleus for a network of scholars and institutions that celebrated regional identity through studies of local geography, history, culture, and hygiene. Miguel Lillo became the preeminent naturalist and botanist of the Northwest, and his vast library and herbarium, filled with specimens he collected throughout the region, served as the basis for the college of natural sciences that now bears his name. Alberto Rougés and Ernesto Padilla—provincial governors, scions of the Tucumán sugar oligarchy, and trustees of the university—created an institute for the study of folklore and traditional music of the Northwest and sponsored the leading compiler of regional folklore, Juan Alfonso Carrizo.[56] The school's Public Extension Department fashioned practical lessons on the public health problems of the Northwest, such as a pamphlet on the prevention of malaria, published in 1914.[57] The regional university thus filled important needs and interests that could not always be met in the country's established centers of higher education.

Leaders of the regionalist movement increasingly heaped scorn upon Buenos Aires, rather than viewing it as a model society worth emulating. Benjamín Villafañe was one of the most avid proponents of this new view. A key political figure in Jujuy, Villafañe served in various capacities, such as president of the provincial Board of Hygiene, governor, and national senator. Villafañe, known as a traditionalist and conservative, claimed that the littoral had been forming a "distinct nationality" from the 1880s onward, an identity that was devoid of patriotism and authenticity.[58] The achievements of Buenos Aires in consolidating political and economic power, he argued, had come at a great cost: a fragmented, soulless identity. The Northwest, on the other hand, was the "true reservoir of the 'national soul.'"[59] The notion of a "reservoir" of nationality was a strong metaphor: the very stillness, silence, and tradition of the region made it the source of authentic and autochthonous national identity. Villafañe and others construed this identity in a language that seamlessly mixed race, history, and geography. The "race" of the Northwest was truly criollo, a mixing of indigenous and Spanish blood in colonial times. Since this initial period of mixing, this alloyed identity had remained fixed, hidden from outside influences, and deeply rooted in place. This biological-cultural criollo identity would serve as a defense against the incursions of cosmopolites and immigrants and as the basic ingredient to reinvigorate national identity.[60]

Villafañe and others also developed a more incisive political-economic critique of the region's chronic underdevelopment. The problems of the Northwest, such as endemic disease, illiteracy and ignorance, unequal land distribution, and lack of agricultural development, were due mainly to the national government's fiscal policies, which left the provinces unable to solve their own problems. He compared the relationship between Buenos Aires and the interior to that between "a bad, powerful older brother who exploits his helpless younger brother" or "an all-powerful stepmother who administers the fortune of a defenseless orphan"; the government seized millions of pesos annually to build palaces to itself in Buenos Aires and watched "distracted and impassively as tropical fevers, tuberculosis, and other scourges devoured" the poor, abandoned people of the Northwest.[61] Simultaneously, Alejandro Bunge, an economist, marshaled demographic and economic data to analyze the problem of interregional "disequilibrium." Inspired by an invitation from Terán to study the economic geography of the northern provinces, Bunge proposed that the pursuit of economic liberalism—the *librecambista* ideology—had made Argentina the breadbasket of the world, yet the production of the interior had virtually no domestic market, with imported goods so cheaply obtained. Foreshadowing Latin American dependency theory, Bunge saw intensification of protectionism as an antidote for regional imbalances. Similar to Villafañe and Terán, he also celebrated the industrious criollo, condemned the cosmopolitan and materialist Porteño, and singled out malaria control as the most important investment that the national government could make in promoting the development of the Northwest.[62]

The inquisitive yet defiant spirit of the new regionalism inspired the development of a school of regional pathology, with concrete connections to Tucumán's new university, local intellectuals, and the Malaria Service. Guillermo Paterson, Salvador Mazza, and Carlos Alberto Alvarado were the pillars of this regionally focused medicine, and all would make vital contributions to malaria science in Argentina.[63] While all of these illustrious physicians were connected with Tucumán and its regionalist institutions, the true locus for this network was Jujuy, the country's northernmost province. Paterson, born in 1871 in Yorkshire, England, settled in Jujuy at the behest of the Leach Brothers, owners of La Esperanza sugar mill in the town of San Pedro. In his capacity as staff physician at the plantation, he carried out important studies of the *Anopheles pseudopunctipennis* mosquito (hereafter, *A. pseudo*).[64] He also served on the University of Tucumán's first board of trustees, taught the very first class of any kind at the university (on the subject of hygiene), and directed Tucumán province's Department of Bacteriology.[65] Mazza, born in the province of Buenos Aires in 1886, would come to know the Northwest only in his late thirties. Yet he would dedicate his life to understanding the endemic diseases of the region.[66] Alvarado (1904–1986), the youngest of the three, was born and died in Jujuy and would eventually lead the most successful phases of the national malaria campaign in the 1930s and 1940s. These three men, separately and in collaboration, put the idea of regional medicine into practice, developing research methods and fostering institutions adapted to the realities of the region. At the same time, their work demonstrated the continued importance of communication and collaboration with foreign scientists.

Mazza is now a legend in Argentine medicine, celebrated for his rigorous, productive research and his passionate devotion to rural health. As with most Argentine medical scientists of his time, Mazza was trained at the Facultad de Medicina of the University of Buenos Aires, where he was well placed in the tightly knit network of hygienists and medical researchers.[67] After World War I, Mazza worked in French North Africa with Dr. Charles Nicolle, who developed important techniques for the diagnosis and treatment of typhus, leishmaniasis, and other zoonoses, all while working in a "public health backwater" far from the European centers of medical research.[68] In Nicolle, a Pasteurian microbiologist and future Nobel laureate, Mazza found a role model and steady collaborator.[69] In 1925, sponsored by the University of Buenos Aires and the DNH, Mazza and Nicolle toured northwestern Argentina for the first time, traveling from the subtropical lowlands to the arid Puna of Salta and Jujuy Provinces, collecting insects, speaking with local doctors, taking blood and tissue samples from people and animals, and observing hospitals and clinics.

Before they returned to Buenos Aires, an important meeting took place between Mazza, Nicolle, Villafañe, then the governor of Jujuy, and Ricardo Alvarado, the head of the province's Board of Hygiene.[70] They discussed an idea that Mazza had for an institute specifically devoted to the study of the region's medical problems, modeled on Nicolle's institute in Tunis. Nicolle himself proposed that the institute should be located in Jujuy, to build on the work of Paterson and to "prevent the commotion of the metropolis [Buenos Aires], with its intrigues and special interests, from stifling the very purpose of the institution and deviating men from their effort."[71]

Mazza quickly put this idea into action with the foundation of a pair of institutions for the advancement of regional medicine. The Sociedad Argentina de Patología Regional del Norte (SAPRN: Argentine Society of Regional Pathology of the North) was founded in Jujuy in February of 1926, with Paterson as its president and Villafañe as its honorary head. The SAPRN connected medical scientists and hygienists from throughout the region, bringing these professionals together at regional medical conferences.[72] The SAPRN held nine meetings in the Northwest (and Mendoza) from 1926 to 1935. With each meeting, its research output grew more prodigious: the proceedings of the first meeting numbered just 75 pages, but by the fifth meeting (Jujuy, 1929) there were a hefty 1,534 pages of papers in two volumes.[73] Affiliated with this group was the Misión de Estudios de Patología Regional Argentina (MEPRA, Argentine Mission for Studies of Regional Pathology), which Mazza also initiated in 1926. This institution was actually a dependency of the Medical School of the University of Buenos Aires, and its origins owed a lot to the interest of the medical school dean, José Arce, and the rector of the university, Ricardo Rojas.[74] Villafañe also played a key role by donating the land in Jujuy's capital to build the MEPRA headquarters. There, Mazza established a laboratory and clinic and taught courses on tropical medicine and regional diseases. The connection of the MEPRA to northwestern culture was symbolized by the group's logo, a drawing of a *huaco* (funerary urn) utilized by the pre-Hispanic cultures of the area.[75] Such symbolism helped to establish the institution's spiritual home in the Northwest, though it still depended on Buenos Aires for funding and personnel.

True to their aims, both the SAPRN and the MEPRA became catalysts for important research in the pathologies that affected the Northwest region, particularly in its poorest and remotest areas. The major research focus for Mazza and his colleagues was Chagas disease and other vector-borne pathologies. Beyond his scientific accomplishments, Mazza's spirit, attitude, and methods inspired a generation of medical scientists in the Northwest to recognize their identity as *regional* scientists. One of his biographers, the Salteño Andrés Cornejo, wrote that this identity evolved from the perception that the doctors of the region were "abandoned and bereft," far away from the universities that had formed them, without resources, and without a clear view of the special problems of the region.[76] While Aráoz Alfaro, Villafañe, and Terán had gestured at ways to remedy this marginal situation, Mazza articulated the problem and created the institutions that joined professional and regional identities.

Also vital to Mazza's mission was "taking medicine to the people": knowing that poverty and distance prevented many people from seeking treatment in the hospitals of the provincial capitals, or even at the more ubiquitous Malaria Service dispensaries, Mazza and his assistants created mobile laboratories and clinics. The MEPRA, for example, used a *vagón sanitario,* a railroad car equipped with a microbiology lab and medical clinic, which allowed them to travel throughout the impoverished interior, collecting samples and treating patients.[77] On journeys by train, by car, or on horseback, Mazza took blood and tissue samples in suspected cases of parasitic disease—even in the field, he was never without his microscope—and treated and vaccinated patients for common illnesses.[78] Fieldwork acquainted the regional pathologists with people and their medical conditions and also with distinctive environments and disease ecologies. The conditions of the natural and built environment and the specifics of the interaction between people and their surroundings, particularly with animals, were central to understanding the nature of zoonoses.[79]

The strong regional identity of the MEPRA and the SAPRN did not translate, however, into parochialism. Mazza sought the best assistance without regard to nationality. He realized early on that in Argentina he would not find people with the technical capacity in bacteriology, hematology, parasitology, or microscopy to allow the MEPRA to carry out advanced work. Thus, Mazza employed a succession of lab technicians, all female, from Germany.[80] Mazza also collaborated with personnel of the Rockefeller Foundation from 1925 to 1929 on various research projects on malaria in the Tucumán area.[81] Mazza and other MEPRA scientists were active in international conferences, received training in foreign countries, and established a working relationship with their Brazilian counterparts.[82]

Yet in later years, Mazza's willingness or ability to collaborate seemed to decline. Mazza could be "gruff and abrupt" and "favored an almost solitary research style," which some interpreted as coldness.[83] Professional rivalries and apathy toward the mission of regional pathology frustrated him.[84] He complained bitterly, "In this region there are no young men who want to study, only those who want to make money."[85] An intense feud with Carlos Alvarado starting in the 1930s limited Mazza's direct role in the malaria campaign, although by then he focused almost exclusively on Chagas disease, a fixation that guided him into the arid highlands and desolate Chaco, mostly outside of the malarious zone.

While Mazza's influence on the distinctive school of regional pathology was unmatched, the development of this cohort reflected a more broad-based project of building regional institutions in science, education, and the arts. The distinctive focus and attitude was inspired, in part, by a rising sentiment that revalorized the humble criollo and the traditions of the interior provinces. At the same time, scientific work responded to the unique conditions imposed by the region's physical geography, the basis for endemic conditions such as Chagas disease and malaria. Indeed, Nicolle's North Africa and Carlos Chagas's Brazilian Sertão served as better geographic analogues for the Argentine Northwest—at least, from the perspective of disease ecology—than Italy's Pontine Marshes. Concern over regional public health was transmitted and understood through an alternative expert network, whose key participants included doctors (Gregorio Aráoz Alfaro, Guillermo Paterson, Salvador Mazza), political figures (Ricardo Rojas, Benjamín Villafañe), and academics (Juan B. Terán, Alejandro Bunge). This network shared a concern for appropriate pathways to regional development and fostered important institutions of research and public health.

At the same time, regional scientists were far from insular: the search for local solutions to local problems did not preclude engagement with notable foreign scientists. In fact, the regional political and scientific elites could be more cosmopolitan in their outlook than their counterparts in Argentina's national government. As we will see in the next section, the Rockefeller Foundation's brief sojourn in Argentina owed much of its success to the support of this local network, but political machinations at the national level ultimately undermined their best intentions.

The Rockefeller Foundation's Malaria Work in Argentina

In the first half of the twentieth century, the Rockefeller Foundation (RF) was the foremost philanthropy dedicated to the improvement of public health around the world. Through its International Health Board (IHB) the foundation sponsored projects dedicated to the control or eradication of major infectious diseases, especially hookworm, yellow fever, and malaria.[86] Many analyses of IHB's infectious disease control action have portrayed a powerful, quasi-imperial organization serving US political, economic, and technological interests. As "missionaries of science," some have argued, the foundation's delegates imposed technology-driven solutions within a reductionist framework that kept the social causes of disease strictly at the margins.[87] Subsequently, through the influence of RF veterans such as Fred L. Soper, the Rockefeller model of disease control served as a template for the global malaria eradication program, whose unwarranted technological optimism seemingly doomed it to failure.[88] Newer historical interpretations, however, suggest that the RF negotiated, rather than imposed, its relationships with national public health establishments. These relations were "complex" and marked variously by "subordination, cooptation, alliance, pragmatism, conflict, or mutual adaptation."[89]

The RF's involvement in Argentina's malaria control program from 1925 to 1929 seems to fit the latter interpretation. Importantly, however, the so-called national group was not homogeneous in relation to the "foreign" scientists of the RF. From the start, in Argentina the RF had to negotiate the conflicting demands and interests of local actors in the Northwest and of the national government. The IHB found that collaboration with regional scientists, such as Salvador Mazza and Guillermo Paterson, was important for establishing local credibility, gaining support for control measures, and improving understanding of malaria epidemiology and vector ecology. Yet such cooperative efforts were no match for the general apathy of DNH bureaucrats or the stridently nationalistic and anti-interventionist attitude of the second Hipólito Yrigoyen presidency, which began three years into the RF's mission. The widespread perception of the RF as a vanguard for "Yankee" imperialism—specifically, as a surrogate for the Standard Oil Company—undermined the whole endeavor. The RF officers found themselves involuntarily embroiled in local political conflicts they barely understood; yet, ironically, the detailed documents they left behind give us a uniquely candid outsider's perspective on the politics of malaria control in Argentina.

Significantly, the first pleas from Argentina for RF assistance in malaria control came not from the National Department of Hygiene but rather from one of the leading forces behind the Northwest's regionalist movement: Terán, the president of the University of Tucumán. In 1919, when Terán wrote to the RF, the foundation had not yet begun overseas malaria control work and had been performing malaria control demonstrations in the southern United States for only three years, building on a successful experience with hookworm control.[90] After a long correspondence, the IHB decided to send two of its representatives to conduct preliminary surveys in early 1921.

As a sign of things to come, political problems immediately complicated the IHB's plans for a preliminary malaria survey. While IHB representatives H. A. Taylor and Jerome Mieldazis were en route to Argentina, President Yrigoyen had replaced Tucumán's governor Juan Bascary with a federal overseer (*intervento*). Upon their arrival, Taylor and Mieldazis found themselves bereft of official support since the overseer refused to recognize them.[91] Faced with this awkward situation, Taylor cabled to the foundation's headquarters in New York, requesting an immediate return home; representatives of the Argentine government, learning of his request, implored them to stay and carry out their work.[92]

Despite the perplexing political circumstances, Taylor and Mieldazis were still able to carry out cursory surveys of the towns of Monteros, Concepción, Lules, and Aguilares, four towns along Tucumán's provincial railroad line. Taylor's account of the province's rural areas dwelled on the character and disposition of the local poor, whom he described with barely restrained contempt. In Concepción, he remarked, "The majority of the people are lazy and indolent, they go about their work with a stupid look in their eyes, thin and pale with little interest in life and their lack of education makes them satisfied with their miserable dwellings." In Monteros things were about the same: "These people, as in all the towns in the malaria zone, are lazy and miserable dragging themselves rather than walking through the streets or sitting at the doors of the huts and houses."[93]

While perhaps unduly harsh, Taylor framed his descriptions in much the same way as Argentina's hygienists, arguing that malaria was the root cause of social and sanitary ills of rural areas. In the town of Aguilares, for example, he reported, "No [other] infectious disease is known in this town, malaria is the only drawback at present and it is believed that practically every inhabitant of the town is under its power."[94] Experience in rural communities in the southern United States no doubt conditioned Taylor's assessments of Argentina since his words echoed the paternalistic, demeaning, and often racist rhetoric of malaria control advocates in the South.[95] The RF officials who followed Taylor to Argentina were, perhaps, less bigoted but shared the perspective of American supremacy in matters related to science and medicine.

With political circumstances having truncated the Argentine survey, the country fell off the IHB's agenda for the next few years. Reassured by the support of a new president (Marcelo T. de Alvear) and the head of the DNH (Aráoz Alfaro), the IHB returned to Argentina in September of 1925, formally establishing a cooperative agreement with the DNH. Rapidly, the IHB mobilized a small staff from its operations in Brazil to begin survey and control work in Tucumán. The IHB's main representatives in Argentina—first, Nelson C. Davis, followed by Elsmere R. Rickard—had scant experience with malaria control and medical entomology, particularly with anopheles mosquitoes. Later on, the IHB's scientists would make key contributions to malariology and the foundation would become a key player in malaria control campaigns throughout the world. But when operations began in Argentina, the situation was different: Argentina was only the second foreign country where the RF undertook a malaria control demonstration project; in the first, Brazil, operations had begun only in 1924.[96]

Neither the foundation nor its personnel could rightly have been called "expert." Davis, who was the first director of the IHB's collaborative effort in Argentina, had only one year's experience in malaria control work when he was posted to the board's Brazil office. Rickard, who replaced Davis in 1927 as field director in Argentina, was also a medical doctor with similarly limited training in malariology; his reports also reveal a greater interest than Davis in local political and social conditions. For a time, entomologist Raymond C. Shannon conducted research with IHB staff on mosquitoes in the Northwest.[97] The IHB personnel, usually stationed in an office in Tucumán, received frequent visits from their supervisors at the Brazil office, first, George K. Strode and then Soper, who would become famous in the annals of malariology for his unprecedented eradication of the *Anopheles gambiae* mosquito in northeastern Brazil (with the notable aid of Shannon) in the late 1930s.[98] The often-domineering Soper tried to orchestrate the Argentina operation, and his diaries and letters leave an invaluably candid (though partial) account of scientific work and political machinations.[99]

By 1925 the RF's model for malaria control was crystallizing around key principles of administration, planning, and control strategy. Mostly oblivious of the then thirty-year history of malaria control in Argentina and the ongoing political debates on the issue, the RF hoped to impose its own model in Argentina without adjusting for the structures and strategies already in place. RF malaria control projects were always predicated on cooperation between the foundation and institutions of the "receiving country"; however, defining the contours of collaboration and cooperation would prove to be a constant challenge. Rather than taking over a country's public health operations, the RF conducted "demonstration" projects in selected locales, which were meant to serve as a template for continued government control work once the RF left the scene. The receiving government's contributions to the demonstrations, in the form of funding, personnel, and equipment, would gradually increase until the government took full "ownership" of the program at the end of an agreed-upon period (five years, in the case of Argentina). In its demonstration projects, the RF emphasized the need for careful epidemiological survey prior to control work, one of many aspects that distinguished RF operations from the status quo in malaria control in Argentina. Following these surveys, the RF focused almost entirely on mosquito control, rather than the "dual strategy" employed in Argentina. Finally, to aid mosquito control the RF conducted extensive entomological research, often in collaboration with local scientists, and these investigations would prove to be the foundation's most important legacy in the region.

Departing significantly from Argentina's approach, the IHB emphasized rigorous epidemiological surveys to accompany control work. The national Malaria Service, as we have seen, relied mainly on changes in caseload at its clinics to assess the severity of the malaria situation. As a result, the directors of the Malaria Service were hard-pressed to determine whether control methods were proving effective. In contrast, the RF employed two fairly rigorous methods for assessing the progress of their demonstrations. First, when beginning work in a locale, the RF would take spleen or blood (parasite) surveys of most of the population, along with mosquito captures, preferably in residences. At regular intervals afterward, as control work progressed, they would repeat the surveys to analyze secular change in malaria intensity.

The other "scientific" method used to prove the effectiveness of malaria control was to use towns with similar health and socioeconomic profiles as "experiment" and "control" locations for the purpose of comparison. For example, the IHB mission in Tucumán decided to begin work in the town of Medinas first and leave nearby Concepción "under observation" for a few months, letting mosquito breeding go unchecked.[100] Even after the IHB began control work in Concepción, it still focused effort on just a handful of towns, leaving the rest of the region to serve as a comparison. By contrast, the Malaria Service tended to spread itself thin, opting for widespread but perhaps mildly effective coverage. Although it was never stated explicitly, the Malaria Service probably felt more of a mandate to cover the whole malarious region, while the RF was under no such obligation.

While the Malaria Service attempted (at least in principle) to employ a mixed method that included both "internal" and "external" strategies, the IHB demonstration was almost exclusively dedicated to anti-mosquito work. The IHB representatives in fact tended to exaggerate this difference in approaches. Davis asserted, inaccurately, "The previous work of the [Argentine] gov't alone had mainly been the distribution of quinine."[101] RF officials mostly ignored the extensive saneamiento work of the Malaria Service, which had only intensified in the 1920s, and the other common ground they shared with their counterparts in Argentina, including a fascination with environmental sanitation as the means of achieving larger development goals. In any event, the IHB's work focused almost exclusively on eliminating mosquito-breeding areas through the construction of drainage works. Davis dismissed other strategies, such as house control of adult mosquitoes, as "never more than a palliative measure."[102] While the IHB did not exactly discourage the distribution of quinine in Northwest Argentina, it sometimes feared that widespread use of the drug confounded efforts to establish a resilient relationship between specific control efforts and a reduction in malaria cases.

Because of their focus on environmental sanitation, the IHB scientists paid very close attention to local topography. Results of field surveys were assiduously mapped on large-scale topographic sheets (usually, 1:10,000 scale). IHB maps contained a much greater depth of information than those of the DNH, conveying a more spatially sophisticated perspective on the malaria problem. Generally, DNH maps of malarious locales, such as those from the Anschütz-Restagnio expedition of 1911, served as an aid to engineering work: thus, visible hazards (areas of standing water) were mapped, along with ditches, canals, and fills (completed or projected). In contrast, IHB maps of a given locale, in addition to such environmental features, also incorporated *epidemiological* and *entomological* data. Locations of individual human malaria cases, adult anopheline captures (mainly in homes), and sites with anopheline larvae were noted. Thus the IHB scientists made an important distinction between potentially hazardous landscape features and known anopheles breeding foci, which did not necessarily coincide in space, whereas the DNH tended to conflate the two. Expressed graphically in maps, and connected to the analysis in their papers and reports, the IHB developed a nuanced understanding of malaria transmission in space and time. However, the practical effect on control work was, superficially, not that different from that of the DNH, except perhaps in the intensity and detail of drainage measures.

Control work in Concepción and Medinas, neighboring sugar mill towns in southern Tucumán, exemplified the RF approach. The use of large-scale topographic maps helped the RF to envision a comprehensive drainage network for each town and its outskirts, parts of which were already in place. A case in point was the Laguna La Palúdica in Medinas, located where the village's drainage system flowed into the Medinas River. The name of this place, literally meaning "malarious lagoon," testifies to its well-known status as a malaria hazard. As Davis diagnosed the situation, a local farmer, Mr. Correa, had diverted water from the village drain into his own canal by throwing up earthen dams. With the outlet to the river obstructed, water backed up to form the lagoon. Davis decided to rectify the situation, literally, by deepening and straightening a derelict canal along its entire length, to more rapidly remove drainage water, and then by constructing a wooden sluice gate at the head of Correa's canal, which was poorly built and overgrown with vegetation. Davis even withheld water from Correa until he could "put his ditch in shape."[103] The visual result of control work on the lagoon was striking: unruly nature, with its stagnant water and overgrown vegetation, was transformed into an orderly, functional, and thoroughly modern landscape. In nearby Concepción, RF photographs showed how malaria control had transformed a wild, forbidding swamp—described as a "prolific focus for A. pseudopunctipennis"—into a farmer's field within months, complete with orderly crop rows and apparently even a new paint job for his humble shack (fig. 3.2).[104]

Such before-and-after photographs graced the pages of the foundation's annual reports on progress from Argentina, as well as contemporary DNH publications.[105] To understand why wetland drainage was such a favored strategy to the RF and national malaria control advocates alike, we should not underestimate the impact of such imagery. These before-and-after series of nature transformed were the most visible, tangible, and quickly grasped icons of the work of malaria control. Other indicators of success—increased health and well-being, lower blood parasite rates, a decline in mosquito activity— were more difficult to express graphically, or else were too abstract. Nothing beat the visceral impact of a photo to show that work was being done.

The IHB conducted drainage works in only a few towns, so the great-

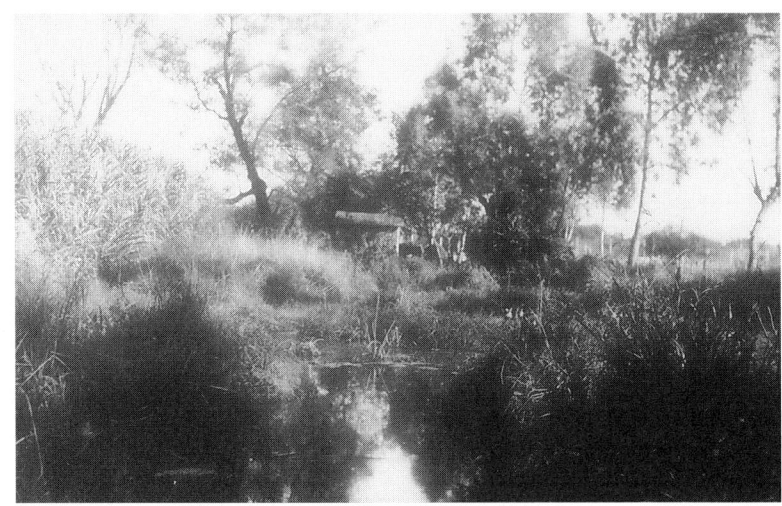

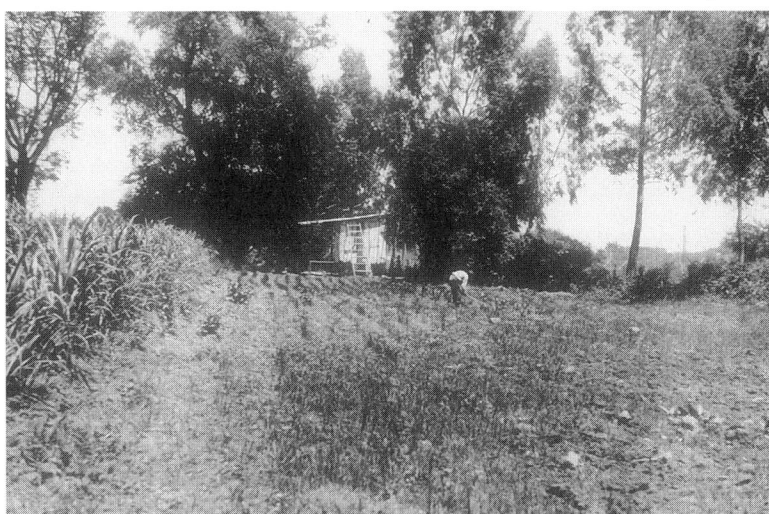

Figure 3.2. A swamp near Concepción, Tucumán, before (*above*) and after (*below*) drainage work carried out by the Rockefeller Foundation in 1927. "Annual Report of the Argentina Malaria Service," 1927 (photo #20095R and #20095S), Folder 1375, Box 105, Series 3, RG5, Rockefeller Foundation Archives, Rockefeller Archive Center. Courtesy of the Rockefeller Archive Center.

est legacy of the IHB's short-lived effort would be original entomological research, frequently in collaboration with Argentine scientists. Strode and Davis, during their September 1925 tour of Argentina, recognized that the "entomological side [of malaria control] has been unduly neglected. Considerable confusion exists in questions relating to classification; the biology of local anopheles is almost untouched; and a considerable number of other problems in medical entomology await the touch of trained hands."[106] For his part, Soper implied that Argentina's malaria chief, Antonio Barbieri, could not even distinguish an anopheles mosquito from its mostly harmless cousins, much less tell apart different anopheles species.[107] The RF's assessment of the Malaria Service's indifference to research on mosquitoes is mostly accurate, though the DNH had sponsored an entomological field mission to the Northwest in 1924, led by Peter Mühlens.[108] Nevertheless, RF officials often listened more closely to local scientists than the Malaria Service did. For example, when Strode and Davis visited Guillermo Paterson in Jujuy, he advised them that *A. pseudo* was the main, if not the only, vector for malaria in Northwest Argentina, an insight not completely incorporated into the DNH designs for malaria control until the 1930s.

Based on the work of Paterson and others, along with their own field observations, the RF increasingly favored a species-specific approach. Experiments in Medinas and Concepción showed that *A. pseudo,* unlike other local anophelines, gravitated toward human settlements, lingered in homes, and preferred human blood meals. Such evidence convinced the RF to confine control work to known foci of this species in July of 1926.[109] As control work proceeded, the RF scientists conducted still more research on the ecology, habits, and bionomics of *A. pseudo.* In the Río Medinas, Davis, with the aid of Dr. Miguel Lillo, the resident naturalist of the University of Tucumán, identified algae and other aquatic plants that seemed to be associated with anopheles breeding.[110] With Salvador Mazza, Rickard investigated the role of rice fields as mosquito breeding areas.[111] Later, in Ledesma, Rickard made an important discovery about *A. pseudo* flight range. By staining mosquitoes near their breeding sites, releasing them, and then identifying them in home captures, he determined that *A. pseudo* had a flight range of four to six kilometers, depending on wind velocity, significantly more than previously thought. This indicated the need for control of mosquito breeding areas far outside of urban zones and helped explain some past failures in malaria control.[112]

As early as 1927, the RF's assistance in malaria control in the Northwest was beginning to bear fruit, with a lowering, generally speaking, of malaria incidence in the towns where work had taken place, as well as a palpable decline in the number of mosquitoes. Moreover, the IHB claimed to have successfully rehabilitated numerous acres of wetlands, turning them into productive farmland.[113] The RF demonstrated, as they had intended, new techniques for malaria control, in particular, a species-specific approach that confined intervention to a smaller number of sites where *A. pseudo* larvae were discovered, making control work potentially more cost-effective.

RF scientists contrasted their selective and meticulous strategies with what they viewed as disorganized, often pointless control methods employed in Argentina. In a letter to Davis in 1928, Rickard ridiculed the DNH for having spent 6,000 pesos to drain and fill brick pits six kilometers outside of the Salta city limits, where only the larvae of harmless culex mosquitoes had been found.[114] Rickard was referring to the ambitious work led by Oscar C. Pickel, an American sanitary engineer, to drain over twenty substantial marshes and lagoons around Salta. In contrast, Barbieri praised the work enthusiastically.[115] Recognizing small differences between mosquito species had enormous implications for control efforts, but Malaria Service officials were, by and large, not impressed with the RF's insights.

The RF would soon discover that a lack of friends in high places had doomed their effort in Argentina. In spite of steady progress and measurable success, along with a fruitful collaboration between the RF and local scientists, the cooperative agreement rapidly unraveled in 1928 due to political instability and a cynical brand of nationalism that had come to permeate the federal government. While Rickard was on leave in the United States, leaving his Argentine assistant in charge, the national political situation changed dramatically with the re-election of Yrigoyen to the presidency. During the interregnum of Marcelo T. de Alvear, a rift had developed in the Radical Party between the supporters and enemies of the party's founder, and Yrigoyen himself had become increasingly nationalistic, paranoid, and ineffective.[116] Meanwhile, Dr. Manuel Bataglia replaced Gregorio Aráoz Alfaro, a staunch supporter of the RF, as the chief of the DNH.[117] Bataglia questioned the terms of the agreement between the two parties, which in 1929 required the Argentine government to pay 80 percent of the cost of the malaria demonstration program.[118] As the situation deteriorated that year, Rickard lamented that the national Malaria Service had failed to reorganize along the lines suggested by the demonstration projects and proposed that the foundation's resources might be better spent in countries with more acute needs and more cooperative governments, such as Brazil.[119]

But according to foundation officers in South America, the real culprit was Yrigoyen: Soper referred derisively to Argentina as a "one man Government" and a "voluntary dictatorship" because of Yrigoyen's zealous and overbearing governing style. No minister could make an important decision without his consent.[120] For several days in December of 1928, Soper and Rickard wandered between government offices, seeking an audience with anyone who seemed to have authority over the cooperative agreement. The minister of the interior disavowed all knowledge of the situation, while Barbieri proved once again to be a non-entity. Aráoz Alfaro offered moral support but, as a political dissident, could do little. Arranging a face-to-face meeting with Yrigoyen proved impossible. Thus for a time the continuation of the cooperative agreement was delayed by indecision, and in the meantime mutual suspicion grew. Soper remarked sardonically, "It is plain that no one will take any responsibility for anything here."[121]

At the time, Soper and Rickard failed to perceive the larger political context: Yrigoyen's nationalism, marked by anti-interventionism and suspicion of foreign institutions in Argentina, became increasingly strident.[122] Standard Oil, the original source of the RF's endowment, played the role of foil in Yrigoyen's anti-foreign rhetoric. While the RF was overseeing malaria control work, Yrigoyen engaged in a complicated battle with Standard Oil over petroleum rights in Salta Province.[123] From the start of RF activity in 1925, Salta newspapers had conflated Standard Oil and the RF; indeed, the IHB did antimalaria work at Standard Oil's operations in Tartagal. Years later, L. W. Hackett would suggest that Yrigoyen suspected that the RF was a front for Standard Oil, but there is no evidence that Yrigoyen explicitly made this connection. Meanwhile, the total absence of reference to Standard Oil in Soper's and Davis's diaries, and in the internal correspondence of the IHB, casts doubt on the validity of the implied claim.[124] In Argentina, the RF and Standard Oil functioned independently. Yet with the seeds of a suspicion of conspiracy planted, Yrigoyen surely saw no incentive to support the RF, and he declared that foreign institutions could not participate in government public health functions.[125] After a few months of vacillation, RF personnel withdrew from Argentina at the end of September 1929. The RF would later return to Argentina in another capacity, as we will see in chapter 5, but its active involvement in the malaria program was finished.

Conclusion

The premature demise of the Rockefeller Foundation's cooperative agreement in Argentina was not a total disaster, but it does illustrate the ironic, diverse impact of nationalism on the campaign against malaria. By the late 1920s, the ideology of conservative nationalism was ascendant: within a year of the RF's departure from Argentina, Yrigoyen would be overthrown in a bloodless military coup. A sense of nationalism had initially validated a burgeoning spirit of regional pride in the Northwest and nurtured the development of new institutions such as the University of Tucumán and the SAPRN. Yet nationalism also encouraged suspicion of foreigners and the institutions they represented. Nonetheless, the academics and scientists of the Northwest had no qualms about seeking out the assistance of the RF, welcoming its arrival, and engaging in collaborative research to improve the malaria situation in ways that the federal government alone obviously could not. Beyond this nucleus of interested individuals, such as Aráoz Alfaro, Terán, and Mazza, there seemed to be little support for the RF's involvement, and many within the Malaria Service and the rest of the DNH seemed to desire the demise of the agreement.

Another irony is that the RF, though a "foreign" institution, paid more attention to local factors in malaria control than any "national" institution had done to that point. Many historians have criticized the RF for importing methods of disease control without regard to local conditions, and to some extent it is true that RF officers in Argentina had rigid ideas of the "right" way to control malaria, particularly from a technical and administrative perspective, and were frequently dismissive of expertise in Argentina. However, during its four years in Argentina the RF engaged actively in research on micro-scale ecological and entomological conditions. Where Antonio Barbieri and others in the Malaria Service saw generic landscapes, their vision occluded by an optimistic embrace of the Italian control model, the RF actually came to know local conditions in intimate detail through careful observation and rigorous experimentation and with the helpful input of local experts. However, political intrigues spoiled, or at least delayed, the impact of collaboration between local and foreign scientists.[126]

After the RF's departure, Argentine scientists took up the lines of inquiry that the foundation had initiated. Research on the bionomics and ecology of *A. pseudo* grew more variegated and complex and eventually the Malaria Service would alter control methods according to these new findings. Many of the methods that the RF had introduced, such as the recording and mapping of malaria cases, mosquito breeding foci, and house captures; staining, releasing, and recapturing mosquitoes to determine mosquito flight range; and introducing an economic calculus to control decision-making, were adopted. Many within the Malaria Service and interested parties outside of it would continue to persist in the notion that Argentina's situation was like that of Italy and that imitation was the best route toward resolving the problem. While these fanciful notions still had currency in some circles, others would face up to the economic and political limitations of the campaign and incorporate new entomological knowledge to propose practical and localized control methods. The leader of this new, more dynamic phase of the campaign was Carlos Alberto Alvarado, the protagonist of the next chapter.

4

"Think like a Mosquito"
Turning the Tide against Malaria

The organization of the antimalaria campaign in our country has already
achieved international prestige; in foreign countries they speak of "the
Argentine school"; long-lasting prestige does not come from repeating
the same things, but rather from increasing knowledge and demonstrating
a perennial capacity for progress and improvement.
                    —Carlos Alberto Alvarado, *Memoria de la*
                    Dirección General de Paludismo 1944

By the early 1930s, four decades had passed since Eliseo Cantón's foundational treatise on the medical geography of malaria in northwestern Argentina, and twenty years since the initiation of the National Department of
Hygiene's malaria campaign.[1] Despite some successes here and there, malaria still reigned as the most important endemic disease of the region, if
not in the mortality tables, at least in the mind of the public, leading sanitarians, and reformist politicians. During this time, malaria was linked to so
many other problems—unproductive agriculture, unsanitary urban environments, an idle workforce, and even the vitality of the Argentine race—that it
seemed to be an indelible marker of the Northwest, along with stiflingly hot
summers, sugarcane, and tradition-bound torpor. Politicians would continue
their fact-finding missions, lamenting the intricate backwardness of the place,
while shedding little light on what could be done about it. For its part, the
Malaria Service struggled to find traction against the one disease that it was
charged with controlling. Its leadership continued to indulge in fantasies of
replicating the transformative scope of Italian *bonifica,* a preeminent example
of the modern state's scientific and technological prowess, despite their own
agency's precarious and marginal existence within Argentina's national government. A confounding politics ruled: senseless nationalism upset a productive collaboration with the Rockefeller Foundation, while parochial rivalries
placed federal bureaucrats against regional scientists such as Salvador Mazza.

Outside of the malaria campaign, demographic and political-economic
circumstances were changing regionally and nationally. As discussed in the
previous chapter, the population of the Northwest continued to grow steadily,

and it further concentrated in the lowlands, foothills, and valleys. While the Northwest still did not attract European immigrants in large numbers, movement within the region was dynamic. Poor criollos and indigenous people from the relatively unproductive highlands and Chaco made yearly pilgrimages to the sugar-growing zone for the *zafra,* and increasing numbers stayed on permanently. At the same time, while Tucumán remained the undisputed hub of economic activity in the region, the center of population shifted slightly northward, with migrants pulled by the relatively newer and larger *ingenios* in the lowlands of Jujuy and Salta, such as Ledesma and San Martín de Tabacal, and the recently discovered oil fields near the Bolivian border.[2] Thus, the so-called malarious zone was actually growing faster than the nonmalarious parts of the Northwest, and population was concentrating in even more tropical areas where malaria risk was presumably higher.[3]

Nationally, the political panorama changed rapidly. The conservative nationalists, already influential ideologically, finally seized power in 1930, overthrowing the already-discredited Hipólito Yrigoyen. Social elites and the public at large welcomed the nearly bloodless coup: with the worldwide economic depression taking hold, Argentines sought order and predictability in government.[4] In this "era of false democracy," rigged elections and heavy-handed political interventions ensured that conservative interests would prevail.[5] Yet, at the same time, to cope with the effects of the depression the longstanding agro-export model of economic development began to change, with the initiation of state-supported industrialization. Rising industrial centers around Buenos Aires proved to be a magnet for newcomers, although increasingly they came the from interior provinces, such as Santiago del Estero and Tucumán, as immigration from abroad slackened.[6] This exodus of rural poor to Buenos Aires and its suburbs would accelerate the transformation of labor politics in Argentina, eventually figuring in the ascent of the populist Juan D. Perón.

Perón, in the 1940s, would provide the resources and authority for the decisive eradication of malaria. The real turning point in the malaria campaign, however, came in the 1930s, when Carlos Alberto Alvarado, a public health doctor from Jujuy, took over the Malaria Service (fig. 4.1). This chapter examines his revitalizing influence. Alvarado instituted a number of key changes, particularly the reorientation of control work toward a single mosquito species, *Anopheles pseudopunctipennis* (hereafter, *A. pseudo*). He introduced a number of administrative innovations, such as the professionalization of agency managers, rigorous epidemiological evaluation of control measures, reorganization of field personnel, spatial zonation of service districts, and cost-benefit analysis of control work. All this was done with an eye toward increasing efficiency, almost in a Taylorist mode, with Alvarado al-

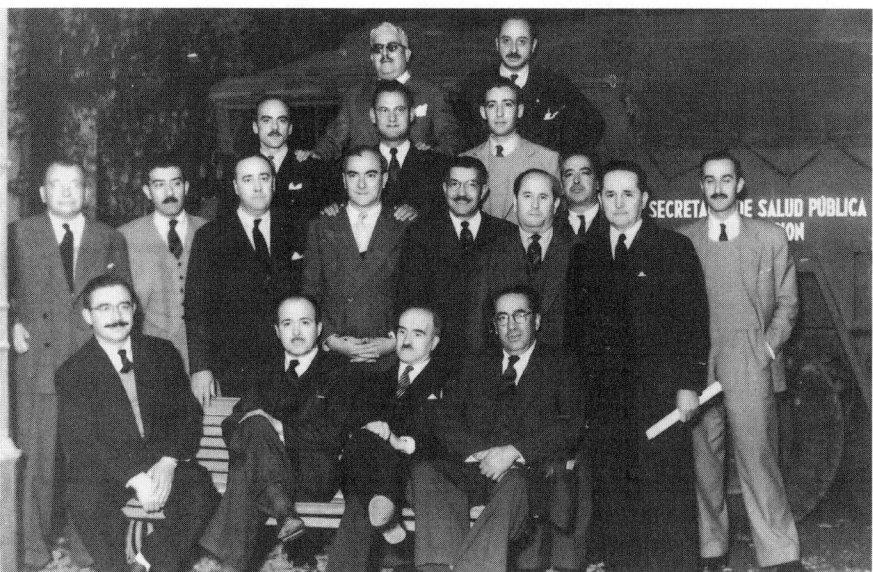

Figure 4.1. Carlos Alberto Alvarado (*seated, second from left*) and other directors of the Malaria Service, June 1947. Photo courtesy of the archives of *La Gaceta* (Tucumán).

ways finding new ways to yield more from the same inputs. Yet he also found creative ways to increase the budget of the service, mainly by inducing the collaboration of private enterprises in the Northwest. Alvarado's knack for management was as important as his role as scientist.

Crucially, Alvarado exposed the flaws of the *saneamiento* model and broke its dominance in Argentina's malaria campaign. As we have seen, the saneamiento model was born in the miasmatic era, when strong conceptual linkages between place and disease prevailed, validated by the successful sanitation of Santiago del Estero in 1902 and encouraged by the success of similar landscape-based techniques in Italy, where *bonifica* works were carried out on a grand scale. Saneamiento was a broadly socio-ecological framework that joined malaria control to other development goals through specific transformations of the environment, especially wetland drainage. Alvarado convincingly demonstrated that malaria was, in Argentina, not strongly associated with swamps, marshes, and other areas of standing water, due to the peculiar characteristics of the local malaria vector. In the process, Alvarado adopted a more reductionist and narrow view of the malaria problem, yet with the aid of concepts from ecological science.

This chapter begins by exploring the early career of Alvarado, including his training abroad and the initial field experiments he conducted in Jujuy. After a successful pilot run of the foci patrol program, Alvarado and Miguel

Sussini, the new president of the National Department of Hygiene (DNH), reassessed previous epidemiological and entomological research to build a counter-narrative to saneamiento.[7] Announced with great fanfare at an international conference of leading sanitarians in Buenos Aires, this new model, called foci patrol, thoroughly discredited previous leaders of the campaign. The new model depended on an original reading of ecology, which cannot be found exclusively in contemporary malariology or tropical medicine. Ascending rapidly in the DNH, first as an aide to Sussini, then as chief of the Malaria Service, Alvarado brought about major changes in the agency's administration and technical approach. Alvarado's reforms were largely successful, not only for their immediate impact on malaria incidence, but also for building the technical capacity and conceptual foundations for another major shift in strategy, based on house-spraying with DDT, in the 1940s.

Carlos Alberto Alvarado and the Jujuy Experiments

Alvarado was at home in the Northwest. He was intimately familiar with the region's landscapes and especially attached to the province of Jujuy, where he was born in 1904. Orphaned at a young age, Alvarado was raised by an aunt and uncle in the countryside near San Salvador, the provincial capital. On his relatives' farm, he developed a love of nature and an intense interest in the problems of rural society, which in turn drove him toward a calling in public health.[8] This career would take him far from the Northwest. First, Alvarado received his medical training at the University of Buenos Aires, where for two years he assisted future Nobel laureate Bernardo Houssay at his Institute of Physiology.[9] During his residency, he was supervised by Gregorio Aráoz Alfaro, president of the DNH, at the Hospital de Clínica in Buenos Aires. From 1929 to 1930, thanks to grants from the province of Jujuy and the University of Buenos Aires, Alvarado received additional training at the Scuola Superiore di Malariologia at the University of Rome and the London School of Hygiene and Tropical Medicine (LSHTM). After the 1924 mission to Italy led by Antonio Barbieri, the directors of the malariology institute in Rome greeted Argentines with suspicion because of their "dissolute lifestyles and lack of devotion to their studies."[10] Yet Alvarado soon assuaged these fears with his acumen and enthusiasm. On a field trip led by the renowned Italian malariologist Alberto Missiroli, Alvarado was the only one of a group of students to accompany the eccentric master on a swim across a river to survey mosquito-breeding sites.[11] His studies at London were, apparently, less eventful, though he profited from the insights of such tropical medicine experts as Patrick Buxton, a renowned entomologist.

After returning to Jujuy, Alvarado initially devoted himself to private practice, since an adverse political situation in Jujuy thwarted his interest in a public health position.[12] In 1932 Sussini, the president of the DNH, called on Alvarado and Eduardo del Ponte, an entomologist, to oversee a yellow fever prevention program in Tartagal, near the Bolivian border, following an outbreak of this disease in Santa Cruz de la Sierra. The successful effort in Tartagal, which sparked a rift with Mazza, also served as a springboard for regular work in public health.[13] In 1933, Sussini named him regional director of the Malaria Service in Jujuy to replace his uncle, Ricardo Alvarado.[14]

Initially, Carlos Alvarado carried on the work of his predecessors, using the mixed strategy of external (saneamiento) and internal (quinine) prophylaxis, while making do with limited resources. However, by virtue of a highly methodical approach to surveying malarious zones under his supervision, he soon made important findings about the mosquito; these findings would serve as the basis for a new model of control. Ironically, budgetary constraints may have actually forced a path toward a breakthrough. The Jujuy office of the Malaria Service covered most of the urban and suburban area of the capital, which included about sixteen thousand inhabitants. Alvarado decided, given the scarcity of personnel, to devote his resources to just one zone at a time, rather than spread efforts too thinly across the whole service area. The area he chose was known as La Viña, on the northern bank of the Río Grande, just across from the city. In Alvarado's division of the Malaria Control's services in Jujuy, he labeled the working-class, semi-rural area of La Viña as Zone 3. E. R. Rickard, of the Rockefeller Foundation (RF), had surveyed the area in 1929; his census showed that La Viña had a population of 174 people over about five square kilometers. Though this was a zone of farms, the population included just 21 agricultural laborers and 31 day laborers; 56 were domestic servants, presumably mostly women who worked in upper-class homes across the river.[15]

By concentrating activity in Zone 3 alone, Alvarado created the conditions for a controlled experiment. His office studied and continuously treated mosquito-breeding areas in Zone 3 while observing how other areas fared without intervention. Due to its position along the north bank of the Río Grande, between the Río Chijura and Arroyo Higuerillas, with steep embankments to the north, Alvarado felt that Zone 3 was relatively isolated from the areas where mosquitoes were left to reproduce unimpeded and malaria transmission continued unabated.[16] As was by then common practice, Alvarado initiated activities with a topographic survey, but at a much finer scale (1:5,000) than had been mapped before. On this map, Alvarado identified all of the areas that had potential to contain water, including canals, ditches, springs, and streams. For several months, Alvarado and his assistants sampled larvae from these water bodies, classifying each site by the anopheline species that predominated, and mapped the results. The vast majority of anopheles larvae found were of the species *A. argyritarsis*. Although it was ubiquitous in La Viña, the species was understood to be zoophilic, and thus not a malaria threat. In baited traps, however, Alvarado was finding many *A. pseudo* adults around homes. Where were they coming from?

Alvarado was surprised to find that *A. pseudo* predominated in pools and springs forming in the bed of the Río Grande bordering La Viña. Based on his cursory observations in Jujuy in 1928 and 1929, Rickard had identified the riverbeds of the area, particularly the wide, shallow Río Grande, as the primary locations of mosquito breeding.[17] From this point forward, Alvarado began to revive and confirm the earlier findings of Rickard, Nelson C. Davis, Guillermo Paterson, and Alois Bachmann, although it appears that initially he was not familiar with all of these studies. Alvarado and his colleagues discovered numerous *A. pseudo* larvae in seepage areas and braided channels of the Río Grande, as well as in nearby canals and springs. Sites tended to be populated exclusively by one species or another (either *A. pseudo* or *A. argyritarsis*), but these sites could be found just meters apart along the same stream or canal. Alvarado noted that *A. pseudo* larvae were found in canals or streams with straight, steep banks, relatively free of vegetation, except for a surface film of spirogyra algae; meanwhile *A. argyritarsis,* and not *A. pseudo,* was found in streams with irregular banks and abundant aquatic vegetation. These associations between the two mosquito species and their respective microenvironments became so obvious that field workers dropping off their larva samples at the lab would guess the species, almost always correctly, based on where they had been taken.

To confirm these microenvironmental differences in species-site associations, Alvarado decided to conduct what we might today call an experiment in ecological restoration. He found a spring-fed stream that had been previously cleaned, straightened, and deepened in saneamiento works populated by numerous *A. pseudo* larvae. He ordered the modified stream "re-naturalized": workers tore apart the straightened banks with picks and shovels, transplanted aquatic vegetation, and widened the stream bed, thus exposing it to shade from trees and shrubs along its margins. This area was left untreated, and before long it was populated by *A. argyritarsis* larvae while *A. pseudo* vacated the area. Soon afterward, in April of 1934, Alvarado found an unexpected opportunity for a complementary experiment, which started with a complaint by a farmer in Villa Gorriti, an area just to the south of San Salvador, across the Río Chico. In years past, the farmer protested, the Malaria Service had always kept the local canals and ditches free of vegetation, but lately this work had been neglected and now his house was full of mosquitoes. The farmer even threatened to take his grievance to the local newspaper. Alvarado explained that the Malaria Service was focused on work in La Viña and challenged him to clear the vegetation in the canals himself. He did so, and a few weeks later *A. pseudo* larvae were found there in abundance, along with a new growth of spirogyra algae.

It was becoming clear that these algae determined *A. pseudo* breeding areas. Bringing together all of his field observations and the evidence from the literature, Alvarado decided that the algae, not water temperature or water chemistry, presented the key explanatory variable: where spirogyra algae predominated, so did *A. pseudo* larvae; if these algae were absent, having been replaced by larger aquatic plants, then so were *A. pseudo* larvae. To explain this association Alvarado offered an elegant succession-and-disturbance model. Algae were always the first plant to develop in clean, vegetation-free water, since algae are excellent and rapid colonizers of disturbed aquatic environments. *A. pseudo* larvae found sustenance and shelter from predators in these algae. Subsequently, algae would compete with watercress, duckweed, and other more complex plants for dominance; and during the season of growth a "biological equilibrium" would be established, which under most circumstances meant the predominance of other plants and the crowding out of the algae.[18] As a result, *A. pseudo* production would decline, while other anopheline species would take over in sites with more mature vegetation. In this cyclical succession model, disturbances of equilibrium (for example, if a farmer cleared canals of vegetation, or seasonal floods stripped vegetation from stream beds) provoked favorable conditions for new algae growth, the production of *A. pseudo,* and the beginning of a new succession sequence.

Alvarado was thus convinced that eliminating *A. pseudo* larvae hinged on controlling the growth of spirogyra algae. Based on a year's worth of experiments, he reoriented the campaign toward what he termed *policía de focos,* or "foci patrol." Infused with the new awareness of the mosquitoes' microenvironments, this strategy was concerned only with finding and treating or eliminating breeding foci for *A. pseudo,* especially through the removal of algae. Workers physically removed mats of algae from streams with picks, shovels, hoes, or brooms; and where removing algae was less feasible, they treated breeding areas with petroleum or Paris green (copper aceto-arsenate). The foci patrol strategy led to some immediately quantifiable results: the blood index of people in La Viña, solely through this method and without the administration of quinine, dropped from 30.0 percent in April 1929 to 7.3 percent in October 1934. In November 1933, seventy-three *A. pseudo* adults were captured in fourteen houses; one year later, only two *A. pseudo* adults were captured in nineteen houses.

Alvarado's program represented an important break with saneamiento. If *A. pseudo* was the only significant malaria vector, and if it was not prone to breeding in stagnant, marshy environments, then why would large-scale drainage be expected to control malaria? Alvarado, a thirty-year-old upstart, could hardly expect to undo the status quo. However, he found an ally in Sussini, the president of the DNH. Together, they decided to lay out the case against saneamiento and present their new approach in a very public forum. There would be no going back after that.

The Case against Saneamiento

While Alvarado and Sussini prepared their indictment against the ingrained model of malaria control, things carried on as usual in the Malaria Service. Barbieri still presided over the agency, which continued its policy of general distribution of quinine, combined, when financially feasible, with saneamiento interventions, while carrying out practically no original research into the disease. In 1933, Barbieri published an article summarizing the campaign's achievements over the previous ten years. He reported that, thanks to a "system that followed the example of the most experienced countries," malaria control was a success, as saneamiento, in combination with quininization, had reduced incidence of the disease in the Northwest, especially in its major cities. Notably, Barbieri took special pride in the ways that malaria work had transformed the landscapes of the region: "All you have to do is visit the populations or cities of Monteros, Concepción, Medinas, Trancas, Aguilares, Famaillá, Rosario de la Frontera, Salta, Jujuy, Santiago del Estero, to comprehend the sanitary work of saneamiento undertaken by the National Department of Hygiene. Open drainage canals and large, small, or subterranean drains, with a total extension of more than 200,000 linear meters, [along with] fills and reclamations, have changed the suburban aspect of those cities and towns."[19] Barbieri advised a continuation and intensification of these successful saneamiento measures, and he also proposed a comprehensive program of rural development in public health, which would include the construction of "hygienic residences" to replace the "miserable shanties" that made rural life so precarious. Thus Barbieri concluded that broadening the idea of saneamiento, which had worked so far, would be "of great importance for the progress and the health of the provinces of the North."[20]

Even so-called new orientations for malaria control rehashed old ideas. In 1934, for example, Nicolás Lozano, a veteran of the campaign, and the engineer Domingo Selva presented such a proposal at the Fifth National Medical Conference in Rosario.[21] Their plan mostly reiterated what had become the standard position in malaria control: "internal prophylaxis" (i.e., quininization), though widely employed, was a second-rate strategy against the disease. To truly solve the malaria problem required more investment in large-scale saneamiento schemes, following the Italian bonifica model. They celebrated once again the achievement of Antenor Alvarez in the Santiago del Estero epidemic, thirty years before, and, similar to the DNH's sanitary reforms of Salta around the same time, lumped malaria control together with projects to supply clean water and sewage systems.

Clearly, the leaders of the Malaria Service were locked into a specific ideology. The saneamiento model had been born in the miasmatic era, put into practice during the Santiago del Estero epidemic, formalized in legislation and the work of the Malaria Service, and validated by Italy's experience. More than just a scientific model, however, it was also a narrative of regional development. By this point, to move in a different direction required not small adjustments, but a new narrative. A genuinely new course for the malaria campaign was made public in November 1934 at the Ninth Panamerican Sanitary Conference in the city of Buenos Aires.[22] Here, with delegates assembled from most of the countries of the Western Hemisphere, Sussini, borrowing from Alvarado's work, presented the case against environmental sanitation and the need for a new approach. They took apart the old narrative by exposing its false analogies and reframing older scientific evidence and offered an alternative model, foci patrol, that fit the geographical and epidemiological conditions of the Northwest.

Sussini devoted most of his paper to reviewing the mounting body of evidence, some of it over twenty years old at that point, that undermined the model. Mostly, these data came from published studies of the distribution, behavior, and ecology of anopheles mosquitoes, readily available to DNH officials. The foundational text of the counter-model was "Las fiebres palúdicas en Jujuy" (Malarial fevers in Jujuy) by Guillermo C. Paterson, published in 1911.[23] Paterson, one of the key members of the network of regional pathologists in the Northwest, was an English-born physician who supervised the medical clinic at La Esperanza sugar mill in San Pedro, Jujuy, from 1894 to 1943.[24] During his tenure there, as early as 1899, he researched the local epidemiology of malaria, which led him to examine the habits of local mosquitoes. In his 1911 publication, Paterson made two points that would eventually come to have great significance. First, he found that *A. pseudo* was the most prominent anopheline species in areas of Jujuy and Salta where malaria was prevalent. Almost invariably, the presence of this species was associated with the disease, while that of other species, such as *Anopheles argyritarsis,* was not. The preponderance of *A. pseudo* in domestic spaces led Paterson to argue that it was "practically *the only species* that acts as an agent to disseminate malaria" in the area.[25]

Second, based on numerous observations, Paterson characterized a typical breeding area of *A. psuedo* in this manner: "Breeding grounds are found in *clear waters,* and preferably in those that contain certain classes of multi-cellular algae, allied with *spirogyrae,* which constitute the favorite food for [*A. pseudo*] larvae."[26] The characteristics of *A. psuedo* breeding areas—clear water and presence of spirogyra algae—were so obvious in 1911 that even the untrained workers of the local branch of the Malaria Service (which Paterson also headed for a while) could recognize them at a glance.[27] For good measure, Paterson had also included a table of the main sites of *A. pseudo* breeding in San Pedro and Ledesma; specific *vertientes* (springs), *arroyos* (creeks), and *pozos* (excavations or wells) predominated, while *ciénagas* (swamps) were rarely mentioned.

In the years that followed, there were sporadic echoes of Paterson's initial findings and additional information about the complex of anopheles mosquitoes in the Northwest. In 1924, for example, Juana Petrocchi, the DNH staff entomologist, described the environmental conditions where *A. pseudo* larvae thrived: "[*A. pseudo* larvae] develop only in clear, well-aerated waters, with a preference for a weak current and especially very shallow waters. The classic locations populated exclusively by anopheles larvae, in Salta and Jujuy, are small *springs.* The water emerges and flows slowly, forming rivulets or brooks among the rocks and sand, only a few centimeters deep, there anopheles larvae pullulate especially among the *lama* (groups of algae that float in the water forming mats among which the larvae take refuge, hiding from predators and feeding on these same algae)."[28]

A few years earlier, Bachmann, head of the Malaria Service office in Famaillá (a sugar mill town southwest of Tucumán), had published findings on the local malaria–carrying mosquitoes.[29] In reference to *A. pseudo,* Bachmann wrote that "on the beaches of the rivers one finds all of the conditions for the survival of larvae, *slightly running water, abundant sunlight, sandy bottom,* and *a mat of algae* that shelters and encloses their food."[30] Although Bachmann had indicated these decidedly un-swamp-like conditions for mosquito breeding, the DNH's 1928 report on progress in malaria control instead highlighted the benefits of large-scale wetland drainage in and around the city: engineering works had created a "complete network of canals for drainage and the hydraulic regularization of Famaillá."[31] Such works were exemplary of *piccola bonifica* or *saneamiento pequeño.* The Malaria Service's saneamiento work, however, barely touched the banks of the Río Famaillá, where Bachmann found *A. pseudo* breeding in seepage areas.[32] In other words, despite his precise understanding of the environmental conditions favorable for *A. pseudo,* Bachmann continued drainage works according to the old model, leaving this species' breeding grounds largely unaffected.

Around the same time, the Rockefeller Foundation began work in Argentina. As discussed in the previous chapter, from 1925 to 1929 the RF pursued saneamiento-style strategies in the towns of Concepción and Medinas predicated on drainage of wetlands. But in conjunction with this practical work RF personnel also carried out key studies of the *A. pseudo* mosquito. In his 1934 presentation to the Panamerican Sanitary Conference in Buenos Aires, Sussini cited the work of RF scientists Davis, Rickard, and Raymond C. Shannon as a crucial improvement in the understanding of *A. pseudo,* particularly in three aspects: host preference, range of flight, and favored breeding places. After beginning work in Medinas, Davis and his colleagues realized that *A. pseudo* was intensely anthropophilic relative to other anopheline species, thus confirming Paterson's 1911 observations.[33] As a result, the RF's environmental sanitation work was quickly reoriented to focus almost exclusively on primary breeding sites for this species, while the Malaria Service continued to be mostly indifferent to inter-species variation.

In terms of flight range, when RF officers arrived in Argentina, they assumed that female *A. pseudo* moved no more than 1.0 to 1.5 kilometers between breeding sites and domiciles.[34] In 1927, Rickard undertook an ingenious experiment in Ledesma to determine the mosquito's flight range; Sussini later termed this as "magnificent research." Rickard found that seepage areas in the bed of the Río Ledesma were primary breeding sites of *A. pseudo* production and wondered if these mosquito nurseries were near enough to the town of Ledesma to represent a threat (fig. 4.2). A few yards from the riverbank, Rickard set up three artificial breeding tanks protected by screens, where previously captured *A. pseudo* eggs and larvae were allowed to develop into adults. Rickard and his assistants then stained and released the newly emerged adults. Later, a tiny proportion of over ten thousand stained mosquitoes were captured in homes in the settlements of Ledesma, Pueblo Nuevo, and Florencia. The results were startling. Just under half of the mosquitoes had traveled at least 2.5 kilometers from their birthplaces, and some had even flown 4–6 kilometers.[35] The implication of this study was huge: the zone of malaria control action around Ledesma and other settlements would need to be widened considerably.

Even as they continued to employ conventional saneamiento techniques— Davis and Rickard wrote in 1928 that drainage, "where practicable, constitutes the best means of extinguishing [mosquito] larvae"[36]—experimental and casual observations began to reveal that characteristic breeding areas of *A. pseudo* were usually not amenable to permanent, landscape-transforming techniques. Shannon labeled *A. pseudo* "primarily a mountain species" with preference, especially early in the breeding season (late winter to early spring), for "the valleys and the gorges in the mountains where it finds springs and streams having a permanent supply of fresh water." *A. pseudo* was also partial to "pools containing an abundance of green algae" that offered the somewhat

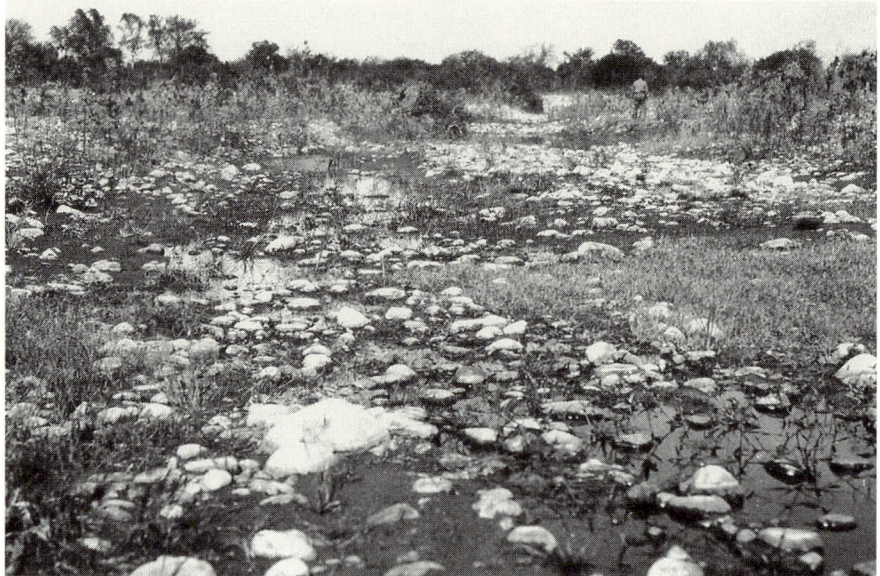

Figure 4.2. "Rocky seepage area in bed of Río Ledesma" (caption from original source). "Annual Report of the Argentina Malaria Service," 1928 (photo #20364), Folder 1379, Box 105, Series 3, RG5, Rockefeller Foundation Archives, Rockefeller Archive Center. Courtesy of Rockefeller Archive Center.

sluggish larvae protection from predators as well as a source of food.[37] It appeared that the presence of green algae was the key variable associated with almost all sites of intense *A. pseudo* production, regardless of other characteristics of the landscape: "whatever class of water [body] that is favorable for the growth of green algae is exceptionally favorable for larvae of *A. pseudopunctipennis.*"[38] Thus, large, shallow areas of standing water were not inappropriate for *A. pseudo* breeding *per se;* rather, in such bodies of water other vegetation types tended to predominate over green algae. In such "dangerous-looking" swampy areas, Davis and Rickard had indeed found countless larvae, but of the *Nyssorhynchus* group, not *A. pseudo.*[39] Meanwhile, in canals that had been cleared of brushy or grassy vegetation during saneamiento works—"in canals as well maintained as possible"—Davis and Rickard *did* find *A. pseudo* larvae from time to time.[40] On one occasion, Davis exclaimed, "believe it or not, the more you clean these canals, the more pseudopunctipennis you find."[41] On a trip through the area in 1927, Fred L. Soper found the algae so remarkable that he included a photograph of himself holding up a dense mat of it, in a letter to F. F. Russell (fig. 4.3).

The RF helped contribute one more piece to the mosquito puzzle through studies of the relationship between malaria and rice farming.[42] Many provin-

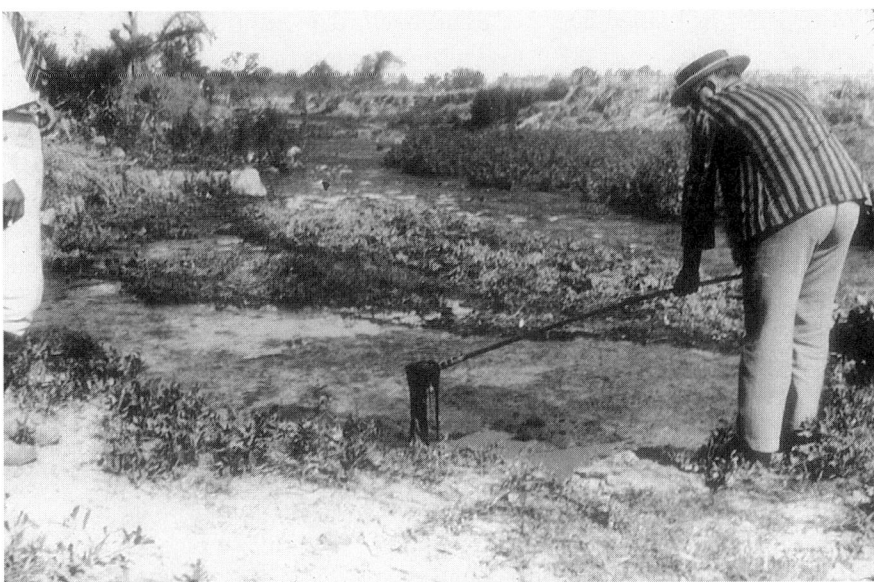

Figure 4.3. Fred L. Soper examining mats of spirogyra algae, November 1927. Photo #19828, originally attached to letter from Soper to F. F. Russell, December 28, 1927 (no. 441), Folder 59, Box 5, Series 301, RG 1.1, Rockefeller Foundation Archives, Rockefeller Archive Center. Courtesy of the Rockefeller Archive Center.

cial and national lawmakers, along with public health officials, had attempted to regulate or prohibit wet rice cultivation due to the entrenched perception that standing water was associated with malaria. But the issue was never studied until the late 1920s, when Rickard and Mazza collaborated on a meticulous, two-year study of mosquito breeding on rice farms in the department of Chicligasta, Tucumán Province. They discovered that the presumed association between rice fields and malaria was spurious. Although *A. pseudo* adults were found in abundance in houses near rice fields, only 4 out of 784 anopheline larvae captured in the rice fields (i.e., just 0.52 percent) were identified as *A. pseudo,* and the rest belonged to the anopheles group *Nyssorhynchus* (predominately *A. albitarsis* and *A. tarsimaculatus*).[43] Rickard and Mazza concluded that the absence of *A. pseudo* in rice fields could be explained by the absence of the algae that was instrumental to their protection and sustenance. While other mosquito species thrived when surrounded by abundant rice plants, *A. pseudo,* on the other hand, predominated in nearby sites. This evidence suggested yet another reason to disassociate wetlands from malaria and, by extension, to distinguish agricultural development from malaria control.[44]

In synthesis, reconsidering all of the evidence, Sussini concluded that saneamiento had failed because it had been focused on the wrong kind of mosquito. *A. pseudo* was the principal vector for malaria, but it did not breed in swamps, marshes, or other large areas of standing water. To drive home the point, Sussini offered a detailed presentation of the findings of Alvarado's La Viña experiments. The historical evidence, now recomposed in a new narrative, seemed to lead to just one logical conclusion: Alvarado's program of foci patrol. This constituted a very public rebuke of the leadership of the Malaria Service. Sussini accused them of not only committing important errors, but also willfully ignoring evidence that was right before them, for years. Making matters worse, many of the aforementioned studies had been published in the National Department of Hygiene's own journals!

With this speech, Sussini declared an end to the era of *bonifica* and permanent saneamiento works, instituting a new motto for the Malaria Service: "to fight against the anopheles vector of malaria in northern Argentina is to fight against algae."[45] Alvarado dramatically changed the optic of malaria control from vaguely defined and potentially innumerable marshes, swamps, and other areas of standing water to only those specific, though still numerous, sites where easily identifiable spirogyra algae flourished. After 1934, the Malaria Service adopted Alvarado's plan of foci patrol (sometimes simply called Plan Alvarado) as the "new model" and explicitly opposed the "old model" of the Italian-inspired saneamiento school. "Our country followed that route [of the Italian school] and for many years effort has been concentrated on the drainage of small marshes, swamps, and quagmires," Alvarado wrote later. "Success did not accompany those efforts of *saneamiento del suelo,* and the redemption of *tierra palustre* brought only an improvement in agriculture with mediocre sanitary results."[46] Or as Sussini put it, "The literal application in our territory of methods that are successful in other parts of the world is not only ineffective, but can become inconvenient, even detrimental."[47] Indeed, over the years the construction of new ditches and the straightening, deepening, and cleaning of old canals for wetland drainage, rather than reducing malaria transmission, may have unintentionally created improved habitats for *A. pseudo* in many locations.

In the end, Alvarado and Sussini had not exactly discovered something *new,* but had reframed what was already known, yet habitually overlooked. Research on anopheles in the Northwest had been *accumulating,* but not *advancing,* because of a lack of cross-referencing, synthesis, and a theoretical structure to make sense of it all. More importantly, research discoveries did not immediately lead to new directions in malaria control strategy.[48] With an ecologically informed lens in place, the causes of the malaria problem and the means of controlling it suddenly seemed crystal clear.

Based largely on the success of the La Viña experiments, in November of 1935 Sussini elevated Alvarado to the position of secretary general in the National Department of Hygiene, making him the second-ranking public health official in the nation. Though thoroughly discredited, Barbieri clung to his position in the Malaria Service for a few more years, but as little more than a figurehead. Now effectively in charge of malaria control, Alvarado began to rebuild the institution in the image of his new approach.[49]

Scientific Ecology and the New Control Model

One of the hallmarks of Alvarado's approach was a strong ecological orientation that had previously been absent in the campaign. As his son Peter said to me, "When he made the plan to control malaria in Jujuy, he did it with an ecological sensibility. . . . [H]e said, 'You have to think like a mosquito to understand its behavior.'"[50] But, what exactly does it mean to "think ecologically" in the context of malaria control? And, given that ecology was unknown at the time in Argentina, where did Alvarado gain his special perspective? Foci patrol applied ecological ideas selectively, strategically, and pragmatically; at the same time, Alvarado eschewed "socio-ecological" perspectives and isolated the malaria problem, analytically, from other social issues. In this way, Alvarado represented a major paradigm in international malaria control, the "species sanitation" school. Yet his highly original framework owed as much to plant and pond ecology as to malariology.

Alvarado's concept of foci control fit within a contemporary, international school of thought in malaria control known as "species sanitation."[51] Advocates of the species sanitation approach argued that the most effective methods of malaria control were based on the elimination of larval habitats of only those mosquito species known to transmit human malaria and found in close proximity to human settlement. The major pioneers of this approach, such as Malcolm Watson, N. H. Swellengrebel, Fred L. Soper, and Lewis W. Hackett, brought a greater awareness of mosquito biology and niche ecology to bear on the malaria problem.[52] As malariologist D. J. Bradley puts it: "The idea of species sanitation depends on there being a localized, specific, and highly predictable habitat for the crucial species of anopheline vector for an area during its larval stages. Implicit is a highly developed concept of the ecological niche. Its geographical location is retained, but there is a concept of multiple features that make the place suitable for a particular species of anopheline."[53] Species sanitation methods, then, targeted only the ecological niches of "relevant" mosquitoes (those that transmitted human malaria) and ignored the environments of "irrelevant" species. Sometimes, in fact, species sanitation strategies altered environments of the harmful species to create a niche more favorable for the harmless mosquitoes.

How was species sanitation distinct from other environmental sanitation approaches? As we have seen, malaria scientists, as well as lay people, had long made associations between malaria and particular places. For the most part, these tended to be weakly understood associations, without strong theoretical foundations, relying on spatial coincidences and vague qualities of place. Bradley, following George Macdonald, calls such superficial associations "circumstantial epidemiology with a geographical component."[54] In contrast, the species sanitation approach viewed a place not as "malarious" per se, but as the site of intersection (and interaction) among environmental characteristics that created favorable conditions for mosquito breeding. Moreover, suitable mosquito habitats varied dramatically between, and even within, species.

Hackett demonstrated the species sanitation perspective in his 1937 classic, *Malaria in Europe: An Ecological Study.* Synthesizing a decade's worth of research in Italy and the Balkans, along with historical evidence, Hackett found not only important variation among anopheline species, but also within "species complexes," most notably that of *A. maculipennis.* The various "races" or subspecies of this mosquito exhibited behavioral differences that belied their morphological similarities. In areas with the perplexing phenomenon of "anophelism without malaria," zoophilic subspecies predominated; over the long span of history, changes in animal husbandry practices drove away anthropophilic subspecies, thus serendipitously reducing malaria incidence. Arriving at such an understanding required attention to the minutiae of mosquito physiology, behavior, and ecology. The intensive focus of species sanitation on discrete microenvironments tended to sever control strategy from larger development goals, such as reclamation to promote agriculture or urban development.[55]

Alvarado's model of malaria control shared many of the elements of species sanitation: an ecological perspective, a focus on specific anopheline species, and a desire to "disentangle" the malaria problem from a larger set of social ills.[56] Species sanitation proponents argued for narrow, entomological interventions and expressed skepticism of "social development" malaria control policies based on multiple, interrelated strategies, such as land reclamation, improved housing and sanitation, and education. The latter type of approach sought to eliminate the "root causes" of malaria within a broad social and environmental framework, but species sanitation scientists doubted that such policies could make much headway against malaria itself. Swellengrebel and Hackett actively questioned the Italians' integrated agrarian development, or *bonifica,* model, as well as social policies sanctioned by the League of

Nations Malaria Commission during the 1920s and 1930s.[57] They also came to see quinine as simply a palliative, not the basis for effective malaria control. At the end of the 1930s, the eradication of the invasive *Anopheles gambiae* from Brazil, led by Soper, validated the species sanitation approach, setting the stage for postwar eradication campaigns using DDT.[58]

Alvarado was probably aware of the debates between the species sanitation and social development approaches, even though the ideological lines were not yet so clearly drawn. In Italy, Alvarado certainly witnessed both sides of the argument. From May to October of 1929, Alvarado was a fellow at the Scuola Superiore di Malariologia in Rome, where he studied under Alberto Missiroli and met Hackett, who was stationed there as an RF officer.[59] Together, Missiroli and Hackett conducted field experiments during the 1920s that demonstrated the effectiveness of species sanitation techniques.[60] Alvarado's arrival coincided with an era of good relations between the RF and the Italian malariology community, with a florescence of original research on malaria vectors. However, Missiroli would have a profound change of heart in the 1930s, moving away from the site-specific approach of species sanitation and embracing the grand-scale *bonifica integrale* strategy, which, of course, resembled the saneamiento strategy that Alvarado later criticized.[61]

In addition to the world of malariology, Alvarado was also engaged in a wider, interdisciplinary scientific network that helped shape his understanding of a pivotal relationship: the ecology of algae and its influence on mosquito development. After his experience in Rome, Alvarado took up residence at the LSHTM, from February to July of 1930, where he was exposed to insights from the emergent science of ecology.[62] The intersection of expert networks in ecology and malariology has not been explored by historians, at least not for this time period, when ecology was still in its infancy. In Argentina, ecological theory had scant influence on the natural sciences until much later in the twentieth century.[63] Alvarado's case suggests that an interesting and innovative cross-pollination of ideas may have been occurring earlier and that studies of vector-borne disease provided an important conduit for the diffusion of ecology to Argentina.

Although the evidence is somewhat circumstantial, the method and substance of ecological and entomological research taking place in London had striking parallels to Alvarado's own work in Jujuy a few years later. Notably, graduate students Lucy J. Howland and Mary V. F. Beattie collaborated on an investigation of the annual cycle of "the succession of the algal flora" and its relationship to mosquito breeding, on a pond in Hertfordshire, over the course of four years (1925–1929).[64] As a recipient of the prestigious Wandsworth Scholarship at the LSHTM, Beattie conducted research for several years there under the tutelage of Patrick A. Buxton. Howland studied under Buxton at the same school and under Felix Eugen Fritsch at the University of London. Buxton was the head of medical entomology at the School of Hygiene and had served in the British colonial administration in Palestine in the 1920s, where he researched local anopheline vectors.[65] Buxton's interest in the relationship between insect species and the dynamics of plant ecology emerged most strongly in his research on tsetse flies in Africa.[66] Fritsch, meanwhile, was an expert in freshwater algae and pond ecology, as well as the president of the British Ecological Society.[67]

In their research, Howland and Beattie were most concerned with explaining why different mosquito species bred in different environments. Reporting results of their work in Hertfordshire in separate articles in the same issue of the *Journal of Ecology* in 1930, Howland and Beattie found associations between certain species of mosquito (including anopheles) and certain species of algae (including spirogyra).[68] Moreover, they concluded, such associations explained the spatial variability of mosquito larvae better than differences in water chemistry; and mosquito productivity was in sync with the seasonal cycle of algae growth. Alvarado took courses with Buxton at LSHTM, just as the results of Beattie and Howland's experiments were being published. While Beattie and Alvarado could not have crossed paths—she was in Trinidad conducting similar experiments on anopheles mosquitoes—he certainly knew Buxton and may have had contact with Howland and Fritsch. It seems warranted to speculate that the influence of this small research cluster, along with Missiroli and Hackett in Rome, enabled Alvarado to synthesize concepts from aquatic plant ecology, entomology, and malariology.[69]

Drawing on these diverse international influences, a reconsideration of Argentine malaria studies starting with Paterson, and his own field observations, Alvarado framed the environmental dynamics of mosquito-breeding areas within what today might be termed a "classic" succession and disturbance model. In the absence of other aquatic vegetation, algae such as spirogyra were the first to colonize spring-fed streams, canals, seepage areas, and river channels, following disturbances such as high-energy flows that scoured vegetation from streambeds and banks. These constituted the "primary" or "preferred" breeding areas of *A. pseudo,* where adult *A. pseudo* mosquitoes were found earliest in the season, in greatest numbers, and with the least competition from other mosquitoes. As *A. pseudo* reproduction overwhelmed primary areas, the mosquito populated secondary or "expansion" sites, including irrigation canals, creeks, and marshes.[70] In such sites, other vegetation types would gradually take over following a classical succession model: first other algae and weedy plants, such as *berro* and *lampazo,* then larger, flowering plants, and so forth. Alvarado identified late-succession marshy environments with diverse plant life as examples of "biological equilibrium," that is, a complex and stable community that made a good niche for many kinds of mosquitoes.

Thus, typical *A. pseudo* environments were subject to frequent disturbances (such as floods), while other mosquitoes favored late succession or "climax" communities of aquatic life, characterized by taller, thicker vegetation. Using this framework to map and plan control efforts, Alvarado classified riverbed environments into four categories in ascending order of time since last flood, inversely related to risk of *A. pseudo* breeding. In effect, Alvarado constructed a model narrative of short-term environmental change that allowed him and his colleagues to identify hazardous areas according to the plant communities found there. Alvarado's insight is reminiscent of that of the pioneering American ecologist Henry C. Cowles. As Donald Worster has written of Cowles's experience at the Indiana Dunes, "A keen observer, walking inland from the water's edge, could trace a pattern of ecological succession *in space* which paralleled the development of vegetation in time."[71] Cowles saw climax communities—the oldest, most diverse, and most stable assemblages of plants—as the natural endpoint of ecological succession for a given climate, topography, and soils. To Alvarado, the "biological equilibrium" of mature plant communities prevented the predominance of any one insect species. Anthropogenic disturbances, such as clearing vegetation from ditches, destroyed "the ecological balance established by nature" and established the conditions for increased *A. pseudo* breeding.[72] His valorization of "natural" wetlands as beneficial to public health—or at least, not detrimental to it—contrasts sharply with the decided antagonism toward them in earlier phases of the malaria campaign. But the crucial point is that Alvarado, as Cowles did, could "see" these ecological processes, with all of their dynamism and complexity, inscribed on the landscape.

Thus refracted through the ideas of his contemporaries, the meaning of Alvarado's "ecological vision" becomes clearer. He did not see society and environment coupled together in the same system, nor did he see society as an "organism" that conformed to the same organizing principles as nature. Rather, as did Hackett, he saw humanity and nature engaged in a faceoff, across a great divide, with forces organized on each side. Ecological principles were useful for understanding the way nature worked, in hopes of subverting or altering its machinery. He knew that malaria control was a boon for humanity, and perhaps for the economic development of the region, but success in this endeavor demanded reductionism—the life of malaria-carrying mosquitoes had to be perceived in its minute detail. Ecology was instrumental: it provided the necessary framework for understanding why certain mosquitoes were associated with certain plant communities; how different species responded to environmental change, whether natural or anthropogenic; and how the vector's spatial distribution changed seasonally. Finally, it offered a way of predicting, more accurately than previous approaches, where mosquito larvae could be found. The ecological complexity of the disease demanded resilient social organization in response. To this end, Alvarado methodically scrutinized administrative techniques, to a far greater degree than his predecessors.

"See and Record": The New Logic of Organization

Alvarado introduced a meticulous attention to *method,* both scientific and administrative, to the Malaria Service. Generally, the methods of his predecessors were poorly developed, inconsistently applied, and rarely scrutinized. In contrast, attention to order, detail, and procedure permeated all of the malaria control work carried out under Alvarado, as demonstrated by several important innovations. Under his direction, the Malaria Service constantly experimented with new control methods, while subjecting them to rigorous evaluation. He reorganized labor resources to correspond to the spatial and temporal dynamics of the *A. pseudo* mosquito. As the malaria campaign grew larger, he increasingly looked to the military as a model for efficient and effective use of scarce resources. He also introduced accounting, even a rudimentary form of benefit-cost analysis, to further streamline the campaign's services. In all, this emphasis on efficiency and effective outcomes furthered his goals of professionalizing the Malaria Service, increasing its technical capacity, and isolating it as much as possible from the vicissitudes of public health politics.

Although the foci patrol program showed immediate, positive results, Alvarado took just as much pride in the empirical methodology that he used to design the program. Knowing how to observe epidemiological and environmental patterns was the underlying basis for any successful plan, he argued, implying that his predecessors in the Malaria Service habitually failed in this respect. In 1938 he wrote:

> In sanitary medicine knowing how to see is a quality *sine qua non,* and I would add: *see and record,* to use an expression of our President [Miguel Sussini] whose experience and intuition in sanitary matters places him today among the most accomplished figures in the history of sanitation in our country. . . . I know intelligent colleagues with years of experience who fail to notice certain facts occurring in the same environment in which they are working, because they do not know how to *record*

what happens in front of their eyes on a daily basis. If someday a school of hygiene is built in this country, I will arrange to have them write on the walls, from the floor to the ceiling, these two words: *see and record*.[73]

While there was nothing revolutionary about these ideas, Alvarado drew a distinction between his approach and that of Barbieri and others who persisted stubbornly with saneamiento-based control without clear signs of success. In contrast to this doctrinaire attitude, Alvarado and Sussini freely admitted that foci patrol was simply the best program under the present circumstances, and open to debate. "These observations represent what has been seen and done in a very short time, less than one year and a half," said Sussini in his presentation of the experiments in La Viña. "We do not expect that these observations have resolved the problem, and these conclusions should be the motive for new, subsequent verifications. In a field as vast as that of malaria, we should always hope for the possibility of finding something new or better."[74] Alvarado reinforced this idea in 1938, stating presciently, "It is logical to admit that tomorrow new possibilities will be discovered that will make anti-malaria programs more perfect and economical."[75]

In keeping with this philosophy, the Malaria Service under Alvarado experimented with new techniques to control *A. pseudo* larvae. Here, Alvarado was clearly in touch with progress in the international field of malaria control, which in the years immediately prior to the advent of DDT expanded its repertoire of mosquito abatement techniques.[76] For example, in the late 1930s, Alvarado constructed *subterráneos biológicos,* roughly "biological tunnels," in many sites. This "naturalistic" method consisted of using layered branches and leaves to cover brooks and canals, thus casting shade on the water below and preventing the establishment of spirogyra algae. A few years later, sanitary engineer Prudencio Santillán, Alvarado's right-hand man, experimented with anti-larval sluicing using automatic siphons. Made of cement, these structures used the natural action of siphonic flow to flush larvae downstream, very similar to the action of a flush toilet.[77] Santillán experimented with several models, in a specially designed hydrology lab and in the field, before finding the appropriate dimensions for the apparatus. Stream shading and sluicing were both subjected to rigorous field testing, with the Malaria Service's now-regularized mosquito sampling (of larval and adult forms) providing the necessary data to test effectiveness of new methods. The results of such techniques were not overly impressive, but Alvarado's Malaria Service demonstrated its openness to new tactics, as the rapid adoption of DDT would later confirm.[78]

In the meantime, through the 1930s Alvarado adjusted the Malaria Service's organization of labor resources to the spatial and temporal dynamics of *A. pseudo* breeding. Under the foci patrol program, the extent of the work area assigned to each technician varied according to the number of potential *A. pseudo* breeding sites he could regularly visit and treat (by removing mats of algae or spraying larvicides) in one week's time. Thus work zones with numerous, densely situated hazards were smaller than zones with fewer, dispersed hazards. Only one worker would patrol each zone, meaning the elimination of gang labor or work teams, as had been the norm under previous leadership. Alvarado reasoned that a team of laborers, making a circuit over a large area from one larval habitat to the next, visited a given hazard only occasionally, perhaps once every few weeks. Such an interval was ineffective for control, since *A. pseudo* mosquitoes took only about ten to fourteen days to grow out from egg to adult. The division of a service area into contiguous zones, with each zone patrolled by just one worker following a weekly itinerary, would theoretically offer complete and uninterrupted coverage of the entire area. In this manner, Alvarado also assigned greater responsibility to each worker and created more transparent criteria for assessing individual performance. This increase in responsibility was reflected in a new job title for the lowly *peón: encargado de sección,* or "section manager," a change that suggested an increase in trust and proprietorship of a well-defined work space.[79] Alvarado also believed that the psychology of the criollo was better suited to solitary work.[80] Moreover, this system streamlined administration at the lowest levels, since fewer foremen would be needed for direct supervision of laborers, thus freeing them for other tasks, such as research.

Alvarado's interest in harmonizing the spatial logics of mosquito ecology and the technical-administrative aspects of malaria control was also reflected in his zonal model for urban malaria control. At a micro-spatial scale, the division of labor of the campaign revolved around the timing and location of *A. pseudo* breeding, but at a more macro scale, such as that of a city and its vicinity, campaign planning hinged on the flight range of the mosquito. Alvarado's general scheme for urban malaria control was based on zones in concentric rings around a city. The underlying rationale was to maximize protection of the most densely populated areas in the center. Using a large-scale map (e.g., 1:20,000), a typical locale would be divided into four zones: A, B, C, and D. The urban area proper corresponded to area A, the zone of "absolute protection," with other zones determined by concentric circles at two-kilometer intervals from the center. These intervals were based directly on the assumption of a two-to-four-kilometer flight range for *A. pseudo,* drawn from Rickard's earlier studies in Jujuy. If all of the potential breeding areas for *A. pseudo* in zones A, B, and C could be completely monitored and systematically destroyed, the probability of transmission within zone A was practically nil.[81]

The foci patrol scheme protected urban areas—where high population densities produced lower per-capita cost of sanitation works—from the inside outward: the concentric ring system buffered the center from invasion of *A. pseudo* mosquitoes on the fringes. The Malaria Service supplemented this strategy, most effective during the season of malaria transmission, with an intensive winter program that sought to control foci as far as twenty kilometers away from cities. Alvarado concluded, just as Shannon and his colleagues had in 1928, that *A. pseudo* production seldom continued unabated throughout the year; there was a sharp decline, if not an absolute cessation, of breeding in the drier, cooler winter months (for the Malaria Service, roughly May to October). During this season, *A. pseudo* mosquito larvae were typically found in a state of suspended animation in their most preferred breeding sites, such as creeks and springs in foothill canyons. Malaria Service investigators occasionally would find frozen or lethargic larvae in icy waters on winter mornings.[82] In the spring, these sites would become origins of the first adults, and mosquitoes would rapidly repopulate other foci and move progressively closer to populated areas. Thus, during the winter dry season, foci patrol turned away from cities, directing control efforts toward the rugged foothills. Though the discovery and treatment of all foci was impossible, by impacting over-wintering grounds the spring expansion of breeding sites could at least be delayed.

For Alvarado, the epitome of efficient social organization was the military. Although bellicose metaphors and military-style planning were hallmarks of malaria and yellow fever campaigns worldwide, from the Panama Canal Zone to Italy and Brazil, the notion of a "war" on malaria or the mosquito was never made explicit in Argentina until Alvarado took charge.[83] With an emphasis on planning, organization, execution, and constant vigilance, his plan bore a striking resemblance to a military campaign, in rhetoric and practice. Alvarado chided the previous directors of the malaria campaign for their lack of initiative and aggression against the "enemy," the anopheles mosquito: "There is a military precept that says he who attacks imposes the rules of combat on his adversary. . . . It is necessary to get out and challenge the enemy, in his own camp, over the rules of combat; it is necessary to attack, and the attack requires movement."[84] Along these lines, Alvarado habitually characterized the mosquito as the aggressor (*agresor*) and the human host as the attacked (*agredido*), a language seldom employed before in the rhetoric of the campaign. Alvarado increasingly ascribed centrality and *agency* to the mosquito vector. He shifted the role of "enemy" from the disease or the landscape to the mosquito, calling malaria control a "war against the mosquitoes."[85] References to "the theatre of operations and the conduct of the aggressor" anthropomorphized the mosquito and defined it as a combatant.[86] At times, Alvarado merged ecology and military strategy: by making the landscape more suitable for *A. argyritarsis*—the harmless mosquito species—he could make a valuable "ally" against the "common enemy," *A. pseudo.*[87]

Beyond these rhetorical maneuvers, Alvarado relied heavily on military ideas about organization, logistics, and, to a lesser degree, tactics. Peter Alvarado recalled his father telling him, "When I have a problem of supply, I look for a military man who knows about planning."[88] The broad geographical scope of active control operations, which after the integration of DDT techniques would cover five provinces, was surpassed only by that of military operations, so Alvarado "conversed often" with army officers for advice on campaign logistics.[89] Even under the relatively low-intensity program of foci patrol, Alvarado imposed military logics of hierarchy, chain-of-command, planning, execution, and individual accountability. As he said in 1938, "Foci patrol is based on unified execution and in the sum of individual performances. One mistake, then, has repercussions for the success of the group. Realization [of foci control] should be militarily conceived and militarily executed."[90] Since foci patrol depended on "100 percent" implementation of control measures within an assigned area, "failures [were] punished severely."[91] This regime of labor discipline, however, was tempered by the autonomy given to each peon, who was evaluated based on completion of individual tasks.

Alvarado also made a greater effort to quantify success or failure of the campaign. Alvarado believed that statistical surveys defined the magnitude of a sanitary problem and thus aided in the design of control strategies.[92] Epidemiological evidence constituted the standard of proof of effective control measures. Before Alvarado took over, baseline epidemiological studies (e.g., blood or spleen indices) were carried out only sporadically; and the DNH before Alvarado was just as likely to define success in other quantifiable, but not necessarily *relevant,* terms: total area of marsh drained, canals constructed, man-hours of labor spent, or quinine distributed.[93] For example, the 1928 DNH publication *La lucha antimalárica en la Argentina* (whose relatively slick production values suggest that it was intended, in part, as a public relations tool) is full of this sort of superficially impressive but not necessarily significant data.[94] Alvarado, in contrast, made the blood index of children under the age of two the baseline measurement in every locale where the Malaria Service was active.

Alvarado used such statistics to make hard choices about the spatial coverage of the campaign. With a dispassionate, utilitarian attitude, he argued that the Malaria Service's action in a given locale had to surpass a threshold of cost-effectiveness. In other words, the monetary costs to society of uncontrolled malaria had to outweigh the costs of malaria control to justify the agency's intervention. To calculate the costs of uncontrolled malaria, Alvarado included "the expense of curative malaria medication, medical attention, loss of life from malaria, loss of life indirectly attributable to malaria (debilitation of the organism), loss of work days, and finally, economic or social depression."[95] Vaguely, he added to this cost a "small percentage more" for "the right to health." Alvarado calculated these costs generically, and more by analogy and estimation than any true formula. He estimated that any program costing less than five pesos per capita per year was "financially practicable" because the British colonialists had stipulated a figure of four shillings, and the malaria works in the Panama Canal Zone cost the United States only about two dollars per capita.[96]

The novelty of Alvarado's approach was to perform a rudimentary cost-benefit analysis at the scale of communities (cities and towns). With careful planning and attention to detail, he wrote, "The cost of a program of 'foci patrol' that maintains community X free from harm can be calculated with the same meticulousness as a work of engineering or architecture (of the well-calculated ones!)."[97] Where the potential cost of malaria control work fell below the fixed baseline of five pesos per capita per year, it was considered viable. This calculus favored urban areas, and the more densely populated, the better. Thus, to protect the sixteen thousand inhabitants of San Salvador de Jujuy cost about 54,000 pesos, or 3.37 pesos per person per year, well under the baseline figure. Protecting Salta was even more economical: only 1.5 pesos per person per year.[98] In those places where the cost would be too high, the Malaria Service would offer only a "rural" control plan, little more than a stopgap measure that entailed minimal expenditure. The more comprehensive urban plan centered on the foci patrol strategy, while the rural plan relied on distribution of quinine, medical attention (when available), and sanitary education. This coldly calculated two-tier system sacrificed the well-being of rural people in favor of city dwellers, yet Alvarado was simply formalizing a situation that was already in place and exhibiting a characteristic willingness to confront budgetary and logistical challenges head-on.

New Approach, Better Results?

During their leadership of the DNH from 1935 to 1937, Sussini and Alvarado restructured the bureaucracy of the Malaria Service. They sought to align administrative functions with the needs of the new foci patrol approach and to increase the autonomy of the agency within the state's public health administration. With such measures, Alvarado set out to transform the nearly moribund Malaria Service into what he called "a technical organization with increasingly specialized personnel," and this redesign was made official policy by the National Congress in April of 1937.[99] Alvarado was made chief of the Malaria Service, now renamed the Dirección General de Paludismo (General Directorate of Malaria), finally replacing Antonio Barbieri, who had retired after almost thirty years in that office. Alvarado made himself and Prudencio Santillán, the inspector general, the first full-time employees of the service.[100] Previous administrators of the Malaria Service, even Barbieri, had served part-time while maintaining their private medical practices, but under the new regulations moonlighting was prohibited.

Agency officials were more likely to directly experience the fierce summers of the Northwest now that Alvarado had moved the headquarters of the agency (and his own office) from Buenos Aires to Tucumán, in the heart of the endemic area. Alvarado also ended the practice of summer vacations for most Malaria Service personnel, which followed the typical custom for professionals in Argentina, starting around Christmas and ending in late January. Though appropriate for other professions, Alvarado argued that it hardly made sense to suspend services during the height of the malaria season, regardless of the oppressively hot conditions. He shook up the lower ranks of the service by shutting down old regional offices and rebuilding them according to the logic of foci patrol. Due to this restructuring, the Malaria Service's coverage initially shrank, leaving only ten locales in the Northwest with functioning offices.[101] Personnel and resources were focused on the few active offices, and then gradually others were created (or reconstituted) and integrated into the new regional directorates.

Alvarado persuaded outside institutions in the Northwest to collaborate in malaria control action. From the early days of the Malaria Service in the 1910s, apathy from local government and private enterprises had constantly frustrated leaders of the agency. This lack of external support, coupled with habitual budgetary shortfalls, significantly narrowed the possibilities of malaria control. Alvarado convinced private and public enterprises to contribute a gradually greater share of the Malaria Service's budget, nearly tripling this value between 1940 and 1945.[102] The vast majority of the value of this assistance came in the form of loaned labor, which was measured in *jornales* (work days), each equivalent to about six and a half pesos. Most of the remaining contributions came in the form of construction materials, such as cement for automatic siphons (used to flush out mosquito larvae). The largest donations came from large, labor-intensive enterprises: the Ledesma sugar mill in Jujuy; YPF (the state-owned petroleum corporation), for their operations in Salta Province; the steel mill and munitions factory of Palpalá (Jujuy);

and the company building the Cadillal dam, which would supply water and power to the growing city of Tucumán. Even Standard Oil, which had a tense relationship with the Argentine government since Yrigoyen, collaborated with the Malaria Service for control work around its School of Nursing in Tartagal by donating the labor of two peons.[103] Other assistance came from hotel associations and local government in the few towns of the Northwest whose economy depended on tourism: Rosario de la Frontera (Salta) and Río Hondo (Santiago del Estero), both renowned for their mineral hot springs.

By offering labor and materials, rather than money, these enterprises could virtually ensure they were helping to improve the malaria situation in their own local area. Thus private collaboration was not really charity, but rather an investment in the local economy or the enterprise itself. Towns or settlements where external collaboration was commonplace received many benefits from malaria control. New Malaria Service offices in Tucumán (Escaba and Cadillal) and Jujuy (Palpalá) originated as cooperative efforts between enterprises and the agency. The Malaria Service was more likely to carry out "special investigation" projects in collaborating communities, such as the sanitation of a mill dam at Ledesma and a hatchery for larva-eating fish in Río Hondo.[104]

Private contributions may also have changed the very nature of sanitation work for some locales. Perhaps because private institutions were footing the bill, in these communities Alvarado appeared more willing to deviate from the foci patrol concept and carry out conventional, drainage-oriented saneamiento works. Ledesma, dominated by the large sugar company of the same name, consistently had far more "open drainage" work than any other community, exemplified by the 1942 reclamation of one hundred hectares of wetland, converted to a plantation of eucalyptus, willow, and poplar trees.[105] Alvarado saw the increasing collaboration of private institutions as evidence of the "formation of a sanitary consciousness" among the populace, but it could also be viewed as increasing an extension of private self-interest.[106] Alvarado, who constantly promoted the economic benefits of malaria control, could hardly be dismissive of his donors' pecuniary motives.

To promote the development of such a "sanitary consciousness," Alvarado redoubled the agency's publicity, education, and outreach efforts. Though he rarely indulged in social commentary during his time as Malaria Service director, the traces of a previous generation of hygienists—Carlos Malbrán, José Penna, Aráoz Alfaro—were evident in his sometimes patronizing and nationalistic rhetoric. Continuing a well-known line of critique, Alvarado was dismayed by the public's ignorance of matters related to health and hygiene. He condemned what he viewed as backward social priorities: families with "adequate resources" to purchase consumer goods, such as automobiles and telephones, nevertheless ate poorly, drank contaminated water, did little to prevent malaria or other infectious diseases, and treated themselves with useless patent medicines. He believed that the social and physical environment exerted a strong influence on individual health and character, even arguing that the country, with its abundant sunlight and fresh air, shaped more capable leaders in business and politics than cities, which bred promiscuity, immorality, and degenerative diseases. Backward and dangerous "customs, beliefs, prejudices, fears, [and] ideals" spread like contagious diseases, especially ravaging those with deficient moral and physical constitutions.[107]

However, exposure to correct ideas of hygiene and sanitation would work like a vaccine to stop the spread of degenerative forces. To this end, in 1939 Alvarado began the dissemination of the *Sanitary Almanac,* an illustrated wall calendar, to households and schools of the region.[108] Illustrations and accompanying text focused almost exclusively on malaria: its causes, impacts, and how to prevent it. The scenes depicted were allegorical and didactic. For April 1939, the illustration shows a school playground, set in an idealized pastoral landscape (yet one unmistakably inspired by Tucumán, with orange groves in the middle ground and the Sierra de Aconquija looming in the distance). All of the children are at play, under the watchful eye of a teacher, except for one, Juancito, doubled over and weary, hidden in the shade. A dialogue between his classmates reveals that Juancito has malaria, but that his real fault lies in not obeying his teacher, who offered him quinine tablets (fig. 4.4). Malaria Service personnel reiterated such lessons in radio broadcasts, pamphlets, newspaper articles, and hygiene courses at the University of Tucumán. By 1944, Alvarado reported confidently that the elusive "sanitary consciousness" was developing, so that fighting malaria was no longer perceived "exclusively as the duty of the state."[109] But, concrete effort came mostly from major enterprises, such as the ones mentioned above, rather than individuals.

In Tucumán, at least, the collaboration of private enterprise in public health was increasingly demanded by the government. Successful labor union activism, a fairly progressive political atmosphere, and industry self-interest had led to marked improvements in sanitary conditions in and around sugar mills. In the early 1900s, the provincial government would attempt, sporadically, to legislate the quality of working and living conditions on sugar mills; but these laws were mostly ineffective, and what little progress there was came from a few high-minded and paternalistic mill owners. Beginning in the 1920s, ingenio workers themselves played a stronger role in agitating for improved conditions, leading to provincial laws for minimum wages, limited working hours, and free medical assistance. The rise of the Radical Party also gave significant aid to the cause of organized mill workers, expressed in

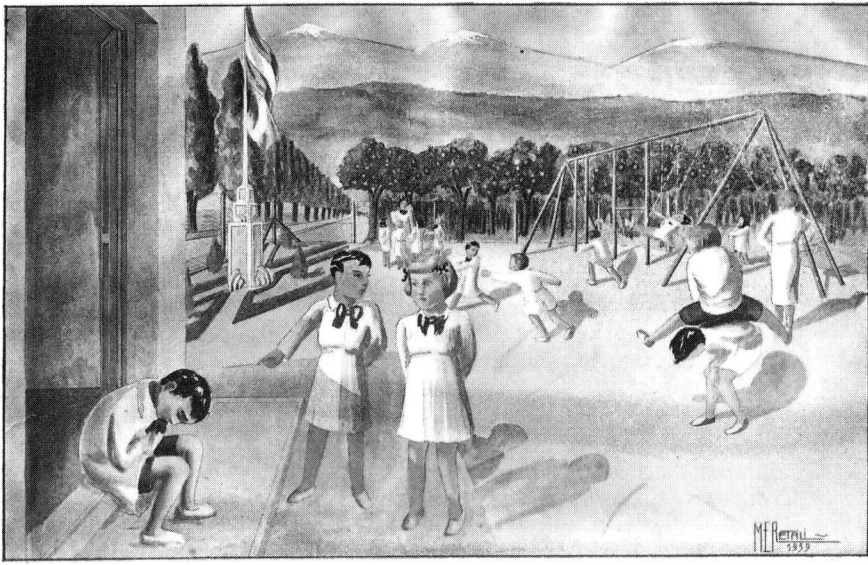

_ Qué le pasa a Juancito que no juega con los otros chicos ?.....

_ Antes de ayer tuvo un amago de chucho y no quiso tomar los comprimidos de quinina
que le ofreció la maestra, hoy le ha repetido mucho más fuerte y yá no pudo tenerse en pie.-

_ Es una lástima que Juancito no haya comprendido el bien que quiso hacerle su maestra,
hoy estaría sano!

Figure 4.4. Detail from *Sanitary Almanac* for April 1939. Dirección General de Paludismo, *Almanaque Sanitario* (Tucumán: Dirección General de Paludismo, 1939).

a landmark strike in 1923.[110] By 1942, sugar mill medical services were more regular and widely established. That year, the clinics of Tucumán's twenty-eight ingenios received almost 238,000 patients, among them 116,000 children.[111] However, there was a substantial gap in health conditions between permanent mill workers and those of seasonal migrants who worked in the fields. It was taken for granted that they would work and live in extremely unhealthy and precarious conditions. On balance, the Northwest's cities were the healthiest place to live, followed by the permanent sugar mill residences, while those living in rural areas continued to be highly vulnerable to malaria and other infections.[112]

In any case, for those lucky enough to receive government support for malaria control, the foci patrol approach showed immediate, positive results; and the Malaria Service under Alvarado had better data, compiled and analyzed in yearly reports, to prove it.[113] Infant morbidity indices, used to model malaria incidence, declined steadily under foci patrol, though with yearly cycles of resurgence each spring. The urban core zones in the malaria campaign (denominated as zone A) consistently showed the lowest intensity of malaria, with incidence increasing, generally, moving from zone B to C to D. Thus, the goal of the control model was met. In addition, there was a broad-based decline in malaria incidence from 1939 until 1942, the year that, according to Alvarado, set the record for fewest malaria cases in Argentina.[114] Subsequently, incidence began to rise again, though erratically. All the while, however, malaria incidence remained extremely low in the core zone of "absolute protection."[115] Bearing in mind that these urban core zones had, by definition, much larger populations than outlying areas, the total suffering from malaria also diminished. Hospital statistics from Tucumán show a similar geographical pattern: malaria incidence, expressed as the proportion of malaria cases among all hospital admissions, declined more quickly in the capital city's hospitals than in other parts of the province.[116]

In the end, it is not easy to proclaim Alvarado's program either a "success" or "failure" simply by tracking malaria incidence. For one, malaria and other health data from this era are somewhat spotty. But more importantly, as social reformers pointed out constantly, malaria did not exist in a vacuum isolated from the broader social environment. Probably much of the long-term decline in malaria came from general improvements in living conditions, including better nutrition and sturdier housing, just as occurred in other regions of temperate-zone malaria, such as the southern United States.[117] Over the short term, public health conditions in the Northwest correlated with economic fluctuations; particularly, as the sugar industry's fortunes rose and fell, so did that of workers and their families, especially in the sugar zone, but also in more distant regions that provided migrant laborers for the harvest.[118] Although the Northwest was developing economically, in the long run and in the aggregate, development was uneven spatially and socially and erratic over time. Such conditions helped structure patterns in infectious diseases, including malaria. Alvarado was not ignorant of these larger structures and processes; rather, as a pragmatist above all else, he knew these forces were beyond his control.

Of Malaria and Morality Tales

Alvarado's "discovery" of the peculiarities of the *A. pseudo* mosquito, dismissal of the older, Italian-inspired saneamiento methods, and subsequent reorientation of malaria control strategy have become part of the lore of Argentina's Malaria Service today. Alvarado is venerated in Argentina's public health and medical communities as a founding hero whose sharp observations and ingenious methods advanced the malaria campaign. In this vernacular historical narrative, Alvarado's predecessors failed to perceive the truth about malaria that was right under their noses. His courage to reject the conventional wisdom set him apart and made him great.

This story has become important. The few official documents that represent malaria control to the public today employ this narrative of genius and discovery. For example, the pamphlet *Malaria in Argentina,* published in 1999 by the Salta Association of Public Health Professionals, begins this way: "Alvarado succeeded in making an important verification: the malaria vector in our country, *Anopheles pseudopunctipennis,* did not develop in habitats in standing water of marshes, swamps, and quagmires, rather it grew in water currents without shade and without sufficient marginal vegetation, where an algae grew that the larvae fed upon. This discovery led to the rethinking of sanitation measures that had predominated up to that time."[119] This story, with a well-defined turning point corresponding to an epiphany about environmental dynamics, has become the received wisdom, persisting within the historiography of public health in Argentina.[120]

The malaria control story has even found a place in larger historical narratives. One of the first comprehensive accounts of Argentina's environmental history puts it this way: "malaria had taken hold in the country thanks to an *ecological error.* . . . The idea that the malaria–carrying mosquitoes bred in swamps was, for a long time, an article of faith, since that is what happened with malaria in Italy. . . . In the 1930s the ecology of the mosquito began to be studied and it was discovered that in Argentina the anopheles species that live in swamps do not transmit malaria. The situation is *exactly the opposite* [of what had been assumed]."[121] The authors conclude with a moral: "We cannot calculate how many deaths occurred because of this *ecological error,* but it is one more example of the risks of ill-founded manipulations of nature."[122] Alvarado's predecessors, the story goes, got it all wrong; and Alvarado was the first to get it all right because he acted according to the principles of ecology. We could also infer that disease control strategies must be in harmony with ecological reality to save lives.

It is easy to succumb to this received narrative. It is a modern morality tale, in which those who act against ecological principles are doomed to failure and condemnation. And, like all good stories, it features a determined protagonist (Alvarado) facing various antagonists (the wily *A. pseudo* mosquito, of course, but also his arrogant, ignorant peers). Yet a major question remains: If saneamiento was so obviously wrongheaded, then why did it persist for so many years before Alvarado's reforms? Was it simply obtuseness on the part of Malaria Service officials? Were their strategies so misguided, after all?

While it's true that Alvarado had great expertise in malariology, ecology, and tropical medicine, it would be a mistake to say that "improved knowledge" or "better science" proved the decisive factor in the malaria campaign's turnaround. Such a narrative of social progress through scientific breakthroughs is commonplace, but not altogether convincing in this case. Lack of scientific evidence casting doubt on saneamiento was never the major issue. After all, most of the important studies on *A. pseudo* had been published in the DNH's own journals. What was missing was a way to put this evidence into perspective by integrating it into a new model or counter-narrative. That is what Alvarado was able to accomplish.

Saneamiento persisted for so long because of its place in a far-reaching and longstanding narrative of regional development. Malaria control depended on a particular diagnosis of regional underdevelopment, in which the defects of nature and society were mutually reinforcing. Saneamiento seemed, if not exactly a panacea, an integrative approach that held the solution to many problems at once. Controlling and transforming nature seemed to hold the key to social progress. Leaders of the DNH, when faced with new scientific evidence, had difficulty seeing outside of the dominant paradigm, which after all had roots going back to the 1890s, to the miasmatic era. The paradigm was reinforced by a famous example of success in the field, in Santiago del Estero, repeated visual rhetoric of before-and-after photo series of drainage projects, and, not least, the mounting success of an extremely ambitious and large-scale bonification program in Italy. In essence, the officers of the DNH, as well as politicians, journalists, and other interested parties, wore conceptual blinders that prevented the incorporation of true alternatives. Similar to the workings of a Kuhnian paradigm, accumulating evidence on the peculiar habits of the *A. pseudo* mosquito did not fit squarely within the prevailing model of understanding and, therefore, was ignored, or at least not integrated into control strategy. The peculiarities of the *A. pseudo* mosquito did not fit the geographical imaginary of the Northwest that dominated the outlook of well-intentioned hygienists and politicians.

Still, there are other plausible explanations for the persistence of the saneamiento model, despite its being obviously ill suited for Northwest Argentina. For one, the scientific evidence—the entomological research, particularly—may not have been so outstanding, and it becomes convincing only in retrospect. The volume of entomological data on *A. pseudo* was never that large, and there would remain many unsettled questions on the mosquito's habits and ecology.[123] In addition, due to historical accident, basic research on malaria epidemiology and vector ecology in Argentina suffered from some important discontinuities. For one, Guillermo Paterson never published again on malaria after 1911; by failing to expand on his pioneering work, he lost an opportunity to insist on the significance of his findings. Juana Petrocchi, a respected entomologist who made important observations on *A. pseudo* and other Argentine anophelines, died suddenly of appendicitis in 1925, at the age of thirty-two.[124] The entomological and epidemiological work of foreign scientists such as Peter Mühlens, or Shannon, Rickard, and Davis of the RF, was not well integrated into the research program of the Malaria Service.[125]

Finally, some enigmas may never be resolved. In particular, why did large-scale drainage work so well in Santiago del Estero in 1902? Were those actually *Anopheles pseudopunctipennis* mosquitoes? If so, what were they doing in such an unusual habitat and so far from their preferential wintering sites in the foothills?

Ultimately, however, an emphasis in the historical narrative on the dichotomy between foci patrol and saneamiento and the ecological differences between *A. pseudo* and other mosquitoes is flawed for a different reason. This framing of the story gives disproportionate centrality to the success or failure of particular malaria control strategies, and thus neglects Alvarado's most important contributions. He should also be recognized for innovations that transcended any specific policy. First, Alvarado introduced an attention to rigorous experimentation and empirical methodology that had previously been lacking in the malaria campaign. In this manner, he established consistent means for the program to evaluate its own success or failure. Second, he brought an ecological perspective to malaria science in Argentina. More than anyone before him—although his intellectual debt to Paterson, Mazza, the RF scientists, and other ecologically oriented scientists is clear—Alvarado understood the environments of malaria-carrying mosquitoes as dynamic and complex; framed these environments in the vocabulary of ecology, such as communities, associations, succession and disturbance, climax, competition, and niches; and, most crucially, married this ecological understanding to the spatial strategies of malaria control.

But perhaps the most important ingredient for Alvarado's success was his unique political style, characterized by pragmatism, professionalism, and strategic networking. He judged the quality of control work by its success in practice, rather than adhering rigidly to preconceived doctrine. Alvarado effectively depoliticized malaria control by severing its connection, as much as possible, to larger projects of social reform. Meanwhile, he focused intensively on improving the Malaria Service, making it a strong, well-funded, and well-respected organization of full-time professionals anchored in the Northwest. This apparently apolitical, scientific temperament allowed him to somehow stay above the fray of everyday politics. Yet, like any bureaucrat who carves out a secure and powerful position for himself, Alvarado was crafty, relying on connections such as Miguel Sussini to rise in the public health bureaucracy and avoiding the internecine conflicts that stymied other scientists such as Mazza. In short, Alvarado's subtle use of power strengthened the organization around him, and this accomplishment would prove resilient even as the Malaria Service altered its course, even more radically, in the mid-1940s.

5

"God Bless General Perón"

The Politics and Technologies of Malaria Eradication

The year 1945 will have historical importance in the fight against
anopheles, since in that year one era ends and another begins. Those who
write the history of malaria in the future will be able to say: before 1945
and after 1945; which is the same as saying before DDT and after DDT.
—Carlos Alberto Alvarado, "La lucha
antimosquito en la América tropical"

With these words, Carlos Alvarado, the director of Argentina's malaria eradication program, captured the heady enthusiasm of malaria fighters in the
postwar era.[1] The chemical insecticide DDT, which had become widely available after the end of World War II, provided a new and qualitatively different
weapon against malaria. With the "magic bullet" of DDT, at last there was the
means of not simply keeping malaria under control, but of eradicating it from
the countries where it was endemic. But for most people in Argentina, 1945
was a watershed year for another reason. That year, the populist army general Juan D. Perón rose to power and brought sweeping changes to national
politics, economy, society, and culture. Inspired in part by Mussolini's Fascism, Perón's governing ideology of *justicialismo* combined displays of military power, nationalist sentiment, and concern for social justice.

With the able and loyal assistance of his minister of public health, Ramón
Carrillo, Perón's administration made health, sanitation, and social welfare
integral elements of the governing ideology. They immediately realized the
long-frustrated project of centralizing national authority over public health
and made a strong commitment to improving the welfare of the masses through
a comprehensive hospital construction program, the establishment of a national social security system, and aggressive campaigns against infectious diseases. One of the most dramatic manifestations of this spirited new state attitude toward public health was the great campaign to eradicate malaria, launched
in 1947. Thanks to Perón's expansion of public health policy, Carlos Alvarado finally had the financial resources, authority, and political backing to
make significant progress against malaria. Before DDT, after DDT; before

Perón, after Perón: for malaria control in Argentina, 1945 represented an un-expected and decisive convergence of the technological and the political.

This chapter develops the theme of historical convergence to understand the rapid mobilization and success of the climactic battle against malaria in Northwest Argentina. The nearly complete eradication of malaria in Argentina resulted from a combination of three factors: the effective organization of the malaria campaign that Alvarado had developed before the advent of DDT; an infusion of new technologies, especially DDT but also motor vehicles; and, lastly, the expansive public health ideology and policy that Perón and Carrillo developed. Each of these was a necessary ingredient, but none was sufficient on its own to effect the eradication of the disease.

As we have seen, during the 1930s Alvarado revitalized a moribund Malaria Service. He redesigned the agency's administrative structure, relocated its headquarters to the endemic zone, trained full-time technical personnel, and continued to invest in basic and applied malaria research. Foci patrol, which targeted very specific mosquito habitats, appeared to be more effective than *saneamiento* in reducing the burden of malaria in the Northwest. Yet all the while, Alvarado eagerly anticipated that a better approach would come along. This solid organizational base, devotion to original malariological research, and a flexible, pragmatic attitude about strategic innovation enabled Alvarado to make a dramatic shift in malaria control strategy. DDT, an insecticide with seemingly miraculous properties, was the key technological element that enabled such a change. Yet ancillary technologies, such as motor vehicles, were also vital to the new phase of the campaign. To carry out the DDT-spraying program required an ambitious infusion of state financial resources, as well as an increase in state authority and support for public health. In a provident coincidence, DDT became universally and economically available at almost exactly the same time as Perón's ascent to power, around the end of World War II.

The ambitious public health policy of Perón and Carrillo provided the final key component to the malaria eradication program. Perón initiated many "great campaigns" to eradicate endemic and/or infectious diseases, such as leprosy, tuberculosis, trachoma, goiter, and syphilis, but the malaria eradication campaign was the most dramatic and successful of these projects. Beyond these specific efforts, however, Perón made public health a central element of his program to transform the relationship between Argentine society and the national state.[2] In Perón's organic vision of society—modeled in part after Italian Fascism, but with obvious antecedents in Argentine political thought—the strength of the nation derived from the health and well-being of its people. Argentina's hygienists of an earlier era had sought to "civilize" the popular classes, but Perón exalted the masses as the authentic embodiment of Argentine national identity. Perón concretized the pact between the adoring masses and their charismatic leader through showy manifestations of beneficent state power, and the malaria eradication campaign exemplified this dynamic. Perón's "social justice" ideology united diverse and interrelated streams of thought, framed in national terms, around the ideas of race, nation, citizenship, science, and health.

While this chapter focuses mainly on national politics and institutions, it should be noted that international events and expert networks continued to influence the policy and practice of malaria control in Argentina. First, the Rockefeller Foundation (RF) returned to Argentina beginning in 1941, after a twelve-year absence; this time, the foundation's purview was more expansive, reaching beyond the issue of malaria and hookworm control. As internal memoranda of the RF indicate, leaders of the foundation were convinced that its activities in countries such as Argentina could act as a bulwark against the Fascist penetration of South America.[3] The RF expanded its scope beyond public health to include promotion of the humanities and social sciences in South America through grants for building institutional capacity and promoting scholarly exchanges with the United States. Similarly, the emphasis of the International Health Division shifted from demonstration projects and research on vector-borne diseases toward making broader improvements in medical education and basic medical research in South American countries.[4] Through grants and scholarships, the RF hoped to increase the influence of the United States on the development of medical researchers, at the expense of Europe.[5]

To promote this new vision, in 1941 the RF established the Río de la Plata and Andean regional office of the International Health Division in Buenos Aires to oversee RF activities in Argentina, Bolivia, Chile, Ecuador, Paraguay, Peru, and Uruguay.[6] Lewis W. Hackett, who had distinguished himself as an RF malariologist in Italy, directed the Buenos Aires office from its inception until 1949. He became the leading administrator of the RF's projects throughout the region. Although Hackett was not officially involved in Argentina's malaria campaign, he nonetheless made frequent trips to the Northwest region to advise, converse with, and learn from his friend Carlos Alvarado. Hackett also created and supervised malaria control programs in the other countries under his watch and shared these experiences with Alvarado. During this time, Hackett kept a highly detailed official diary, and his candid commentary offers a valuable outsider's view on science, politics, and culture in Argentina during a decade of great turmoil.[7] Though Hackett had a productive relationship with Alvarado, interactions between the RF and the Argentine government were fraught with tension.

There is another important element of the international situation to consider: the aftermath of World War II and the technologies and institutions that it produced. The war became the proving ground for the insecticide DDT, and because of these origins and its destructive force, a strong rhetorical connection between warfare and DDT was created. As Edmund Russell has argued, chemical warfare gave rise to modern insecticides, and in the post–World War II era, pest control became a veritable "war on nature," both materially and metaphorically.[8] These bellicose associations appealed to Argentina and other Latin American states where the influence of the military in politics and culture was expanding. At the same time, the aftermath of World War II witnessed the founding of UNICEF and the World Health Organization, both of which would become deeply involved in the organization of malaria eradication efforts around the world.[9] Meanwhile, the Pan American Sanitary Bureau (PASB) took on much greater prominence after the war, thanks in part to increased US interest and funding.[10] In many ways, these institutions would adopt the roles that private philanthropies, especially the RF, were gradually abandoning. Through international conferences and publications sponsored by such organizations, a more fluid and rapid exchange of techniques and technologies of malaria control developed, and what had been disconnected, national-level programs were increasingly orchestrated at an international level. Alvarado was an active and influential participant in this international network, and even more so after malaria had been effectively eradicated from Argentina.

The next section explores how Perón and his chief aide, Carrillo, developed the "new public health" ideology in the 1940s. I then turn to a discussion of the convergence of sanitary organization, national politics, and technological innovation that led to the great campaign to eradicate malaria in Argentina's Northwest, starting in 1947. In the final section I detail the swift action of the campaign and the effect it had on the society and environment in the Northwest.

Perón, Carrillo, and the New Public Health

Perón's public health policy, while innovative in many respects, particularly in the sometimes spectacular character of its execution, represented a convergence of diverse ideological threads that characterized social debate in Argentina since the early 1900s. These often contradictory political impulses included conservative nationalism, the scientific construction of biological races, the revaluation of the figure of the criollo (creole) of the interior as the basis for national identity, and use of social justice as a rationale for state interventions to promote public health. Argentina was also influenced by the social welfare politics of Europe and the humanitarian ethos of the post–

World War II era, reflected in the charter of the United Nations, which institutionalized the notion that health was a basic "human right" and that states should be responsible for the health and well-being of their citizens. Under the leadership of Perón and Carrillo, all of these diverse streams of thought coalesced in the concept of social justice, which featured a stronger state role in protecting a more broadly defined concept of national public health. The Peronist project of social justice meant to spread and redistribute the fruits of wealth and modernity to improve Argentina—the national organism—as a whole. This program was put into operation through specific policies tailored to appeal to Perón's key constituencies (the unionized, industrial working class and the rural poor) and to antagonize his political opponents (the much-vilified oligarchy).[11]

Ramón Carrillo was the principal organizer of Perón's program of public health. Like Carlos Alvarado, a native of Jujuy province, Carrillo came from Northwest Argentina, and these common roots helped cultivate a friendship as well as a shared interest in the health problems of their home region. Born in 1906, two years after Alvarado, to a prominent and conservative family of Santiago del Estero, Carrillo demonstrated a keen intellect, inchoate humanitarianism, and a passion for social justice.[12] Even as a teenager, he condemned Argentina's regional inequalities in wealth, health, and welfare.[13] As a young physician, Carrillo lamented the profound "cultural and technological dependency" of Argentina, the cause of which was simple: "we have taught ourselves to see ourselves in the mirror of Europe or the United States, to envy the dominant empires and to be ashamed of our Hispanic-Creole origin."[14] Thus Carrillo foreshadowed one of the fundamentals of Perón's nationalism, namely, the desire for scientific and technological self-sufficiency, the search for "Argentine solutions" to Argentine problems. Carrillo rose rapidly within the medical profession, becoming chair of neurology at the University of Buenos Aires in 1942, at the age of thirty-six. Meanwhile, he continued as a specialist in neurosurgery at the Central Military Hospital, a post he had held since 1939.

Changing political circumstances would allow Carrillo to enter the realm of public health policy. Soon after Carrillo assumed his prestigious university position, Juan Perón, then an army colonel, took part in the coup that initiated a military government in June of 1943.[15] This regime used force and repression to provide for "social order." The government censored the press; intimidated and dismissed dissident academics at the national universities, including Bernardo Houssay, a friend to Carlos Alvarado and supporter of the RF; incited anti-Semitism; abolished political parties; claimed mystical or sacred political legitimacy as "defenders of the faith" for the Catholic Church; and fomented paranoia about a possible US-backed invasion by

Brazil.[16] Perón participated in all of this, but as historian José Luis Romero has remarked, he also began to put "a more subtle plan" for seizing power into action.[17] Perón tied his political fortunes to establishing relationships of patronage with the country's labor unions. From his position as labor secretary in the military junta, Perón negotiated lucrative contracts for the unions; this generosity was either a preventive measure against the infiltration of communism or a clever way of co-opting labor politics. Regardless of his motives, however, Perón was undoubtedly building a solid and loyal political base among the masses, especially poor criollo migrants from the interior flocking to Greater Buenos Aires.[18]

Perón made social justice a central feature of his populist rhetoric, and he conveyed his concern for the welfare of the masses through flamboyant demonstrations of state benevolence. With the irreplaceable assistance of his legendary wife, Eva, Perón elicited not simply the loyalty but also the adulation of the masses of humble *descamisados* (the shirtless ones). Perón, once nearly forced out of the governing junta by increasingly suspicious and jealous officers, was elevated to the position of indisputable leader by the mass demonstrations of October 17, 1945, in Buenos Aires. This popular support was ratified by a legitimate presidential election in February of 1946. Immediately, Perón established a policy agenda meant to appeal to the working class, including an inflationary economic policy that kept unemployment low and salaries high. Just as importantly, Perón developed a charismatic and populist style of leadership that established an emotional bond with the masses. Peronism was not simply populist, but exhibited many of the hallmarks of Italian and Spanish fascism: militarism, political repression, biological conceptions of national identity, the cult of personality, sublimation of individualism to the necessities of the social body, and a utopian vision of the national destiny. And, following Benito Mussolini, Perón made a show of his concern for the welfare of the masses.[19] A sophisticated system of political propaganda communicated the latest actions of the state, increasingly synonymous with Perón himself, on behalf of the poor.[20] Eva Perón played an instrumental role in building the paternalistic state, for example, by using her eponymous charitable foundation, funded by the government, to hand out clothes, food, and medicine to the needy.[21]

Expanding the state's role in public health became a key piece of Perón's populist social politics, and Carrillo coordinated this effort. Carrillo and Perón had met in 1943, at the military hospital where Carrillo specialized in neurosurgery, while Perón was still a colonel.[22] In June of 1946, now-president Perón elevated Carrillo from an informal advisor to the official role of leading the new Secretaría de Salud Pública (Secretariat of Public Health), with cabinet-level authority equal to that of any other ministry.[23] This new organism superseded the old, substantially weaker National Department of Hygiene.[24] Through this new entity (soon to become a full-blown ministry after Peron's constitutional reform of 1949) Carrillo began to implement the principles of Peronism in matters of public health.

In a series of public addresses and publications in the late 1940s, Carrillo proclaimed, developed, and explained the Peronist public health doctrine. Drawing on diverse sources of inspiration—such as previous generations of Argentine hygienists, the eugenics movement, nineteenth-century Cuban nationalist José Martí, Roosevelt's New Deal, papal encyclicals, the British National Health plan, and the United Nation's Universal Declaration of Human Rights, to name just a few—Carrillo postulated a socially broad view of health. He defined health in the same expansive terms as the new World Health Organization did in 1946: "as a state of complete physical, social, and mental well-being, and not just the absence of conditions or illnesses."[25] Carrillo argued that medical science had become increasingly microscopic in a search for the causes of disease but, in so doing, "could not see the forest for the trees" and "had forgotten the 'macrocosmos,' that is, the *social environment*."[26] Improvement of *social conditions,* such as wages, housing, and nutrition, could have greater impacts on health than purely medical interventions.[27] Echoing the sentiments of turn-of-the-century hygienists such as Emilio Coni, Carrillo proposed that social policy and sanitary policy were inseparable and that the traditional distinction between "private" and "public" hygiene should become obsolete since the state had a vested interest in, and natural authority over, the health of its subjects.[28]

Within the national imaginary of public health and welfare, the government's view included a special role for the people of the interior provinces. If the public health ideology of Carrillo and Perón had an archetypal subject— that is, an idealized recipient of the state's humanitarian aid—it was the impoverished, forgotten, rural criollo of the Northwest. This figure, who suffered from malnutrition, infectious diseases, "starvation wages," and social dislocation, became the "descamisado" whose migrations populated the outskirts of Buenos Aires and swelled the ranks of Perón's party.[29] The idea that people could live under such conditions in a country of such wealth appalled the Peronist conscience, not simply as a question of basic human rights, but also because this dissonance made a mockery of the idea of a unified *nation*. "It is no secret that in this land of such abundance and prosperity," wrote Carrillo in 1949, "a third of our people do not eat enough to live in health."[30] One-fifth of the country's population, located in the rural interior, lived "in the prehistory of hygiene and social medicine."[31] Carrillo, echoing Perón, wondered, What good were the wonders of modern medicine, such as penicillin or vaccines, if there were no doctors, nurses, hospitals, clinics, and ambulances to take it to the people who needed it? For Carrillo and Perón, then, public health problems stemmed not from a lack of development per se, but from an unequal (and sometimes irrational) distribution of medical and sanitary services.[32] Though the Peronists were hardly the first to lament interregional disparities in health conditions, they succeeded in centralizing sanitary authority under a strong national government, precisely for the sake of equalizing health services across the country.[33]

Carrillo believed that eugenics, public health, and social welfare could elevate the criollos to their rightful place within the national society. As did many contemporary nationalists, such as Ricardo Rojas, Carrillo located the wellspring of national identity in the interior provinces rather than the morally corrupt metropolis. He held up the criollo of the interior as the model of authenticity, vigor, and strength—the basic material for the development of an ideal Argentine race. Influenced by the mystical racial thought of Hermann Graf Keyserling, a Baltic German political philosopher, Carrillo believed that a coherent "national essence" was the key to a country's greatness. This essence was located in those creole populations, uncontaminated by European immigration, that carried on Hispanic cultural values and traditions.[34] Carrillo saw tangible demographic shifts as evidence of creole strength. In 1940, he contended that foreign immigration no longer accounted for most of Argentina's population growth, and natural growth rates in Buenos Aires and other cities of the Pampas had also declined. In the northern provinces, however, there was "a great capacity for fertility" with an average of three to five children per couple; given this, the people of this region served as a key population "reserve" for the entire country.[35] Carrillo later characterized the rural poor of the provinces as "the biological reserves of the nation" and further argued that sustaining the reproductive power of the rural poor through improvements in public health guaranteed the labor necessary for the continuing process of industrialization in the large cities.[36] In his inaugural address as secretary of public health in 1947, he proposed the establishment of an "Institute of the Argentine Man" to study the "ideal, somatic, visceral, and psychological biotype that we must approach to be able to say one day, proudly, that we have a healthy and strong people."[37]

Such ideas echo an earlier generation of hygienists, but unlike his predecessors in public health, Carrillo was able to transform his nationalistic, racialized, and organicist ideology into concrete action. With Perón's support, Carrillo began to implement his ambitious plan for public health. The construction of general hospitals and clinics increased the number of hospital beds and expanded availability of medical care. Laboratories administered by the government increased production of vaccines, serums, and other drugs. A national health census was conducted in 1954, and the government promoted hygiene and nutrition through radio broadcasts and public exhibitions. Investment in vaccination programs and campaigns to control endemic diseases helped to reduce incidence of smallpox, diphtheria, goiter, and malaria.[38] Perón's government also launched a major, though not completely comprehensive, program of national health insurance, tailored to satisfy his political base, the labor unions.[39]

In sum, Perón and Carrillo significantly expanded the state's role in providing for the health and welfare of its citizens. This was evident in the more prominent position of public health administrators within the government, increased investment in health from the public purse, and the integration of health concerns into a broader, redistributive political platform of social justice. The partisanship of Perón's populist politics should not overshadow the coherence of Carrillo's public health ideology, which offered moral, biological, sanitary, demographic, and economic rationales for protecting Argentina's masses. Reflecting his own origins, and the ideology of nationalists like Perón, Carrillo felt a special duty to provide for the rural poor of the interior provinces, especially the Northwest. At the same time, Perón, who understood the propaganda value of bold and massive demonstrations of benevolent state power, promoted "great campaigns" to bring rapid improvement to public health and welfare. This propagandistic motive, along with a patriotic concern for the "forgotten" citizens of Argentina's interior, help to explain the special urgency of the malaria eradication program that Perón, Carrillo, and Alvarado launched in 1947.

The "Great Campaigns" and the Eradication of Malaria

Looking back at the state of things at the beginning of 1945, few could have predicted that Alvarado, Carrillo, and Perón would collaborate to nearly eradicate malaria within just four years. In early 1945, Alvarado believed that his professional situation was becoming increasingly precarious. Political intrigues within the rancorous military regime, in which Perón was still battling for supremacy, worried him. Alvarado was not a nationalist, nor a Peronist, nor even a Radical, but rather an old-fashioned conservative in the traditional mold of Jujuy politics, quite similar to Benjamín Villafañe, whose contributions to regionalism and public health were discussed in chapter 3. His political worldview made him something of a relic and, potentially, a dissident.[40] Alvarado complained to his friend Lewis W. Hackett that the director of national health, Dr. Manuel A. Viera, had surrounded himself with his clinician friends, men with little interest in public health and limited knowledge of infectious disease.[41] In September, Alvarado and his staff abstained from attending the first National Conference on Public Health in

Buenos Aires, organized by Viera, and Alvarado anticipated his imminent firing.[42] Hackett remarked in his diary that Alvarado "may lose his position at any moment because of his political opinions."[43] Adding to his difficulties, the malaria campaign itself experienced a serious setback in 1945, with a sharp recrudescence of the disease after years of steady decline.[44] It is noteworthy that in the midst of this turmoil and disappointment, Alvarado casually asked Hackett about the price of DDT.[45] Despite his troubles, Alvarado was still attending to his duties.

Alvarado's rapidly deteriorating situation took an unexpected and auspicious turn on October 17, 1945, the milestone day that mass protests in Buenos Aires brought Perón back from the brink of exile and made him the country's unrivalled leader. With Perón came Carrillo, who offered Alvarado almost total support because of their immense mutual respect and longtime friendship, dating back to medical school. Carrillo let Alvarado continue as the director of the malaria program while defending him against attacks from those who questioned his devotion to the Peronist cause and pointed out his suspicious affiliations with political dissidents, such as Houssay, and foreign institutions, such as the RF.[46] Carrillo, one of Perón's most loyal and ardent followers, was willing to ignore Alvarado's politics because his expertise was irreplaceable. As proof of this, Alvarado's Malaria Service was one of the few old sanitary agencies to survive intact after Carrillo's comprehensive reorganization of public health after 1946, and Alvarado was one of only four high-level bureaucrats to maintain his old position.[47] I also speculate that Carrillo saw Alvarado as a political ally because he was not a political threat. Carrillo's rivals came from within Perón's inner circle: for example, Alberto Tesaire, the navy admiral who would engineer Carrillo's dismissal from his post and exile from Argentina in 1954, was the president of the Peronist party.[48] Since Alvarado had no connection to the party, he would not rise to challenge Carrillo. In any case, after having served directly under the president of the DNH in the early 1930s, Alvarado had lost interest in seeking higher political posts.[49] He clearly relished directing the Malaria Service.

After Perón became president in 1946, Alvarado drafted a plan for malaria control (known to insiders as Plan 46) that was incorporated into Carrillo's five-year national sanitary plan, detailed in the massive volume *Analytical Plan for Public Health*.[50] Plan 46 entailed substantial new investment (10 million pesos between 1947 and 1951) to gradually expand the coverage of foci patrol, in combination with increased dispensation of quinine and general improvements in medical treatment. In Plan 46, Carrillo—probably borrowing liberally from Alvarado's original report—argued for a holistic and integrated understanding of malaria: "Malaria as a social fact is the result of a *series of factors:* biological, climatic, economic, and political; as a result, without approaches and solutions that correlate all such factors, it is not possible to achieve an *integrated* focus and solution to the problem."[51] This view was evident in a diagram that showed how the biological fight (*lucha biológica*) against malaria served as the central node of a whole suite of environmental improvements, including afforestation of riparian zones and stocking of streams with fish that fed on mosquito larvae.[52] This integrated, ecological framework for malaria control reflected Carrillo's broad yet intricate view of public health policy.

In any case, by the time that Carrillo's vast *Analytical Plan* was released in 1947, Plan 46 was obsolete: Alvarado had been working on an entirely different strategy, one that would revolutionize malaria control in Argentina and around the world. The chemical agent DDT (Dichloro-diphenyl-trichloroethane) had been developed in the late 1930s by the J. R. Geigy Company of Switzerland, originally for use against clothes moths.[53] During World War II, with Italy as the principal proving grounds, DDT was used widely as an insecticide, first in the "successful delousing of Naples" (in 1944) and then against anopheles mosquitoes for malaria control (an effort that was spearheaded by the Rockefeller Foundation and its officers serving in the Allied army).[54] House spraying with DDT proved to be incredibly effective against mosquitoes, and by 1946 DDT was employed in malaria control, at least on an experimental basis, in Sardinia, the southern United States, and parts of Latin America (Mexico, Venezuela, and Panama).[55] As Edmund Russell discusses in his book *War and Nature,* DDT also became almost instantly popular as a household and agricultural insecticide after the war.[56] When Alvarado began experimenting with the insecticide, he apparently had never observed DDT-based control efforts, but gleaned what he could from published articles and conversations with the RF's representative in Argentina, Hackett.[57] In 1945, Alvarado first used DDT as a larvicide, substituting it for Paris green while otherwise conserving the foci patrol approach, with mediocre results.[58]

Alvarado, aware of DDT programs in other countries, decided to change targets, from larval to adult mosquitoes, which would require intensive house spraying. He turned to the private sector for help. The Ledesma Company was a familiar contributor to, and beneficiary of, the Malaria Service's efforts. This massive sugar plantation in Jujuy Province, which employed thousands of workers during the harvest season (*zafra*), was the largest private supporter of the Malaria Service, beginning in the 1930s. Typically, the company would lend its workers and donate materials to the Malaria Service to conduct sanitation-related labor on the plantation and adjacent mill towns. Other sugar mills and large enterprises in the region (such as the government-owned oil company, YPF) also offered such support. As historian Daniel

Campi suggests, the sugar mills of the Northwest increasingly took on such obligations and looked after the health of workers to guarantee the productivity and reproduction of their labor force. In addition, provincial governments, labor unions, and prominent social critics applied pressure to mill owners to provide for the safety and health of their workers.[59] In July of 1946, Alvarado asked Ledesma for a gasoline engine, a pump, pulverizing machines, tanks, and small, hand-held sprayers, similar to those used by house painters, along with three or four peons to assist in the spraying.[60] The company agreed to help, and house spraying with DDT began in September.

While the trials in Ledesma were ongoing, Alvarado traveled to Caracas, Venezuela, in January of 1947 for the Panamerican Sanitary Conference, and subsequently to Panama, Mexico, Cuba, and Peru, where he was able to observe firsthand the effectiveness of house spraying for mosquitoes with DDT.[61] After his Latin American tour, and observing that the trials in Ledesma were already showing positive results, Alvarado decided to scrap foci patrol and devote the Malaria Service's resources almost entirely to a strategy based on elimination of adult mosquitoes with DDT. As a larvicide, Alvarado commented, DDT was "just another chemical" with no great advantage over Paris green or petroleum. However, when used against adult mosquitoes, "DDT is not just another weapon in the malaria campaign, it is a *revolutionary factor* in the strategy, methods, and techniques of the fight."[62] In 1947, Hackett remarked, "Alvarado is shutting the door on the past" and "staking everything on DDT."[63] Starting in March of that year, Alvarado convened regular meetings of his regional directors to elaborate a DDT-based campaign. Around that time, Alvarado traveled to Buenos Aires to confer with Carrillo. Alvarado proposed spraying houses at three-month intervals, and promised coverage of 40 percent of the endemic area the first year, and 80 percent by the end of the second year, 1948. Alvarado was proposing a colossal effort, with hundreds of workers covering over seventy-five thousand houses every twelve weeks, over an area of 150,000 square kilometers. To accomplish this would require an infusion of cash and equipment, especially motor vehicles for rapid mobilization of the DDT "brigades."

By endorsing Alvarado's radical plan, Carrillo was taking a great risk: the Perón administration, though powerful, was still quite new; and Carrillo had other ambitious plans for public health, detailed in his *Analytical Plan* and public speeches, such as establishing a network of hospitals and clinics, integrating hygiene into the regular school curriculum, promoting proper childhood nutrition, and reforming the care of the mentally handicapped. Alvarado himself had never undertaken anything like such a massive effort, but then again, there was really no precedent for a national-scale malaria eradication campaign anywhere in Latin America. If Alvarado's gamble should fail, it could embarrass the government and jeopardize other projects. But Carrillo had "blind faith" in his old friend and offered him complete support.[64]

Together, they went to Juan Perón. Alvarado later recalled giving a twenty-minute presentation, complete with tables, charts, and maps. After a brief round of questioning, Perón was convinced. He turned to Carrillo and said, "Give this kid anything he asks of you."[65] Alvarado, only nine years younger than Perón, may have later exaggerated the casualness of their exchange; but, indeed, Perón and Carrillo gave their full endorsement and, with their commitment assured, eradication of malaria became more than just a theoretical possibility.

Carrillo and Perón may have perceived that the enormous propaganda potential of the eradication campaign outweighed other political risks. Some observers compared Perón's propaganda machine to that of Fascist Italy, where every great act of the populist government, especially its assistance to the poor and the sick, presented an advertising opportunity. A cynical Hackett, who had resided in Italy before the RF transferred him to Buenos Aires, remarked in 1947:

> The thing that strikes me as familiar after my years in Italy under Mussolini is the prodigious advertisement of each new plan which the group in power conceives to impress the people and which is launched with spectacular ceremony—the 60 day campaign to lower the cost of living, the heavy industry program (without iron or coal), the declaration of economic independence, Evita's farewell to "her" descamisados, the cavalcade of 90 trucks loaded with hospital supplies to succor the people of the provinces, the new holidays, . . . The common people watch this kaleidoscope as spectators. They no longer have to worry, or think or act in their own behalf.[66]

Through the great campaigns—which included programs to eradicate trachoma and tuberculosis, massive vaccination efforts, and rat eradication in Buenos Aires—Perón sought to demonstrate that the power of the state, including its military might, could be harnessed to massively and swiftly deliver services for humanitarian ends.[67]

Carrillo, for his part, had a more subtle motive for heavy investment in malaria control. He wanted to address persistent infectious diseases first in order to move onto what he saw as more fundamental issues of social welfare, such as improving working conditions, nutrition, child-rearing, and education for Argentina's lower classes. While he sometimes painted a fearsome picture of infectious diseases, at other times he was dismissive of their danger. He believed that modern medical science and sanitary technology offered easy means of eliminating these diseases, making them little more than nuisances; but in the absence of social organization and political will, they persisted.[68] Thus, he hoped to eliminate diseases such as plague, tuberculosis, and malaria swiftly, through massive and decisive campaigns, so that health policy could move onto confronting broader and more complex issues of social welfare.[69]

The monumental malaria campaign bore a striking and calculated resemblance to a military campaign, another reason why it might have appealed to Perón, who after all was a product of army training. Perón undoubtedly appreciated the militaristic flourishes of the proposed campaign. Moreover, new technology, especially military technology, captivated Perón. Few scholars have analyzed the role of technology in Perón's ideology and policy, yet he spurred an increase in industrial output through Soviet-style five-year plans, continued the expansion of state-owned military industries, and sponsored a covert (and ultimately unsuccessful) effort to develop a nuclear power plant in Patagonia.[70] A malaria eradication "army" deploying the "weapon" of DDT fit well into this overall program.

The notion that the campaign represented a "war" on malaria was taken seriously by its participants; the war metaphor permeated the discourse of the campaign as well as its visual appearance and logistics. When he inspected the progress of the great campaigns, Carrillo, who had no military experience other than his work in the army hospital, would don a khaki uniform and beret.[71] Carrillo saw the fight against infectious diseases as nothing less than a war:

> Germs and microbes, this whole army of enemies, lie in wait for us, surround us, and blockade us everywhere—the air, soil, water, etc.,—and try always to penetrate our organism and destroy it. Sanitary medicine has to combat, with precision, this powerful and invisible enemy. Unfortunately, the forces of this army are very well organized. Sometimes, better organized than the Ministries of Public Health, and they sometimes beat us in battle. For that reason, when an epidemic or endemic appears with all of its virulence, it is truly difficult to fight and defeat it, because the organization of microbes on the attack is better than our organization of defense against microbes. In this, just as in military strategy, the best defense is always to attack.[72]

Alvarado, too, had used military rhetoric and logistics even in the days of foci patrol.[73] Later, Alvarado would observe that spraying a house with DDT was simple, analogous to a "sniper" firing a "rifle." But if a "sniper" was sufficient for just one house, to spray the three hundred thousand houses of the endemic area would require an "army."[74] Thus Alvarado set about creating

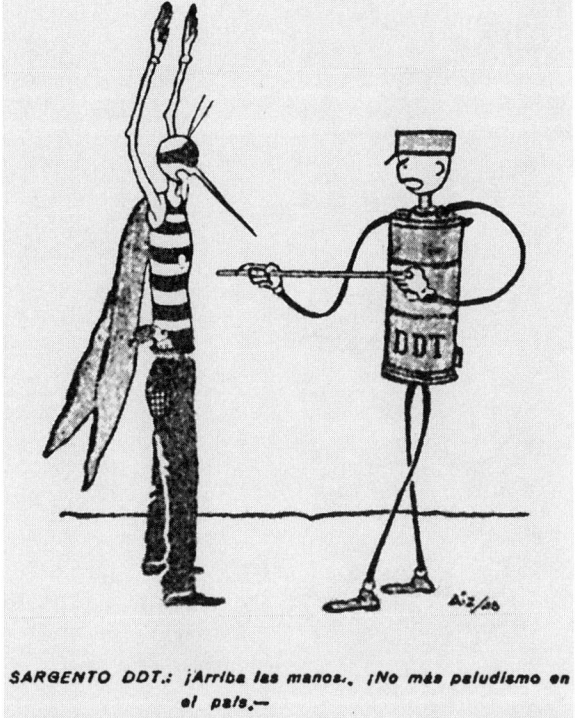

SARGENTO DDT.: ¡Arriba las manos-, ¡No más paludismo en
el país.—
ANOPHELES PSEUDOPUNCTIPENNIS: ¡Me rindo! ¡Han ganado
la partida!.—

Figure 5.1. Cartoon of Sergeant DDT, by Moisés Aizenberg, a physician and amateur cartoonist from Rosario, circa 1948. Text reads: "Sergeant DDT: 'Hands up! No more malaria in this country.' Anopheles pseudopunctipennis: 'I give up. You've won the game.'" Jobino Pedro Sierra Iglesias, *Carlos Alberto Alvarado: Vida y obra* (Salta: Comisión Bicameral Examinadora de Obras de Autores Salteños, 1993), 205.

an army whose weapon of choice was DDT, not bullets, bombs, or grenades. On a lighter note, but still demonstrating the prominence of the bellicose discourse, Alvarado commissioned the creation of a cartoon character, "Sergeant DDT"—part soldier, part DDT canister—for use in campaign publicity and to maintain the morale of his own staff (fig. 5.1).[75] All of this verbal and visual rhetoric exemplifies what was becoming an increasingly prevalent modern perspective: technology could not simply control but annihilate the microbial and insect "enemies" of humanity, turning disease control into a "war on nature."[76]

After DDT, the most important weapon in the eradication campaign's arsenal was the truck, specifically, war surplus trucks, jeeps, and tankers. A caravan of trucks bearing the logo of the Ministry of Public Health became one of the key visual tropes of the great campaigns, symbolizing modern transportation, military might, and the rapid and massive deployment of supplies. The caravans also symbolized the mobile munificence of the national state, distributing vital resources from its seat in Buenos Aires to the far-flung provinces.[77] Perón's government had acquired a fleet of Canadian army sur-

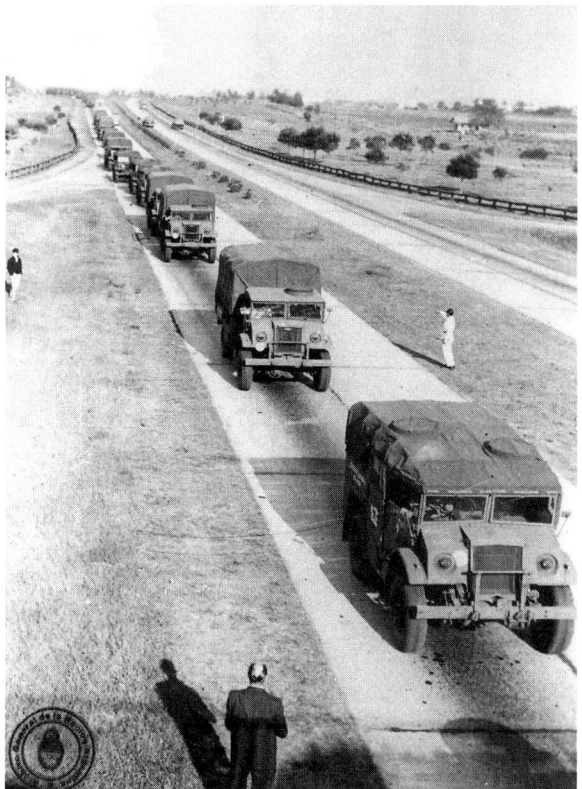

Figure 5.2. Caravan of Ministry of Public Health trucks on highway, 1947, for malaria campaign. Photograph courtesy of the Archivo General de la Nación, Buenos Aires, Argentina.

plus vehicles—which Hackett recorded as fifty-eight trucks, twenty-two jeeps, and six tankers—at the end of World War II.[78] In a well-publicized spectacle, Perón and Carrillo watched as the caravan, manned by teams of doctors and soldiers, departed from the presidential palace for the interior.[79] Alvarado's son Peter, who was just a child at the time, later recalled the emotional day in June 1947 when the long-awaited trucks arrived: "it was a caravan of something like sixty trucks—impressive—still painted in war colors. We waited in Termas de Río Hondo [on the border between Santiago del Estero and Tucumán]. I was with my father and I got into one of the trucks with the driver and we came back to Tucumán" (fig. 5.2).[80] In Tucumán, the trucks were paraded around the main plaza of the city. Alvarado and his regional directors proudly posed for a photograph in front of one of the trucks; the picture was published in the local Tucumán newspaper (see fig. 4.1 in chapter 4).[81]

With the addition of the trucks, the key components were in place for the start of what would prove to be the decisive phase of malaria control. Alvarado had acquired a sure supply of DDT, contracting with the Geigy Company for one hundred tons a year, at five pesos (US $1.25) per kilogram, to be manufactured in Argentina.[82] Pumps, hand-held sprayers, stainless-steel tanks, protective masks, and gloves were acquired for the spraying of DDT. The Malaria Service constructed tanks to store the kerosene that would hold the DDT in solution and the gasoline needed to run the trucks. The personnel, about 250 in total, were already in the service. Everything was ready to go and in working order, but these were merely the raw ingredients for a successful campaign. To spray thousands of houses at three-month intervals throughout the entire Northwest presented new logistical challenges. In the months that followed, Alvarado would show his knack for maintaining a strong yet flexible organization and once again make good on his own maxim: an effective malaria campaign "should be militarily conceived and militarily executed."[83]

Thus, in just two short years, Carlos Alvarado went from nearly losing his livelihood to supervising a well-funded antimalaria "army" on the verge of eradicating this fearsome disease from Northwest Argentina. This turn of events depended, to a large degree, on political changes beyond his immediate control. Alvarado also benefited from the sudden availability of a powerful new insecticide and war surplus vehicles. Without Perón and Carillo's interest in making a bold statement in favor of public health, the prospect of an eradication campaign would likely have been neglected, or at least delayed. Yet at the same time, Alvarado had built a reputation—during the pre-DDT era—as a diligent researcher, public health administrator, and energetic organizer of collective effort, always under conditions of scarce financial resources. Alvarado's reputation helped assure Perón and Carrillo of the viability of the eradication effort, and all three would benefit from the spectacularly effective execution of the campaign.

Eradication: Practice and Impact

Generally, scholars have emphasized how DDT revolutionized malaria control and portrayed the new phase of control as a decisive break with the past.[84] I believe that this perspective is mostly accurate but perhaps overstated. The basic underpinnings of Alvarado's new strategy represented a continuity of the general philosophy, if not the specifics, of the foci patrol model, which Alvarado himself called "the era of organization."[85] Many elements helped bridge the old and the new models: military-like planning, hierarchy, chain of command, and spatial strategizing; a division of labor that charged personnel with specific tasks and avoided repetition of effort; species-specific attention to mosquito biology; use of quantitative methods for rigorous confirmation of results; and meticulous cost accounting, predicated on the quest for always-greater efficiency. On the other hand, a DDT-based strategy created new requirements in terms of timing of effort, labor distribution, and supply. So while Alvarado carried over general concepts or attitudes from the old model, he also made specific and sometimes drastic changes to the campaign's organization. For example, within two years he eliminated all twenty-eight of the Sanitation Services, the units occupied with foci patrol, and suspended all works of sanitary engineering.[86]

Alvarado superimposed a new system on the old one. In the new system, the basic unit of operation was the brigade (*brigada*), usually consisting of five members (chief, driver, and three operators) aboard the all-important truck. Each brigade covered a demarcated zone, within which it was responsible for the spraying of each and every home over a set schedule, and mobilized from a base, which was meant to serve as supply depot, repair shop, meeting place, and domicile—not unlike an army base. Many of these bases were built on the fly while the campaign was underway, by improvising structures out of scrap materials. Staff on the base provided logistical support for the brigades working in the field. Alvarado reported that there were 250 men "on the battle front"—that is, in the brigades—"and an equal number in the rear-guard."[87] Alvarado took great pride in the complex and comprehensive supply chain he developed to keep operations moving.[88] As in military logistics, timing was everything with *dedetización* (literally, DDT-ization): failure to spray houses at planned intervals, usually three times a year, could allow for re-infestation. A network of forty-four primary and secondary bases (expanded to fifty-two the second year), connected and serviced by support personnel, served to ensure that the whole operation would run like clockwork.[89]

The scope of this new organization was impressive, and there were also important differences in practice between the old foci patrol services and the new dedetización brigades. In foci patrol, each Malaria Service operator spent most of the day working alone, responsible for controlling mosquito-breeding areas in his own zone; in dedetización brigades, teamwork was fundamental. Alvarado had originally justified the labor system of foci patrol because he felt that it was the criollo preference to work alone, and Alvarado feared that the new approach would require "a difficult job of psychological conversion" of these laborers.[90] By all accounts, however, the workers adapted well to their new circumstances. The two strategies also differed significantly in their respective key spaces of labor activity. The foci patrol units tended to move in urban (or peri-urban) spaces while focusing on what were mostly natural environments (albeit modified by humans), such as springs, creeks, and seepage areas of riverbeds. Their main task, the search for anopheles mosquito larvae, never took them inside people's homes. The work of DDT brigades was quite different. As the focus of control shifted completely from mosquito larvae to adults, domestic spaces (sometimes peri-domestic spaces as well, such as stables or barns) became the exclusive locus of activity. At the same time, however, dedetización brigades were more likely to be assigned to remote, rural areas than to cities and their suburbs. To reach remote places in their zones, brigades had to deal with the difficulty of driving along muddy, unpaved roads and crossing swollen streams. For the most inaccessible and mountainous zones, brigades often shifted to more nimble jeeps and, when necessary, relied on horses, mules, or their own feet.[91] Thus, a focus on house spraying did not signify the end of contact with "raw nature" for DDT brigades.

Chemically, DDT differed from other insecticides both in its high toxicity to insects and its unique action. DDT was a *residual spray:* that is, its effective action continued long after spraying. Brigades sprayed a solution of 5 percent DDT dissolved in kerosene on walls; and after the kerosene evaporated (this occurred almost immediately), DDT crystals continued to hold to the surface, in a concentration of about two grams per square meter.[92] This invisible residue and its effectiveness against insects would last for three to six months.[93] Since DDT was not used as a fumigant (an aerosol "bomb"), it did not repel insects from entering homes. As it happened, the habits of *A. pseudo-punctipennis,* the local vector that Alvarado understood thoroughly thanks to his earlier and ongoing research, made it particularly vulnerable to the effects of DDT. For one, it was highly anthropophilic and domestic, tending to bite people in their homes, generally while they were asleep at night. Moreover, after taking a blood meal, the female *A. pseudo* tended, almost always, to repose immediately on a nearby wall to begin digesting the blood meal. Since DDT almost always killed mosquitoes on contact, by attacking the insect's nervous system, the chances of a mosquito surviving multiple visits to houses sprayed with DDT was practically nil.[94]

Over the course of months, DDT spraying reduced *A. pseudopunctipennis* densities in treated locales to nearly zero, and before the effectiveness of the DDT wore off completely, another round of spraying would take place.[95] With the mosquitoes effectively eliminated (for as long as the spraying lasted), the cycle of malaria transmission would be broken. Barring the introduction of new human cases from outside, locales could become free of malaria. Thus DDT was unlike the insecticides of old: as Gordon Harrison has commented, it was "in action rather like a vaccine applied to the environment to make it unsuitable for the transmission of parasites."[96] Alvarado, for his part, saw the whole project as having little to do with malariology: he considered the application of DDT little different in method from the application of spray paint.[97] For this reason, once he had established the norms of dedetización, he placed a civil engineer, Luis Silvetti Peña, in charge of the whole operation.[98]

The other key institutional component of the DDT strategy was the Servicio de Vigilancia, or Monitoring Service. Confident in the effectiveness of DDT, Alvarado transformed the mission of the old quinine dispensaries, which for more than thirty years had attended to the majority of malaria patients in the endemic zone. By the middle of 1948, about ten months after spraying had begun, the dispensaries were receiving fewer than one thousand patients per month (by comparison, in the preceding decade, consultations had ranged from five thousand to almost twenty-five thousand per month; see fig. 5.3).[99] Alvarado recognized that the success of DDT was leaving doctors, nurses, and other dispensary staff with time on their hands, so he remade these clinics, now called Puestos de Vigilancia (Monitoring Stations), into the key nodes of the new Monitoring Service. Personnel had two major new responsibilities. First, the Monitoring Service was charged with checking recently sprayed houses for the presence of mosquitoes. Second, and more importantly, these monitors were responsible for epidemiological surveillance: they had to investigate and treat each new suspected case of malaria within their zone. The very possibility of having such a service was proof of DDT's success, since for the first time, malaria incidence had been reduced to such negligible levels that it was feasible to investigate every single case of the disease.

The main purpose of these surveillance activities was to provide data to test the effectiveness of the DDT program. In the first half of 1949, only 134 malaria cases were registered in the whole area covered by the campaign. Of these, 76 (or about 57 percent) were patients whose homes had not received DDT spraying at all. While this number was negligible, Alvarado used the figure to expose the major fault of the campaign, the failure to diligently spray every house, as well as other problems, such as DDT whose effectiveness wore off too quickly or the difficulty of spraying houses made of traditional materials, such as sticks, thatch, and mud. Surveillance also revealed that in a few cases, residents themselves undid the work of DDT by covering sprayed surfaces with mud or plaster, for example, or by sleeping outside.[100]

The work accomplished by the DDT program in its first few months was nothing short of impressive. Between September 1, 1947, and April 17, 1948, the Malaria Service sprayed 170,235 houses in the endemic zone, in the process consuming about forty-three tons of pure DDT, and almost one million liters of kerosene and gasoline.[101] The DDT sprayed in this time covered 22,543,000 square meters of interior surfaces (i.e., over 22 square kilometers), and brigades had covered a distance of over 168,000 kilometers.[102] Such figures add to the story of the endgame of malaria control, but in another sense, the numbers themselves *are* the story. Published reports by Alvarado

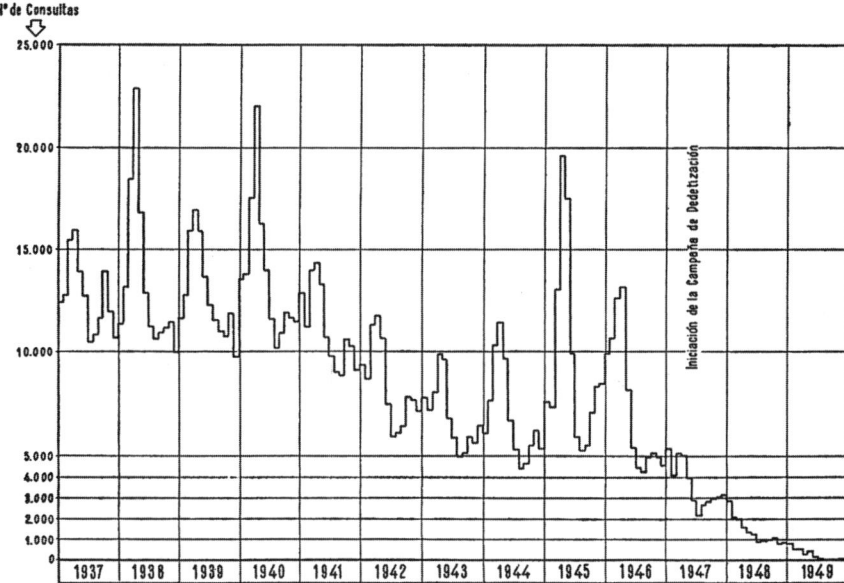

Figure 5.3. Patients consulted in Malaria Service offices, 1937 to 1949. Note the already low number of cases in early 1947, before DDT spraying activities began. Carlos Alberto Alvarado and Héctor A. Coll, "Organización y resultados de la campaña antipalúdica," in *Primera Reunión Panamericana sobre Enfermedad de Chagas* (Tucumán: UNT, 1949).

and other officers of the Malaria Service began to read more like civil engineering reports than public health work, and the disease itself practically left the frame of reference, which instead had cost accounting squarely at its center. Alvarado argued that in the era of foci patrol, precise economic calculations had been complicated and elusive because of the very heterogeneity and complexity of nature, represented by the *criadero* (mosquito-breeding habitat). With DDT, however, "the breeding ground is substituted by a person's house, *a homogeneous unit,* easily accessible and measurable, where in general a basic formula of treatment is sufficient: that is, to apply 2 grams of DDT for every square meter of surface. This revolutionary change in technique also revolutionizes administration, since it permits the calculation of the cost of a *national* malaria campaign, with as much ease and precision as one calculates the cost of the construction of a road, a dam, or a twenty-story building."[103] Even before the campaign proper began, Alvarado had used elaborately calculated cost projections in his proposal to Carrillo and Perón; and as DDT work continued he refined these models, essentially building formulas to predict the cost of a campaign. These formulas relied on factors that were more or less constant (e.g., the estimated two grams of DDT per square meter, number of personnel in a brigade, cost of material needed to equip each brigade, etc.) and many variables (the number of inhabitants of a malarious zone, housing density, labor costs, supply costs) to figure out precisely how much labor, material, and time would be required for a campaign, as well as its bottom-line cost.[104] These models could also be used to compare the cost-effectiveness of DDT spraying vis-à-vis other techniques, though by the late 1940s the superior economies of DDT became practically self-evident.

Why did Alvarado's discourse increasingly take a turn toward mathematics and accounting and away from malariology, biology, and sanitation? For one, he was convinced of the extraordinary potential of DDT in the context of an efficient campaign. As a result, he believed that Argentina's experience could serve as a universal model for malaria control. A decade before, in dismissing the Italian model for Argentina's malaria campaign, Alvarado had cautioned against the hasty transfer of malaria control techniques from one country to another, arguing that it was essential to understand the biology, ecology, and behavior of local mosquito vectors. In Argentina, he had once contended, the uniqueness of *A. pseudo* required uniquely Argentine solutions. While Alvarado did not abandon this position completely, he saw DDT as leveling the differences between mosquito species (since it was effective against all domestic mosquitoes) and, as such, the closest thing to a universal weapon against malaria. Alvarado was not alone in thinking this, of course, as the international meetings of the PASB became something of an echo chamber for the supremacy of this perspective.[105] Given that the efficacy of DDT as a chemical was becoming rapidly accepted in the malariology community, Alvarado may have perceived that his greatest contribution would be to elaborate norms for efficiently delivering DDT, and this project depended on the language of accounting. There are other, more subtle reasons for this turn, however. Alvarado had always railed against the obtuseness of Argentina's obstructionist government administrators, and he viewed careful accounting as his defense against the arbitrariness of bureaucracy. Finally, while Perón and Carrillo granted vast sums to the great campaign, perhaps obviating the need for good bookkeeping, Alvarado had other responsibilities besides malaria control.[106] Carrillo gradually expanded the purview of the Malaria Service, extending it into control of other diseases (such as Chagas disease) and expanding its geographical scope. The burden of these other projects may have been another reason for Alvarado's close attention to the costs of the campaign.

How did the public react to this campaign at the time? Apparently, the public viewed the campaign favorably, but firsthand accounts are scarce. Tulio Ottonello, a businessman and local historian from Monteros, Tucumán Province, related to me that there was "no resistance" to DDT spraying, which began when he was ten years old.[107] DDT spraying was beneficial not only for reducing malaria incidence, but also for eliminating all kinds of insect pests. The public may have perceived this incidental outcome as one of DDT's principal merits. DDT spraying for malaria control coincided with another of Perón's ambitious programs, the aerial spraying of insecticide to eliminate locusts on crops.[108] During this time, according to Ottonello, "there wasn't a single insect."[109] The public assisted in this war on insects by purchasing widely available DDT-based products, sold under such brand names as "Pestroy" and "Nebulair."[110]

In rare instances, the work of the Malaria Service provoked emotional reactions. In 1950, Alvarado recounted how one woman in rural Catamarca had conveyed her gratitude for the campaign a few years earlier. Alvarado and other officials of the Malaria Service were inspecting the work of one dedetización brigade, which they had followed, on foot, to an isolated canyon. After learning that Alvarado was in charge, an old woman approached him and said:

> I'm over ninety years old, sir; during my long life I've listened to promises from politicians and government people, and I've heard stories from many others, but they never came to our house to bring any benefit or to leave us with any improvement, up to now; thanks to what these men are doing, our life has changed, especially that of the poor women, mothers and wives, who spend our lives at home. Now we enjoy a great benefit; we can live and sleep peacefully, without having to think constantly about fleas, bedbugs, lice, or mosquitoes, and above all, because our children have ceased suffering from malaria. That's why I ask that you allow me to kiss your hand in gratitude.

Alvarado deflected her praise and gave Perón the credit for the campaign. All the woman could say in response was "God bless General Perón."[111]

As this anecdote implies, the eradication campaign encountered little public opposition. Historically, government programs of disease control have provoked resistance due to the high-handedness of state officials, cultural differences, perceived racism, and denials of civil liberties. Marcos Cueto, for example, has explored such patterns of resistance in Peru and Mexico.[112] If anything like this occurred in Argentina's malaria eradication program, it was never mentioned in the hundreds of newspaper articles and other documents I reviewed or in the many interviews I conducted. There are probably many factors behind the relative lack of resistance, but I speculate that the mass popularity and adulation of Perón facilitated the labor of the Malaria

Service. Alvarado was also known for maintaining good relations with rural people of the Northwest, and it's also possible that effective eradication took place so rapidly that "resistance" to the campaign never had time to develop.

As a result, Perón and Carrillo easily made political capital out of the success of the malaria eradication campaign. While the results of the campaign were indeed dramatic, and even more than promised, the government's propaganda tended to exaggerate the severity of the malaria problem before the DDT campaign began, thereby overstating how much malaria had declined after DDT. Carrillo, for example, boasted that the number of cases of malaria had declined from 300,000 in 1946 to 137 in 1949.[113] The first number seems to be far off base but unfortunately became widely disseminated in propaganda. The official statistics of Alvarado's Malaria Service (which recorded patients visiting the service's clinics or quinine dispensaries) account for only 87,853 cases in 1946, dropping to 3,164 cases in 1949; from 1937 to 1950, in no year did this figure exceed 165,000 cases.[114] Carrillo also claimed that by eliminating malaria in the north, over 2 million work days had been saved, equivalent to 40 million pesos a year in salary; since the campaign cost only 4 million pesos in three years, Argentina had "made a magnificent bargain."[115] Public health propaganda also used extreme rhetoric to describe the severity of malaria before Perón; the 1950 book *The Argentine Nation: Just, Free, Sovereign,* a massive compendium of the Perón government's early accomplishments, includes a reproduction of a propaganda poster entitled "One Less Enemy" (referring to malaria).[116] The poster's text proclaims that malaria was once an "obsession" for Argentina, a "terrible, implacable enemy" of health. The graphics of the poster accentuate such claims, with an outline drawing of the "rebel mosquito" appearing to threaten the entire country. Interestingly, there are no people in the poster; the heroes of the campaign appear to be the famous army surplus trucks. This propaganda seemed to fulfill its purpose, as Perón was given more than his due credit for executing the campaign. Even Félix Luna, a historian and constant critic of Perón, declared that the success of this campaign alone almost (but not quite) made up for all of the errors of his government.[117]

Conclusion

There is a saying among many public health professionals in Argentina: "malaria was eradicated by decree."[118] Indeed, in July 1949, less than two years after the massive DDT spraying effort had begun, and while there were still sporadic cases of malaria in the country, Perón issued a presidential decree that abolished the Malaria Service (by then, known as the Division of Malaria and Tropical Diseases). His logic was simple: since malaria had been eradicated from Argentina, the agency no longer served a purpose.[119] In its place, this decree created a new agency, the General Directorate of Sanitation for the North (known by its Spanish abbreviation, Digesnorte), still headed by Alvarado. Carrillo formed this and other regional health agencies as part of his plan to expand the effective power of the federal government over public health.

Despite this decree, Argentina's public health ministry continued to attend to malaria eradication, maintaining control in malaria-free zones and snuffing out new epidemics. In reality, malaria has never left Argentina, not completely. During the 1950s, there were only a few hundred cases a year in the Northwest; Tucumán, once the heart of the endemic zone, averaged only about twenty cases a year. But, with the expansion of the resource frontier in the northern borderlands for agriculture, ranching, logging, and oil exploration, malaria resurged in 1959, with 2,623 cases in the area around Orán and Tartagal. That same year, partly in response to this alarming rise in incidence, Argentina joined the global malaria eradication program, led by the World Health Organization and UNICEF.[120] By the 1970s, even as the global campaign faltered, incidence of malaria in Argentina declined once again to negligible levels, although constant vigilance was required to prevent new outbreaks spreading from neighboring countries. As the book's epilogue explains, the Malaria Service continues to operate today, employing a control model that depends on house spraying for adult mosquitoes. This is one concrete legacy of the efforts of Perón, Carrillo, and Alvarado.

In the years following 1949, the architects of malaria's demise in Argentina met different fates. By the end of 1955, Perón was overthrown in a military coup and sent into exile. A year later, Carrillo died of complications from a cerebral hemorrhage in Belém, Brazil. He, too, had been forced into exile, but by rivals within the Peronist party in October of 1954.[121] By that time, his hopes for a comprehensive overhaul of national public health had been frustrated due to budgetary issues, political intrigues, and a geographically uneven implementation of policy that failed to overcome the disadvantages of the impoverished interior.[122] Alvarado was much more fortunate. Beginning in 1950, Alvarado served as an advisor to malaria eradication campaigns in other countries of Latin America and the Caribbean under the auspices of the PASB.[123] At the end of 1954, sensing that Carrillo's ouster had complicated his own professional and political situation, Alvarado sought a way to leave Argentina on his own terms. In November, Alvarado accepted an offer from Fred L. Soper, director of the PASB, to become a permanent consultant on malaria control in the Americas; he relocated to Mexico City and, later, Washington, DC From 1959 to 1964, Alvarado served as director of the World Health Organization's global malaria eradication program, in Geneva, Switzerland.[124]

The experiences of a long career changed Alvarado's outlook on major aspects of malaria control. In the 1930s, he had cautioned against the transfer of malaria control models between countries with different environmental, social, and political circumstances; in the 1950s and 1960s, as a leader in international malaria policy, Alvarado helped enforce the eradicationist perspective, with well-known, tragic consequences. (It should be noted, however, that Alvarado's views were not completely orthodox: for example, he argued that continued entomological research and epidemiological surveying remained important in the secondary phases of eradication campaigns, while Soper believed that DDT had made these activities mostly superfluous.[125]) Yet Alvarado would discover that the success of his campaign in Argentina was hard to duplicate in other countries. The inability to consistently unite three factors—sanitary organization, technology, and strong political support for public health—may provide a partial explanation for the failure of the eradication model in other countries.

Finally, how did malaria eradication impact the Northwest more broadly? In contrast to the expectations of hygienists and other elites of the early twentieth century, the effective elimination of malaria did not have much of a perceptible effect on the prospects of the region. Other kinds of improvements—potable water and sanitary sewers, improved nutrition, the elimination of most epidemic diseases, and a general increase in the standard of living—arguably made a bigger impact on the public health. While malaria was still prominent in the early 1920s, general and infant mortality had already begun to decline steadily. From that point, life expectancy in the Northwest increased at about the same pace, before and after the eradication of malaria, and by the early 1990s was just two years shorter than for the country as a whole. Despite this achievement, the breach in economic development between the Northwest and the rest of Argentina persisted long after the 1940s; while the development "gap" did close somewhat over the years, the peripheral economic status of the region persists.[126] Thus, malaria control represented an important yet incremental improvement in the quality of life for the region, rather than the sweeping social transformation its proponents had once predicted.

Conclusion
Malaria, Geography, and Lessons for Today

In a reversal of the usual formula, malaria is forgotten but not gone in Argentina. "Eradication" is something of a misnomer; the disease was never completely eradicated from the country, with a few dozen to a few hundred cases every year in the northern borderlands. While the malaria campaign may never have achieved total eradication, nearly everyone has forgotten that malaria ever existed in Argentina. Indeed, to those who identify Argentina with tango, beef, and Borges, the thought of malaria, past or present, would seem absurd. What would a tropical disease like that be doing in such a "European" country? The historical erasure of malaria is, then, another achievement in the long and uneven process of building the country's modern national identity.

Still, Argentina was one of the first countries, for all practical purposes, to eradicate malaria from within its borders, and so we might ask if there are any lessons to be learned from its experience. After all, malaria continues to kill millions around the world each year and sicken countless more. This scourge does not show any signs of going away soon; and, in fact, malaria is a bigger problem, on a global scale, than it was a generation ago.[1] It would be a mistake to think that a specific method or strategy could be drawn directly from the Argentine experience and transplanted easily in sub-Saharan Africa, the Brazilian Amazon, India, or other areas where malaria continues to exact a heavy toll. It must be admitted that the eradication of malaria in Argentina, while still a long, difficult, and tortuous process, was facilitated by non-tropical climatic conditions. An interruption or attenuation of malaria transmission, albeit briefly, during the subtropical winter months, offers an invaluable assist to control work. The geography of Northwest Argentina, the southern United States, Italy, or other places where malaria was controlled most decisively cannot simply be picked up and plunked down in the lowland tropics. As one malaria fighter said half a century ago, "The first axiom of malariology, that lessons learnt in one part of the world may not be applied to other parts of the world, without local verification, is as true as ever; it is unfortunately as often neglected as ever."[2]

No, the relevant lessons of Argentina's malaria campaign have less to do with identifying and replicating the ingredients of a successful strategy and more to do with how we might fruitfully understand malaria as a geographical problem, that is, one that represents the relationship between people and the environments they live in, in particular places. Certainly, this book is not the first attempt to analyze malaria as a geographical problem. But the vital lessons here pertain more to how public health problems are framed, which actors play a key role in constructing such frames, the importance of historicizing geographical scale, and the clarification of the meaning of ecology in malaria control.

First and foremost, geographical imaginaries have social power, becoming dominant narratives that shape public health policy on the ground. These framing devices are necessary for simplifying complex reality and enabling action in the world. At the same time, however, the ideological, political, and cultural concerns of the day influence these imaginaries. In other words, they develop in a broader social context from which public health professionals cannot easily isolate themselves, in spite of their best efforts. But more crucially, I have shown how geographical imaginaries may take on such prominence and power that they actually distort a problem, undermine solutions, and become counterproductive.

Malaria first became a prominent social problem in the Northwest around the turn of the twentieth century. Political ideas and scientific frameworks from this era would exert a strong influence on the malaria campaign for years to come, helping to establish a dominant discourse on the malaria problem that worked both for and against productive efforts to fight the disease. During this time of flux in scientific thought, microbiological theories of disease causation shared the stage with older ideas that malaria sprang from insalubrious landscapes, especially wetlands and other areas of standing water, in the subtropical setting of the Northwest. The convincing discovery that malaria was caused by a parasite spread by anopheles mosquitoes did not really change the old model but rather validated the role of the environment in malaria transmission. Thus the systematic science of medical geography, predicated on detailed topographical survey of malarious zones, persisted alongside the modern bacteriological frameworks, rather than being suddenly replaced by them.

The seemingly inexorable association between malaria and particular landscapes—malaria as a disease *of place*—allowed malaria control to be enveloped in broader schemes to promote the development of the Northwest. Drainage, filling, channelization, reclamation for parks, and other modifications of the hydraulic landscape in urban and rural areas were viewed as general improvements to the economy and health of the region. With these improvements, elites of the Northwest hoped to initiate a virtuous circle, whereby development would promote investment and immigration from abroad, and gradually improve (or replace) the deficient criollo stock that predominated in the region. Hygienists in the capital, enamored with theories of racial improvement through public health measures and preoccupied with Argentina's status relative to other "civilized" countries, began to develop the rationale for government involvement in malaria control. Painting malaria as a mobile threat, after an epidemic in Santiago del Estero, and establishing the province's lack of capacity for safeguarding health sealed the national government's role in malaria control.

Environmental sanitation, or *saneamiento,* became the preferred strategy for malaria control because it corresponded to the logic and goals of these larger development schemes. The positive experience of Italy, using similar, even more expansive environmental sanitation techniques, offered encouragement to the leadership of the National Department of Hygiene (DNH) and led to complacency. Only when the Northwest's peculiar disease ecology was understood on its own terms, largely due to the work of a network of regional scientists, was substantial progress made. To understand saneamiento's persistence despite its defects in practices requires an appreciation of the geographical imaginary's role as a dominant discourse or narrative. Thinking outside of the dominant paradigm was challenging, and it took years to undo. So, we might ask ourselves, Are there other grand narratives about disease, social development, and environment that require undoing, or at least critique?

A second lesson is that state actors have a special role in fashioning geographical imaginaries of health and disease. As Richard Peet and Michael Watts have argued, discourses are laden with power; they are produced and reproduced, made to represent a region's problems, and transmuted into policy, not necessarily because of their wisdom or accuracy, but because of the social power of the institutions that stand behind them.[3] As I have shown throughout this book, it was mainly state actors who fashioned the discourse on malaria control in Argentina. Conventionally, and perhaps naively, we might view the state's role as one of responding to problems that develop outside of its domain. Yet, in creating a malaria control program, the Argentine state did not merely respond to a given "social fact" (that is, the presence of endemic malaria), but rather was the key participant in constructing the malaria problem—its causes, impacts, and territorial parameters.[4] The state did not contrive malaria into being, but it may as well have—such was its role in framing the problem. Argentina's malaria campaign exemplified a style of scientific statecraft that aimed to transform the " backward" society of the Northwest through control of space and rationalization of unruly landscapes.[5]

State agents themselves behaved as *geographical actors,* not just according to political, technical, or scientific precepts. Tangibly, from Eliseo Cantón and DNH survey teams to the Rockefeller scientists and Carlos Alvarado, the geographic tools of surveying and mapping were essential for diagnosing the scope of sanitary problems and planning malaria control efforts. But perhaps less obviously, these actors also imagined development futures in spatial terms and operated based on particular models of the relationship between people and the environment. In a more general sense, the inertia of bureaucratic state power helps explain why geographical imaginaries often become so persistent, or "sticky."

A third lesson is that historians of infectious disease and public health should not take geographical scales for granted. The construction of global, national, and regional scales is often a key part of the story, not merely the backdrop to the story. The "geographical imaginary" that framed reformers' models of malaria in the environment revolved around the co-constructed identities of the Northwest and Buenos Aires. The intervention of the national state to combat malaria rested on the fulcrum of perceived regional difference. To hygienists, malaria served to symbolize the danger, backwardness, and decay of northwestern environment and society. It was a localized but potentially mobile threat to the national race and the national organism. The persistence of malaria, as a symbol of regional disequilibrium, was an affront to the cherished idea of a coherent national community. It is telling that malaria, among all other public health problems, rose to such prominence: other diseases and conditions were much greater killers, but malaria served as a unique marker of disparate regional identities.

The Northwest and the interior provinces, more generally, have received short shrift in Argentine historiography.[6] Buenos Aires and the Pampas region that surrounds it—the littoral—are generally accepted as the "core" of the nation; and as a result there is a Pampas-centric bias in political, social, cultural, and intellectual histories, not to mention histories of public health. Many would argue that this bias is simply a reflection of the actual strength and power of the core; insofar as the ontological reality of Argentine history revolves around that center, so should histories of the nation. Without disputing the centrality of this region, there are two problems here. First, the idea that Buenos Aires is representative of Argentina as a whole is a commonplace assumption that deserves deeper scrutiny; indeed, the exceptional qualities of Buenos Aires in relation to the rest of the nation are so profound and obvious that few Argentines, except the most chauvinistic Porteños, could uphold such a claim. Unfortunately, however, Buenos Aires is implicitly representative of Argentina as a whole in most historical studies. Many so-called national histories never leave the boundaries of the capital city.[7]

Yet, as I have sought to demonstrate in this book, such a geographically narrow focus is wrong, not simply because it dismisses the lives and interests of a broad swath of Argentine society, but also because it paints a historically inaccurate portrait of public health politics in the country. While Buenos Aires was the center of scientific learning and public health policy-making, hygienists and social reformers from the capital had an expansive, not narrow, view of the nation and its social and sanitary problems. Figures such as Alfredo Palacios were often fixated on the sanitary conditions of Argentina's interior regions. Furthermore, many of the outstanding figures in the malaria story, by birth or by relocation, were northwesterners, including Carlos Malbrán, Eliseo Cantón, Guillermo Paterson, Gregorio Aráoz Alfaro, Juan B. Terán, Benjamin Villafañe, Salvador Mazza, Ramón Carrillo, and Carlos Alvarado. A northwestern identity—and sometimes even an antagonism toward Buenos Aires—shaped their outlook and actions. Moreover, these regional actors were often far from "provincial" in their outlook, as they were often more engaged in international scientific networks in malariology, tropical medicine, and disease ecology than their Porteño counterparts. Thus knowledge and innovations did not necessarily flow through the capital to the far-flung provinces, but often bypassed Buenos Aires, as the episode with the Rockefeller Foundation so clearly demonstrates.

In effect, I am not arguing for an either-or approach—that is, *more* histories of the interior as a corrective to the vast majority of historical works centered on Buenos Aires. This would be regionalism for its own sake, not a promising basis for critical historical analysis. Instead, I contend that we derive a clearer picture of Argentina's history and identity by "reading" the nation-state not from its center, but from its margins. Regional, national, and global scales, and the identities attached to them, are not preordained; rather, they are co-constructed in a historical process. Histories of health and disease offer one entry point into this new narrative of the nation-state.

Finally, in this book I have also aimed to develop a more nuanced understanding of the role and meaning of ecology in malaria control. Mainly, I believe that it is important to distinguish between a "socio-ecological perspective" on public health and the role of "ecological science" in disease control. To understand the distinction, first we have to recognize that ecology carries a lot of ideological baggage, with multivalent and sometimes conflicting meanings. Today, for example, ecological thinking is almost synonymous with a progressive view on environmental conservation, even though the latter, as a political project, may revolve around fuzzy notions (say, of "stable" and "harmonious" nature) that should give pause to ecological scientists.[8] The geographer Karl Zimmerer makes a useful distinction between ecologically informed approaches that "cast human-environment relations within a unified field of concepts" and those that "have demanded the analytical separation of the environment . . . from human behavior and society."[9] I draw on this notion to make a broader distinction between, on the one hand, social theory infused with an ecological perspective and, on the other hand, a circumscribed (though never "pure") ecological science, analytically separate from the social realm, applied to questions about the natural dynamics of malarial environments.

The first perspective generally corresponds to the "socio-ecological" or "organicist" thinking of such figures as Gregorio Aráoz Alfaro, Antonio Barbieri, or Alfredo Palacios, or to Italian *bonifica* under Fascism. This mode of thinking legitimizes, perhaps even necessitates, the integration of disease control (and promotion of public health more broadly) with social development goals. It also places defects of human biology, the natural environment, and society in the same frame. As we have seen, the socio-ecological perspective often lapsed into a racialized discourse of national destiny. In his public health philosophy, Carrillo seized on similar metaphors of the interconnectedness of human and biological systems. Carrillo and Juan D. Perón's sanitary policy was expansive, comprehensive, and coherent, favoring measures to address the systemic causes of ill health. This mode of social analysis and political action is inherently holistic.

In contrast, Alvarado used ecology in the latter, more reductionist mode: Alvarado apparently had little patience for the grand developmentalist narratives that made malaria control into something bigger than it really was. Though certainly cognizant of the social context of his project, he sealed off malaria control, as much as possible, from other ideological agendas. Thus he defined malaria as a scientific and technical-administrative problem, retreating from the "social problem" discourse that promised sweeping changes but delivered few results. In this respect, Alvarado personified the mid-twentieth-century school of malariology known as "species sanitation," which took a narrow *yet* ecologically informed view of the causes and solutions to the malaria problem. But who would label Alvarado an ecologist, given his later embrace of DDT?

Indeed, in the post-DDT, post–*Silent Spring* world, critics often lament reductionism and celebrate holism. The DDT-based eradication program that Alvarado helped create would eventually be perceived, in many quarters, as a great debacle; it illustrated the harmful consequences of reducing vector-borne disease to a single factor (the mosquito) and of framing disease control as a technology-driven "war" between people and nature. For example, in his book *The Making of a Tropical Disease,* medical historian Randall Packard laments that the "human ecology of malaria"—the dynamic interaction among social and environmental factors, such as the role of human migration, poverty, warfare, education, agricultural development, forest clearing, urbanization, and other large-scale land-use change—"has tended to disappear from view in the face of expanding scientific knowledge of the biology of malaria."[10] Anthony McMichael, representing a new generation of medical scientists adopting an ecological framework in reaction to emerging infectious diseases, argues that "humans and microbes are not 'at war'; rather, both parties are engaged in amoral, self-interested, coevolutionary struggle."[11] All of this is true, so far as it goes. But should we draw the conclusion that holism will be more effective than reductionism as a concrete basis for malaria control?

Argentina's experience, at least, suggests that the answer is "no." The socioecological perspective, as has already been established, did little to further the cause of malaria control. Alvarado, a pragmatist above all else, saw that quick, direct, decisive action against malaria was the best route to take and left it to people such as Carrillo to develop high-minded ideas about social justice and the systemic roots of sanitary problems. While using DDT, Alvarado never discarded the knowledge he had attained through an ecological science perspective on malaria. His understanding of mosquito behavior, gained from previous experience with foci patrol, served him well in the DDT program. Ultimately, whose ideas had more influence? Carrillo's or Alvarado's? Carrillo's visionary exposition of Peronist sanitary philosophy, in the end, was mostly left on paper. Its impact on social justice in Argentina, or on the development of a sanitary consciousness, is hard to gauge. We might say that Alvarado's social vision was less ambitious and all-encompassing, but his accomplishment, while modest, was more concrete. All of the grandiose ideas about malaria control in Argentina since the 1890s—its connections to developing the Northwest, attracting foreign immigrants, making agricultural landscapes productive, creating a more productive and civilized working class—had little impact on the disease. Alvarado's reductionist strategy set aside such concerns and in two years accomplished, for all practical purposes, what all of those sweeping ideas could not: the elimination of malaria.

Epilogue

It is seven o'clock on a November morning in 2002. Today I travel with one of the Malaria Service's brigades.[1] We gather at the agency's base in the city of Orán, just fifty kilometers from the international bridge that joins Argentina and Bolivia. The Orán station is one of only two active bases for malaria control in the Northwest, one of the last remnants of the network of *dedeticización* bases that Carlos Alvarado developed in the late 1940s. Just as Alvarado had envisioned, the station serves as launching pad and support system for control efforts in the field. Inside the base's simple main building, two office workers compile weekly and monthly epidemiological progress reports for the head office in Salta; in the back, the staff microscopist works in a rudimentary but tidy lab space shared with a kitchenette. Thousands of typewritten epidemiological reports, going back to the 1970s, fill the cabinets; each of these sheets traces the surveillance and treatment of a single malaria case. Behind the main office, in the back of the lot, are the garage, supply shed, and mechanic's shop. The brigade's driver backs out a white Ford pickup truck, devoid of detail except for the Malaria Service logo stenciled on each door. At the end of the driveway, I join the driver and the brigade chief in the cab while three *operadores,* or "spray operators," pile in the bed with their backpack sprayers, boxes of insecticide powder, and a small crate containing enough food to get us through the day.

We head north from Orán, toward Bolivia, on a two-lane highway to a place called El Pelicano, a small rural settlement. El Pelicano is one of about fifty or sixty locales in the Malaria Service's Orán district. Some of these settlements are so tiny and remote that they do not figure on the government's official 1:250,000 scale topographic maps. During the month of November—as the hot, rainy, potentially malarious season begins—this brigade's schedule takes them, on a daily basis, from the base in Orán to the zone of plantations on the fertile plain near the confluence of the Bermejo and Pescado Rivers. In each locale, the brigade works according to a specific itinerary, portrayed on a *croquis* (sketch map), which includes major landmarks, plantation boundaries, and, most importantly, the approximate location of every single house, each identified with a unique number. Every year, as new houses are built or old structures are demolished, the brigade chief, Bernardo Carrazán, edits his own map to ensure a complete inventory. On his first map, from 1978, he sketched the location of 205 houses in El Pelicano; today, there are 443 of them, which shelter mostly seasonal migrant workers from Bolivia.

The brigade's task, over the next two weeks, is to spray all of these houses with insecticide. Today, brigades use synthetic pyrethroid chemicals instead of DDT, but in most other respects, the way they work is a legacy of Alvarado. In organizing the DDT-based campaign, Alvarado saw the house as the "homogeneous unit" that allowed for precise planning, accounting, and monitoring of control efforts. In many ways, the Malaria Service's progress continues to be measured by multiples of this basic unit. As he goes on his rounds, each operator keeps a tally on a small card of the houses he sprays, and at the end of each day these figures are entered into a daily report. Such ledgers are meant to ensure comprehensive coverage and efficient use of labor and to monitor the amount of insecticide sprayed. These numbers are the foundation for the agency's reports, one of the principal means by which the upper echelons of the state may remotely judge the work of this agency.

In the field, however, the Malaria Service is far from the embodiment of a single-minded state imposing its policies on powerless subjects. When the brigades come in contact with the ordinary people of the region, control work becomes a negotiated process. To perform their work, the brigades must enter the private spaces of poor families to transfer most of their belongings outside, including furniture, clothing, and kitchen utensils. Theoretically, the brigades have legal authority to enter homes to complete these invasive tasks. Generally, however, the Malaria Service prefers to work through persuasion and cooperation rather than coercion. In El Pelicano, the migrant workers live in precarious conditions and are used to dealing with the indignities of poverty and powerlessness. Yet Carrazán, the spokesman for the brigade, treats all of the families with perfect respect and asks their permission to enter and perform control work.

Ironically, the Malaria Service accomplishes its work not by capitalizing on its authority, but rather by diminishing its affiliation with the rest of Argentina's government. In dealing with the public, Malaria Service personnel articulate a clearly demarcated and narrowly defined mission: to protect people from malaria and to prevent its spread through the use of consistent, established methods. The image they project to the public is that of professional technicians working in a sphere *apart from* other agents of the state (tax collectors, judges, police, soldiers, border guards, and so forth). This neutral positioning and narrow technical focus allow the Malaria Service to gain the trust of the public, which is essential to getting its job done smoothly. In El Pelicano, the brigade's driver, Enrique Laci, also has the task of taking thick blood smear samples of suspected malaria sufferers. If samples test positive for plasmodium parasites at the lab in Orán, Laci must return to treat patients with chloroquine and ask them a series of questions for epidemiological surveillance: Where are you from? Where have you been since you came down with malaria symptoms? Where have you been in the last two weeks? Most of the time, truthful answers to these questions reveal illegal movements of migrant workers between Bolivia and Argentina.

Yet people tend to answer truthfully: the Malaria Service has the reputation in the area of being disinterested in people's activities or reporting them to other authorities. Malaria Service personnel in Orán and Tartagal (the other active base, about one hundred kilometers to the northeast) report encounters with fever-stricken young men in the uncontrolled back roads between Bolivia and Argentina: they are *mulas* (drug traffickers). Even under these circumstances, personnel claim to merely treat the patient and avoid asking questions. The narrowly defined mission and house-oriented control strategy of the Malaria Service, "disentangled" as much as possible from broader social problems and political issues, helps the agency to get its work done.

In the geographical imaginary of malaria control today, these sparsely populated borderlands between Argentina and Bolivia loom large. Back in the early twentieth century, when malaria was endemic throughout the subtropical lowlands, foothills, and valleys of the Northwest, Alvarado and other Malaria Service officials seldom mentioned Bolivia. Yet after Argentina effectively eliminated the disease and entered the "consolidation" phase of malaria eradication, the border became much more significant. Bolivia was far less successful in the eradication effort, so the border became an epidemiological ecotone, a frontier marking radically divergent public health realities. Malaria Service personnel on the Argentine side see themselves as defenders of a porous boundary, along which they maintain a tenuous *cordon sanitaire,* a two-hundred-kilometer-wide buffer of insecticide-treated houses and constant vigilance. Occasionally, malaria seems to break through this barrier, for example, in a 1979 outbreak around the Cadillal dam, just outside of San Miguel de Tucumán.[2] But the vast majority of cases occur in Salta Province, near the Bolivian border, and in the agency's epidemiological reports almost every outbreak of malaria is traced back to an "imported" case—a migrant from Bolivia.

Indeed, there is pressure to find Bolivian origins for new malaria cases in Argentina. Rather than thinking of the Yungas borderlands as one epidemiological system with shared ecologies and the constant circulation of people—and the parasites they carry—within it, Malaria Service officials tend to view the international boundary as a line of demarcation. To the extent that Argentina can demonstrate to the Pan-American Health Organization (PAHO) and the World Health Organization (WHO) that sporadic outbreaks have foreign origins and that they can be rapidly extinguished, the country maintains its malaria-free status. Anxiety over slipping back into the category of a malarious country, along with an outbreak of cholera along the Argentina-Bolivia border in 1992, helped drive the ARBOL II project, a cooperative public health agreement between the two countries from 1995 to 2001. For malaria control, the project focused mainly on the Bermejo Triangle, the southernmost extension of Bolivian territory, bounded on two sides by the Bermejo and Tarija Rivers, which come to a point just north of Orán, appearing on a map like an arrow penetrating Argentine territory. Though wide and in some places treacherous, the rivers present little resistance to those wishing to cross; in fact, settlements on the Argentine side, especially along the Tarija River, have regular contact with their Bolivian counterparts.

Yet on the Malaria Service's maps before ARBOL II the Bermejo Triangle looked like the Bermuda Triangle: a geographic void, featureless and unpeopled. The cooperative agreement allowed Argentina's Malaria Service access to this enigmatic area, and a clearer picture of the malaria situation along the border emerged: the district around the Bolivian city of Bermejo was intensely malarious, with almost 12 percent of the population testing positive for malaria parasites in 1996. By 2001, thanks to the infusion of funding, labor, and technique under ARBOL II, incidence had been reduced to just 0.6 percent, with a concomitant decline of new cases on the Argentine side.[3] ARBOL II lasted only a few years, however, and binational cooperation on sanitary issues is the exception, not the norm.

While the strategy based on house spraying and epidemiological surveillance seems to work well, malaria control has lost sight of the environment around the houses. What anopheles mosquitoes do outside of the house—for example, where they breed—matters little to the personnel of the Malaria Service. They have only a vague idea of where in the local landscape the mosquitoes come from. Malaria Service personnel know how to distinguish anopheles larvae from those of other mosquitoes, and their standard equipment includes ladles and test tubes for collecting larvae. Yet they have no systematic model of vector ecology, and explanations of malaria transmission revolve around the movement of human beings, not mosquitoes. People transporting malaria parasites in their blood are the potential hazards, while the mosquito vector is assumed to be always present, and in any case not amenable to control beyond domestic spaces. When the malaria campaign began a hundred years ago, transforming the natural environment was viewed as the linchpin of controlling the disease and reshaping society. Today, the dynamics of the natural environment are opaque and practically irrelevant to controlling malaria.[4]

One might wonder, So what? As long as malaria control is effective, what difference does it make if the Malaria Service has a hazy understanding of local ecology? For one, the disease problems of the area go far beyond malaria. In the area around Orán and Tartagal, local environmental change appears to be affecting the ecology of malaria and other diseases in ways that are not well understood or, in some cases, downright mysterious.[5] The tiny hamlet of El Oculto, about thirty kilometers west of Orán, has in recent years been afflicted with outbreaks of several vector-borne diseases. Malaria has always been intense there, to such a degree that El Oculto is the only place where the Malaria Service has regularly prescribed chloroquine prophylactically during the malaria season. El Oculto, which has only about seventy residents, also experienced the first known deaths from hantavirus in the Northwest in the late 1990s. Although it is believed that rats and other rodents are the reservoirs of this disease, the precise ecological dynamics of the disease locally are unknown, and its arrival to the area is equally shrouded in mystery.

There are also cases of American cutaneous leishmaniasis, which produces unsightly skin ulcers and disfigures the palate. The first outbreak of leishmaniasis in Salta Province occurred only in 1985.[6] This disease is caused by a protozoan carried by tiny phlebotomine sand flies between people and other animals, particularly dogs. The recent convergence of these vector-borne illnesses in El Oculto—whose name, appropriately, means the "mysterious" or "hidden" place—has perplexed the Malaria Service and local infectious disease experts. One eminent local expert in infectious disease, Nestor Taranto, believes that the occurrence of leishmaniasis in El Oculto and throughout the Yungas has "something to do with the ecosystem and the anthropophilia of the vectors," but no one has really studied the broader ecological dynamics of this disease.[7]

But everyone speculates about the relationship between these diseases, ecology, and anthropogenic environmental change. In Argentina, leishmaniasis tends to impact people whose work takes them outdoors and far from nucleated settlements, such as livestock herders, foresters, hunters, and fishers. Many associate the disease with *desmonte,* the clearing of forests and other vegetation for the expansion of farms, ranches, and settlements. Nery Vianconi, one of the head officers of the Malaria Service's base in Orán, thinks that *desmonte* also creates habitats favorable for the expansion of rodent populations, favoring the transmission of hantavirus. Indeed, some speculate that the continuing deforestation of the Yungas region threatens to make all of these diseases more commonplace.

The emergence of this panoply of diseases in a context of rapid environmental change and degradation calls for an ecological perspective to understand and potentially control these new disease threats. Already there are signs of a change in the Malaria Service's perspective, demonstrated by its response to dengue fever. After having been eliminated through DDT spraying after the 1940s, the *Aedes aegypti* mosquito has re-colonized Salta and Jujuy Provinces. This mosquito's return after a long absence has enabled the transmission of dengue fever, which is potentially as deadly as malaria. Initially, the Malaria Service—which is now one of many government agencies occupied with dengue control work—responded slowly to the spread of dengue because personnel found it hard to adjust to new control strategies. Control work for dengue is different because the ecology of the disease differs greatly from that of malaria. Dengue is mainly an urban disease and the *Aedes aegypti* mosquito is characteristically peri-domestic and anthropophilic. Yet since this species generally does not repose on walls or other hard surfaces, indoor spraying of residual insecticides—the favored strategy against *A. pseudo*—is practically useless.[8] Aedes mosquitoes lay their eggs principally in receptacles that people produce and maintain in their yards, such as pools, buckets, jars, tires, cisterns, barrels—in short, anything that can hold water. *A. pseudo,* as we know, breeds in natural water features, often far from where people live.

Following the lead of other countries with a longer experience of dengue, such as Brazil, control strategy depends on monitoring and treating aedes breeding foci, *not* house-spraying. The work is more labor and time intensive than insecticide spraying for malaria and requires much closer contact with local residents and their collaboration. Interestingly, the language used in training dengue control personnel often recalls the bygone rhetoric of malaria control, before DDT came along (though today the training is done through slick PowerPoint presentations). One training document states that "it is of fundamental importance that we get to know our enemy [the mosquito] if we wish to combat it effectively," echoing Alvarado. Meanwhile, drainage-and-filling operations to eliminate mosquito-breeding areas will not only reduce vector populations, but also "bring better harvests and better agricultural products, preserve the land, and reduce the number of work days lost to illness."[9] Such an argument represents an almost perfect reproduction of the discourse of *saneamiento;* whether such arguments are any more pertinent to dengue control work remains to be seen.

Flash forward to 2009: Argentina suffers its worst-ever epidemic of dengue fever, with over twenty thousand cases nationally, although a precise figure may never be known. Starting in northern Argentina, with a particularly intense outbreak in the Chaco, the disease spreads into the littoral and, by April, into Greater Buenos Aires, inspiring panic and recriminations. The impoverished northern borderlands appear once again as the breeding ground of epidemics and as the porous frontier that allows "foreign" diseases into Argentina. A blogger travels into the "heart of the dengue epidemic," producing this report: "The adolescents lift up the metal sheet and a cloud of a mosquitoes flies out of the hidden pool of infested waters. 'How many of these insects are carriers of dengue?' I thought with alarm, as I ran towards the boys, waving the can of insect repellent. It was too late: the insects had already started to bite, like a squadron of combat planes, on the arms, faces, calves of those kids."[10] Similar to Alfredo Palacios's testimony from the 1930s, the blogger offers a firsthand account of the squalid and unhygienic conditions in the slums on the outskirts of a major city. In the 2009 story, however, the city is Buenos Aires, not Tucumán. Palacios, Ramón Carrillo, and likeminded reformers dreamed of equalizing living standards between the shining capital and the rest of Argentina through sanitary improvements such as malaria control. While greater equality has been achieved, it is perhaps not what hygienists of a bygone era envisioned for Argentina, as public health conditions seem to have eroded all over the country, especially among the growing ranks of the poor, in the last few decades. As one writer for *Clarín,* a major newspaper in Buenos Aires, puts it: "The country is exposed to all sorts of epidemics and there is neither sufficient prevention, nor adequate sanitary infrastructure, nor economic means to confront them"—that is exactly the same situation described in the newspapers of Salta and Tucumán, cities embattled by infectious disease a hundred years ago.[11]

True, standards today are higher than they were in 1905, so the threshold for calamity is correspondingly lower. No matter what is said about dengue and the other ills afflicting Argentina, people live longer and more healthful lives today. But one thing does not change: disease figures strongly in the national geographical imaginary. A porous border channels disease threats; the dangerous, subtropical provinces incubate new outbreaks; the environment—natural, social, and built—must be sanitized. And every comment about dengue is a commentary on Argentina's viability and strength as a nation. Is our government working? Are we a rich nation or a poor one? Are we different from the rest of the world or more like everyone else? Protecting and promoting the nation's health—in every sense of that word—is never a finished project.

Notes

INTRODUCTION

1. Alfredo L. Palacios, *El dolor argentino* (Buenos Aires: Editorial Claridad, 1938). This book was a compilation of Palacios's speeches and bills that he sponsored in the senate. He followed this up with a book on similar themes, derived from an even more extensive tour of the Northwest in 1944, called *Abandoned Peoples*. See Palacios, *Pueblos desamparados: Solución de los problemas del Noroeste Argentino* (Buenos Aires: Editorial Kraft, 1944). Palacios's contribution to debates over public health, generally, and malaria control, specifically, are explored in more detail starting in chapter 3.

2. Palacios, *El dolor argentino,* 84–85.

3. Palacios, *Pueblos desamparados,* 105.

4. Ibid., 13.

5. Victor Garcia Costa, *Alfredo Palacios: Entre el clavel y la espada. Una biografía* (Buenos Aires: Planeta, 1997).

6. Other historians and geographers in Argentina have offered detailed yet partial accounts of the country's history of malaria control. See Susana Isabel Curto de Casas, "Geografía de los complejos patógenos en el territorio argentino" (doctoral thesis, Universidad de Buenos Aires, 1983); Eduardo H. Martine and Raul A. Jorge, "Se acabó el chucho. Carlos Alberto Alvarado y la lucha contra anófeles," *Todo es Historia* 17, no. 198 (1983): 70–88; Jobino Pedro Sierra Iglesias, *Carlos Alberto Alvarado: Vida y obra* (Salta: Comisión Bicameral Examinadora de Obras de Autores Salteños, 1993); Alfredo G. Kohn Loncarica, Abel L. Agüero, and Norma Isabel Sánchez, "Nacionalismo e internacionalismo en las ciencias de la salud: El caso de la lucha antipalúdica en la Argentina," *Asclepio* 49, no. 2 (1997): 147–63; Asociación de Profesionales de la Salud de Salta, Central de Trabajadores Argentinos, and Asociación Trabajadores del Estado, *El paludismo en la Argentina* (Salta: Editorial MILOR, 1999); Federico Pérgola, "Lepra, paludismo y otras endemias," *Todo es Historia,* no. 444 (2004): 48–58; Adriana Alvarez, "Malaria and the Emergence of Rural Health in Argentina: An Analysis from the Perspective of International Interaction and Co-operation," *Canadian Bulletin of the History of Medicine* 25, no. 1 (2008): 137–60.

7. In the last couple of decades, there has been an explosion of scholarship on the role of scientists, especially in the fields of medicine and public health, in constructing a modern Argentine identity, especially for the late nineteenth and early twentieth centuries. See, for example, Donna J. Guy, "Public Health, Gender, and Private Morality: Paid Labor and the Formation of the Body Politic in Buenos Aires," *Gender and History* 2 (1990): 298–317; Eduardo A. Zimmermann, "Racial Ideas and Social Reform: Argentina, 1890–1916," *Hispanic American Historical Review* 72, no. 1 (1992): 23–46; Zimmermann, *Los liberales reformistas: La cuestión social en la Argentina, 1890–1916* (Buenos Aires: Editorial Sudamericana Universidad de San Andrés, 1995); Diego Armus, "Salud y anarquismo. La tuberculosis en el discurso libertario argentino, 1890–1940," in *Política, médicos y enfermedades: Lecturas de historia de la salud argentina,* edited by Mirta Zaida Lobato (Buenos Aires: Biblos, 1996), 91–116; Vera Blinn Reber, "Blood, Coughs, and Fever: Tuberculosis and the Working Class of Buenos Aires, Argentina, 1885–1915," *Social History of Medicine* 12 (1999): 73–100; Gabriela Nouzeilles, *Ficciones somáticas: Naturalismo, nacionalismo y políticas médicas del cuerpo (Argentina, 1880–1910)* (Rosario: Beatriz Viterbo, 2000); Diego Armus, "El descubrimiento de la enfermedad como problema social," in *Nueva Historia Argentina, Tomo 5: El progreso, la modernización y sus límites (1880–1916),* edited by Mirta Zaida Lobato (Buenos Aires: Editorial Sudamericana, 2000), 507–52; Armus, "Tango, Gender, and Tuberculosis in Buenos Aires, 1900–1940," in *Disease in the History of Modern Latin America from Malaria to AIDS,* edited by Diego Armus (Durham: Duke University Press, 2003), 101–29; Julia Rodriguez, *Civilizing Argentina: Science, Medicine, and the Modern State* (Chapel Hill: University of North Carolina Press, 2006); Jens Andermann, *The Optic of the State: Visuality and Power in Argentina and Brazil* (Pittsburgh: University of Pittsburgh Press, 2007); Victoria Lynn Garrett, "Dispelling Purity Myths and Debunking Hygienic Discourse in Roberto Arlt's 'El jorobadito,'" *Hispania* 93, no. 2 (2010): 187–97. The relationship of this scholarship to my research is explored in more detail in chapters 1–3.

8. Nancy Leys Stepan, *"The Hour of Eugenics": Race, Gender, and Nation in Latin America* (Ithaca, NY: Cornell University Press, 1991); Marisa Miranda and Gustavo Vallejo, eds., *Darwinismo social y eugenesia en el mundo latino* (Buenos Aires: Siglo XXI de Argentina Editores, 2005).

9. The term "geographical imaginary" has been used by many geographers and other scholars. Doreen Massey, in one of her books on urban centers and economic globalization, defines the geographical imaginary as "an implicit geography that organises our social understandings." Doreen Massey, *World City* (Cambridge: Polity, 2007), 87. Matt Miller uses the geographical imaginary to capture the artistic amplification of regional identity in his study of rap music in the southern United States. See his "Dirty Decade: Rap Music and the U.S. South, 1997–2007," *Southern Spaces,* June 10, 2008, *http://www.southernspaces.org/contents/2008/miller/1a.htm.* Accessed July 1, 2009. In her exploration of the Indonesian transmigration program, Rebecca Elmhirst sees the geographical imaginary as the foundation for a bureaucratic structuring of space imposed by the Javanese majority in the national center over ethnic minorities in the periphery. Rebecca Elmhirst, "Space, Identity

Politics and Resource Control in Indonesia's Transmigration Programme," *Political Geography* 18, no. 7 (1999): 813–35. The concept of the geographical imaginary borrows heavily from the ideas of Edward Said and Benedict Anderson; see Derek Gregory, "Edward Said's Imaginative Geographies," in *Thinking Space,* edited by Mike Crang and Nigel Thrift (London: Routledge, 2000), 302–3. These are not the only uses of the geographical imaginary, to be sure. To clarify, a geographical imaginary is not the product of pure imagination or synonymous with worlds constructed in fictional works (e.g., C. S. Lewis's Narnia or J. R. R. Tolkien's Middle-Earth); it refers to places or regions that exist in a realist epistemology.

10. Richard Peet and Michael Watts, "Liberation Ecology: Development, Sustainability, and Environment in an Age of Market Triumphalism," in *Liberation Ecologies: Environment, Development, Social Movements,* edited by Richard Peet and Michael Watts (London: Routledge, 1996), 15–16. Peet and Watts also use the term "environmental imaginary," quite similar in meaning to what I call the "geographical imaginary," to emphasize the almost "primordial role" of "the discourse on nature" in constructing regional discursive formations. This is particularly the case in critical environmental histories of African drylands, which form an important school of thought in contemporary political ecology. See Emery Roe, "Development Narratives, or Making the Best of Blueprint Development," *World Development* 19 (1991): 287–300; Jeremy Swift, "Desertification: Narratives, Winners, and Losers," in *The Lie of the Land,* edited by M. Leach and R. Mearns (London: International African Institute, 1996), 73–90; James Fairhead and Melissa Leach, *Misreading the African Landscape : Society and Ecology in a Forest-Savanna Mosaic* (Cambridge: Cambridge University Press, 1996); Jesse Ribot, "A History of Fear: Imagining Deforestation in the West African Dryland Forests," *Global Ecology and Biogeography* 8 (1999): 291–300; Diana K. Davis, "Indigenous Knowledge and the Desertification Debate: Problematising Expert Knowledge in North Africa," *Geoforum* 36, no. 4 (2005): 509–24; Peter A. Walker, "Political Ecology: Where Is the Policy?," *Progress in Human Geography* 30, no. 3 (2006): 384–85; Diana K. Davis, *Resurrecting the Granary of Rome: Environmental History and French Colonial Expansion in North Africa* (Athens: Ohio University Press, 2007); William G. Moseley and Paul Laris, "West African Environmental Narratives and Development-Volunteer Praxis," *Geographical Review* 98, no. 1 (2008): 59–81. Taken together, this scholarship suggests that dominant narratives frame or delimit scientific and bureaucratic perspectives, setting the rules for what is permissible in the discourse on a development problem. Specifically, dominant narratives explain the environmental problems of Africa broadly as a consequence of irrational resource use and overpopulation, which in turn legitimates colonial and neocolonial governance of natural resources. My perspective on the power of narrative to frame social and environmental problems is also inspired by the work of historian William Cronon. As he has suggested, narratives have the power to naturalize that which is actually socially constructed, for example, Western perspectives on nature. See, especially, William Cronon, "A Place for Stories: Nature, History, and Narrative," *Journal of American History* 78, no. 4 (1992); Cronon, "The Trouble with Wilderness; or, Getting Back to the

Wrong Nature," in *Uncommon Ground: Toward Reinventing Nature,* edited by William Cronon (New York: W. W. Norton & Co., 1995).

11. On how space becomes pathologized, and its consequences, see Susan Craddock, *City of Plagues: Disease, Poverty, and Deviance in San Francisco* (Minneapolis: University of Minnesota, 2000), 10–12.

12. Ibid.

13. J. Ettling, *The Germ of Laziness: Rockefeller Philanthropy and Public Health in the New South* (Cambridge: Harvard, 1981); Margaret Humphreys, *Malaria: Poverty, Race, and Public Health in the United States* (Baltimore: Johns Hopkins, 2001); J. O. Breeden, "Disease as a Factor in Southern Distinctiveness," in *Disease and Distinctiveness in the American South,* edited by Todd L. Savitt and James Harvey Young (Knoxville: University of Tennessee Press, 1988).

14. Charles L. Briggs and Clara Mantini-Briggs, *Stories in the Time of Cholera: Racial Profiling during a Medical Nightmare* (Berkeley: University of California Press, 2003). The same cholera pandemic produced a similar racialized and spatialized scapegoating in Peru; see Marcos Cueto, *El regreso de las epidemias. Salud y sociedad en el Perú del siglo XX* (Lima: Instituto de Estudios Peruanos, 2000), chapter 5.

15. Susan Craddock, "Beyond Epidemiology: Locating AIDS in Africa," in *HIV and AIDS in Africa: Beyond Epidemiology,* edited by Ezekiel Kalipeni et al. (Malden, MA: Blackwell Publishing, 2004), 1–10.

16. James C. Scott, *Seeing like a State: How Certain Schemes to Improve the Human Condition Have Failed* (New Haven: Yale University Press, 1998). Along similar lines, see Raymond B. Craib, *Cartographic Mexico : A History of State Fixations and Fugitive Landscapes* (Durham: Duke University Press, 2004); Timothy Mitchell, *Rule of Experts: Egypt, Techno-Politics, Modernity* (Berkeley: University of California Press, 2002). See also, Eric D. Carter, "State Visions, Landscape, and Disease: Discovering Malaria in Argentina, 1890–1920," *Geoforum* 39, no. 1 (2008): 278–93.

17. Craddock, *City of Plagues,* 8–9.

18. James Ferguson, *The Anti-politics Machine: "Development," Depoliticization, and Bureaucratic Power in Lesotho* (Cambridge: Cambridge University Press, 1990); Craddock, *City of Plagues,* 4, 12–13; Rodriguez, *Civilizing Argentina,* 29–50.

19. M. S. Meade and R. J. Earickson, *Medical Geography.* 2nd ed. (New York: Guilford Press, 2000), 26–33.

20. For a good discussion of this scholarly trend, see Diego Armus, "Disease in the Historiography of Modern Latin America," in *Disease in the History of Modern Latin America from Malaria to AIDS,* edited by Diego Armus (Durham: Duke University Press, 2003), 3–6.

21. These recent historical studies of malaria control programs of the early twentieth century have been particularly influential to the argument of this book: Cueto, *El regreso de las epidemias,* chapter 4; Humphreys, *Malaria;* Nancy Leys Stepan, "The Only Serious Terror in These Regions: Malaria Control in the Brazilian Amazon," in *Disease in the History of Modern Latin America: From Malaria to AIDS,* edited by Diego Armus (Durham: Duke University Press, 2003); Warwick Anderson, *Colonial Pathologies: American Tropical Medicine, Race, and Hygiene in the Philippines* (Dur-

ham: Duke University Press, 2006); Frank M. Snowden, *The Conquest of Malaria: Italy, 1900–1962* (New Haven: Yale University Press, 2006); Linda L. Nash, *Inescapable Ecologies: A History of Environment, Disease, and Knowledge* (Berkeley: University of California Press, 2006); Federico Caprotti, "Malaria and Technological Networks: Medical Geography in the Pontine Marshes, Italy, in the 1930s," *Geographical Journal* 172, no. 2 (2006): 145–55; Marcos Cueto, *Cold War, Deadly Fevers: Malaria Eradication in Mexico, 1955–1975* (Baltimore: Johns Hopkins University Press, 2007); Randall M. Packard, *The Making of a Tropical Disease : A Short History of Malaria* (Baltimore: Johns Hopkins University Press, 2007); Sandra M. Sufian, *Healing the Land and the Nation: Malaria and the Zionist Project in Palestine, 1920–1947* (Chicago: University of Chicago Press, 2007).

22. Humphreys, *Malaria,* 55.

23. Craddock, *City of Plagues,* 14.

24. Briggs and Mantini-Briggs, *Stories in the Time of Cholera,* 283.

25. See, for example, Packard's and Cueto's studies of malaria control in different national contexts of the twentieth century (note 21 above).

26. Briggs and Mantini-Briggs, *Stories in the Time of Cholera.*

27. On the notion of "relational" identities, see Peter Wade, *Race and Ethnicity in Latin America* (Chicago: Pluto Press, 1997), 14.

28. This dual outlook of national elites was widespread in Latin America at the time. See Nancy P. Appelbaum, Anne S. Macpherson, and Karin Alejandra Rosemblatt, eds., *Race and Nation in Modern Latin America* (Chapel Hill: University of North Carolina Press, 2003); Virginia Q. Tilley, *Seeing Indians: A Study of Race, Nation, and Power in El Salvador* (Albuquerque: University of New Mexico Press, 2005), 189–217.

29. Larry Sawers, *The Other Argentina: The Interior and National Development* (Boulder, CO: Westview Press, 1996). Julia Rodriguez suggests that elites' search for the "internal other" was an important part of the nation-making process in Argentina, but that the figure of the other changed over time; the European immigrant, especially, played this role of foil to national identity. Though she does not mention the Northwest, or really any of Argentina's regions outside of Buenos Aires, I will argue that the creole (*criollo*) of the Northwest also played this "othering" role in a general way, but also in ways specific to malaria control. This line of argument is developed in more detail in chapter 3. See Rodriguez, *Civilizing Argentina,* 6. On the regionalization of a nation's internal other, see David R. Jansson, "Internal Orientalism in America: W. J. Cash's *The Mind of the South* and the Spatial Construction of American National Identity," *Political Geography* 22, no. 3 (2003): 293–316.

30. According to geographer Silvina Quintero, the official category of "North" to describe a sub-national region originated with the first national census in 1869; then, the region included Tucumán, Salta, and Jujuy. In Alejandro Bunge's important 1922 treatise on regional political economy, *Las industrias del Norte,* which presaged state-sponsored industrialization and regional development programs, the region of the "North" corresponded roughly to what is called the Northwest today; what were then the territories of Formosa, Chaco, and Misiones and the prov-

ince of Corrientes, though clearly located in the north, were considered a separate and less coherent region. In 1944, the socialist national senator Alfredo Palacios also used the term "Noroeste Argentino" in the subtitle of his book *Pueblos desamparados* (Abandoned peoples). Silvina Quintero, "La interpretación del territorio argentino en los primeros censos nacionales de población (1869, 1895, 1914)," in *El mosaico argentino: Modelos y representaciones del espacio y de la población, siglos XIX–XX,* edited by Hernán Otero (Buenos Aires: Siglo Veintiuno de Argentina Editores, 2004), 279; Gregorio Caro Figueroa and Eduardo M. Ashur, *El NOA como región* (Salta: Centro Unico de Estudiantes de Humanidades, 1974), 2–3; Palacios, *Pueblos desamparados.*

31. Marcelo Lagos, *La cuestión indígena en el Estado y en la sociedad nacional. Gran Chaco, 1870–1920* (Jujuy: Unidad de Investigación en Historia Regional, Fac. de Humanidades y Ciencias Sociales, U. Nac. de Jujuy, 2000); Gastón Gordillo, *Landscapes of Devils: Tensions of Place and Memory in the Argentinean Chaco* (Durham: Duke University Press, 2004).

32. A. R. Bianchi and C. E. Yañez, *Las precipitaciones en el Noroeste Argentino,* 2nd ed. (Salta: Instituto Nacional de Tecnología Agropecuaria and Estación Experimental Agropecuaria Salta, 1992), 288. These figures are for 1884 through 1990 and constitute probably the longest reliable climate record for any locale in the Northwest.

33. Alejandro Diego Brown and Héctor Ricardo Grau, *La naturaleza y el hombre en las selvas de montaña,* Colección Nuestros Ecosistemas (Salta: Proyecto GTZ, 1993).

34. Carlos E. Reboratti, *La Quebrada : Geografía, historia y ecología de la Quebrada de Humahuaca* (Buenos Aires, Argentina: Editorial La Colmena, 2003).

35. Simon Romero, "In Bolivia, Untapped Bounty Meets Nationalism," *New York Times,* February 2, 2009.

36. Patricia Isabel Juarez-Dappe, *When Sugar Ruled: Economy and Society in Northwestern Argentina, Tucumán, 1876–1916* (Athens: Ohio University Press, 2010), 9–11.

37. Carlos E. Reboratti, *El alto Bermejo: Realidades y conflictos* (Buenos Aires: La Colmena, 1998), 178–79; Laurie Occhipinti, "Being Kolla: Indigenous Identity in Northwestern Argentina," *Canadian Journal of Latin American and Caribbean Studies* 27, no. 54 (2002): 319–45.

38. Harry Alverson Franck, *Working North from Patagonia; Being the Narrative of a Journey, Earned on the Way, through Southern and Eastern South America* (New York: Century Co., 1921), 58.

39. Daniel W. Gade, "Andean Definitions and the Meaning of *lo Andino,*" in *Nature and Culture in the Andes* (Madison: University of Wisconsin Press, 1999), 31–41; Scott Whiteford, *Workers from the North: Plantations, Bolivian Labor, and the City in Northwest Argentina* (Austin: University of Texas Press, 1981).

40. Ariel De la Fuente, *Children of Facundo: Caudillo and Gaucho Insurgency during the Argentine State-Formation Process (La Rioja, 1853–1870)* (Durham: Duke University Press, 2000).

41. David Rock, *Argentina, 1516–1987: From Spanish Colonization to Alfonsín* (Berkeley: University of California Press, 1987), 119.

42. Juarez-Dappe, *When Sugar Ruled,* 16.

43. Ibid., 28.

44. Daniel Campi, "Economía y sociedad en las provincias del Norte," in *Nueva Historia Argentina, Tomo 5: El progreso, la modernización y sus límites (1880–1916),* edited by Mirta Zaida Lobato (Buenos Aires: Editorial Sudamericana, 2000), 87–89.

45. Ibid.; Daniel Campi and Marcelo Lagos, "Auge azucarero y mercado de trabajo en el Noroeste Argentino, 1850–1930," *ANDES: Antropología e historia* 6 (1994); Juarez-Dappe, *When Sugar Ruled;* Donna J. Guy, *Argentine Sugar Politics: Tucumán and the Generation of Eighty* (Tempe, AZ: Center for Latin American Studies, Arizona State University, 1980); John A. Kirchner, *Sugar and Seasonal Labor Migration: The Case of Tucumán, Argentina* (Chicago: Department of Geography, University of Chicago, 1980).

46. In Argentina, there is a distinct epidemiological zone of malaria in the north-central and northeastern provinces that border Paraguay and Brazil. In this zone, malaria has generally occurred in the form of sporadic epidemics, but even during outbreaks the number of cases is relatively low—a few hundred in a year—and rarely fatal. There, malaria is carried almost exclusively by *Anopheles darlingi,* the predominant tropical lowland vector of South America. J.F.R. Bejarano, "Areas palúdicas de la República Argentina," in *Primeras Jornadas Entomoepidemiológicas Argentinas* (Buenos Aires: n.p., 1959), 275–304; Juan J. Burgos et al., "Malaria and Global Climate Change in Argentina," *Entomologia y Vectores* 1, no. 4 (1994): 123–35; Curto de Casas, "Geografía de los complejos patógenos"; Stepan, "The Only Serious Terror."

47. S. Manguin et al., "Characterization of *Anopheles pseudopunctipennis* larval habitats," *J Am Mosq Control Assoc* 12, no. 4 (1996): 619–26; Bejarano, "Areas palúdicas de la República Argentina," 284; Daniel W. Gade, "Malaria and Settlement Retrogression in Mizque," in *Nature and Culture in the Andes* (Madison: University of Wisconsin Press, 1999), 75–101; Maria Julia Dantur Juri et al., "Malaria Transmission in Two Localities in North-Western Argentina," *Malaria Journal* 8, no. 1 (2009). In the 1920s, *Anopheles pseudopunctipennis* was responsible for transmitting malaria at 3,400 meters above sea level, in the town of La Quiaca on the Argentine-Bolivian border, but in this case the mosquitoes did not develop there naturally, but rather arrived by train. See S. Mazza and F. Calera Vital, "Consideraciones sobre un caso autóctono de paludismo a 3442 metros de altura," in *Quinta reunión de la Sociedad Argentina de patología regional del norte : Jujuy del 7 al 10 de octubre de 1929* (Buenos Aires: Imprenta La Universidad, 1929), 718–23.

48. My understanding of the Northwest's environmental history and disease ecology was enhanced substantially by field observations and interviews that I conducted in northern Salta Province in November 2002 and March 2003, which is discussed in some detail in the book's epilogue.

CHAPTER 1

1. The historiography of Argentina—whether written by Argentines or by foreigners—has scarcely treated the issue of regional disparities. There is a consid-

erable and well-known bias toward Buenos Aires and the littoral region. For book-length, English-language, scholarly treatments of the Argentine interior, see James R. Scobie and Samuel L. Baily, *Secondary Cities of Argentina: The Social History of Corrientes, Salta, and Mendoza, 1850–1910* (Stanford: Stanford University Press, 1988); Guy, *Argentine Sugar Politics;* James P. Brennan and Ofelia Pianetto, *Region and Nation: Politics, Economics, and Society in Twentieth-Century Argentina,* 1st ed. (New York: St. Martin's Press, 2000); Gordillo, *Landscapes of Devils;* Juarez-Dappe, *When Sugar Ruled.* This is not a comprehensive bibliography of Argentine regional history, by any means, but I have highlighted works that are most influential to this study.

2. James R. Scobie, *Argentina: A City and a Nation* (New York: Oxford University Press, 1964).

3. Rock, *Argentina, 1516–1987,* 118.

4. Alejandro E. Bunge, *Las industrias del Norte. Contribución al estudio de una nueva política económica argentina* (Buenos Aires: n.p., 1922).

5. The idea that "malaria blocks development" also prevailed in other parts of the world around the same time. See, for example, Humphreys, *Malaria;* Randall Packard, "'Malaria Blocks Development' Revisited: The Role of Disease in the History of Agricultural Development in the Eastern and Northern Transvaal Low-veld, 1890–1960," *Journal of Southern African Studies* 27, no. 3 (2001); Packard, *The Making of a Tropical Disease.*

6. David William Foster, *The Argentine Generation of 1880: Ideology and Cultural Texts* (Columbia: University of Missouri Press, 1990); Rodriguez, *Civilizing Argentina,* 25–33.

7. Armus, "El descubrimiento de la enfermedad," 514, 546; Zimmermann, "Racial Ideas and Social Reform," 23–46.

8. Armus, "El descubrimiento de la enfermedad," 546.

9. See, for example, Norma Isabel Sánchez, *La higiene y los higienistas en la Argentina (1880–1943)* (Buenos Aires: Sociedad Científica Argentina, 2007).

10. See introduction, note 7.

11. Nicolas Shumway, *The Invention of Argentina* (Berkeley: University of California Press, 1991).

12. Rodriguez, *Civilizing Argentina,* 32.

13. Oscar Chamosa defines *criollo* as "a flexible ethnic term that Argentines used to describe both the descendents of colonial Spanish settlers, and people of mixed indigenous and European background, or mestizos." In the colonial period, "criollo" had a very specific meaning, those of pure Spanish blood not born in Spain; as Benedict Anderson has famously argued, these "creole pioneers" initiated Spanish American independence movements since the structure of colonial government prevented the ascendancy of creoles to positions of authority, despite their economic power. However, in the mid-1800s, Alberdi and Sarmiento used criollo more pejoratively, as a marker of the defects of Hispanic culture. Lowly gauchos were criollos, but then again, so were caudillos such as Juan Manuel de Rosas. In the Northwest, criollos were a type that could be understood for what they were

not: they were not *indígenas* or *Indios,* particularly not the newly subjugated tribes of the Chaco, nor were they new European immigrants. Even the later generation of immigrants from Spain, prominent in the late 1800s, were not criollo. Among the working classes, criollos occupied a similar in-between position. For example, according to Gastón Gordillo, at San Martin de Tabacal, a sugar plantation in Salta Province, criollos occupied the best positions among workers, above indigenous people, but still below the managers and owners. Some early twentieth-century commentators under the influence of eugenics, such as Roberto Levillier, tried to define criollos as a racial type. By the 1930s and 1940s, as later chapters discuss, the status of the criollo was widely reappraised and elevated by the ideology of conservative nationalism, which reacted against the excessive influence of recent European immigration on the elusive "Argentine character." Criollo has another, usually positive connotation to describe traditional and authentic aspects of Argentine culture, as in the phrase *"es bien criollo."* Oscar Chamosa, "Indigenous or Criollo: The Myth of White Argentina in Tucumán's Calchaquí Valley," *Hispanic American Historical Review* 88, no. 1 (2008): 71; Gordillo, *Landscapes of Devils,* 113; Roberto Levillier, *Orígenes argentinos: La formación de un gran pueblo* (Paris, Buenos Aires: E. Fasquelle, 1912), 314–16. See also Adolfo Prieto, *El discurso criollista en la formación de la Argentina moderna* (Buenos Aires: Siglo Veintiuno, 2006).

14. Domingo Faustino Sarmiento, *Civilización y barbarie: Vida de Juan Facundo Quiroga* (1845; repr., Mexico City: Editorial Porrúa, 1977), 159; cited in Shumway, *The Invention of Argentina,* 146.

15. Juan B. Alberdi, *Bases y puntos de partida para la organización política de la República Argentina* (1852; repr., Buenos Aires: Editorial Sudamericana, 1969), 250; quoted in Shumway, *The Invention of Argentina,* 147.

16. Carl E. Solberg, *Immigration and Nationalism, Argentina and Chile, 1890–1914* (Austin: University of Texas Press, 1970).

17. Gabriel Carrasco, in Argentina Comisión Directiva del Censo, *Segundo censo de la República Argentina, levantado el 10 de mayo de 1895,* 3 vols. (Buenos Aires: Taller Tipográfico de la Penitenciaría Nacional, 1898), 2: xlv, xlviii. Cited in Zimmermann, "Racial Ideas and Social Reform," 30. (Carrasco wrote the introduction to the census.)

18. Thomas E. Skidmore and Peter H. Smith, *Modern Latin America,* 5th ed. (New York: Oxford University Press, 2001), 71.

19. Armus, "El descubrimiento de la enfermedad," 507–52; Rodriguez, *Civilizing Argentina.*

20. Rodriguez, *Civilizing Argentina,* 32.

21. José Luis Romero, *Las ideas políticas en Argentina* (1956; repr., Buenos Aires: Fondo de Cultura Económica, 2001), 193.

22. Rodriguez, *Civilizing Argentina,* 33.

23. Abel L. Agüero, "Prólogo," in Sánchez, *La higiene y los higienistas,* 24.

24. Andermann, *Optic of the State;* Hernán Otero, "La transición demográfica argentina a debate. Una perspectiva espacial de las explicaciones ideacionales, económicas y político-institucionales," in *El mosaico argentino: Modelos y representa-*

ciones del espacio y de la población, siglos XIX–XX, edited by Hernán Otero (Buenos Aires: Siglo Veintiuno de Argentina Editores, 2004); Otero, *Estadística y nación: Una historia conceptual del pensamiento censal de la Argentina moderna, 1869–1914* (Buenos Aires: Prometeo Libros, 2006); Quintero, "La interpretación del territorio argentino en los primeros censos nacionales de población (1869, 1895, 1914)."

25. Stepan, *Hour of Eugenics.*

26. Zimmermann, "Racial Ideas and Social Reform."

27. Ibid., 39–41.

28. Stepan, *Hour of Eugenics,* 85–86; Rodriguez, *Civilizing Argentina,* 185.

29. Rodriguez, *Civilizing Argentina,* 40–41.

30. Ibid., 41.

31. Emilio Quevedo and Francisco Gutiérrez, "Scientific Medicine and Public Health in Nineteenth-Century Latin America," in *Science in Latin America: A History,* edited by Juan José Saldaña (Austin: University of Texas Press, 2006), 165–85; Marcos Cueto, *The Value of Health: A History of the Pan American Health Organization* (Rochester, NY: University of Rochester Press, 2007).

32. Armus, "El descubrimiento de la enfermedad," 509; Miguel Angel Scenna, *Cuando murió Buenos Aires, 1871* (Buenos Aires: Ediciones La Bastilla, 1974).

33. Armus, "El descubrimiento de la enfermedad," 519–20.

34. Sánchez, *La higiene y los higienistas,* 92–108. A separate but closely allied federal agency took charge of public sanitation works. Buenos Aires, of course, was the first city in Argentina to develop potable water and sewage systems, as early as 1870, and by 1906 about 90 percent of the city had access to potable water, while only about 26 percent had access to the sanitary sewer system. Armus, "El descubrimiento de la enfermedad," 524.

35. Armus, "El descubrimiento de la enfermedad," 534.

36. Karina Inés Ramacciotti, *La política sanitaria del peronismo* (Buenos Aires: Editorial Biblos, 2009), 23–38.

37. I adapt the term "Gospel of Hygiene" from Nancy Tomes; it evokes the practically religious fervor of both Argentine and North American hygienists of that era. Nancy Tomes, *The Gospel of Germs: Men, Women, and the Microbe in American Life* (Cambridge: Harvard University Press, 1998).

38. Eliseo Cantón, *El paludismo y su geografía médica en la República Argentina* (Buenos Aires: Imp. La Universidad, 1891), vi; José Penna and Antonio Barbieri, *El paludismo y su profilaxis en la Argentina* (Buenos Aires: D.N.H., 1916), 18; Gade, "Malaria and Settlement Retrogression in Mizque," 86; James L. A. Webb, *Humanity's Burden: A Global History of Malaria* (Cambridge: Cambridge University Press, 2009), 66–67.

39. Academia Argentina de Letras, *Diccionario del habla de los argentinos,* 1st ed. (Buenos Aires: Espasa Calpe, 2003).

40. Gregg Mitman and Ronald L. Numbers, "From Miasma to Asthma: The Changing Fortunes of Medical Geography in America," *History and Philosophy of the Life Sciences* 25 (2003): 391–92; Nash, *Inescapable Ecologies,* 52.

41. Here, Argentina's malaria control campaign may be an exception to Diego

Armus's general assertion that in Latin America, "miasmatic and environmentalist approaches dominated medical perceptions of health and disease without producing major changes in the sanitary infrastructure or overall mortality. Toward the end of the century, modern bacteriology took center stage and profoundly shaped the dynamics of many public health undertakings." For malaria control, bacteriological frameworks did not simply replace the older approaches, but rather they coexisted, at least for a time. However, it is fair to say that the confirmation of the parasite-mosquito etiology of malaria spurred hygienists such as Carlos Malbrán to action since it allowed them to fit malaria within their preferred bacteriological model. See Armus, "Disease in the Historiography," 9.

42. Frank A. Barrett, *Disease and Geography: The History of an Idea* (Toronto: Atkinson College Dept. of Geography, 2000); Conevery Bolton Valencius, "Histories of Medical Geography," in *Medical Geography in Historical Perspective (Medical History, Supplement No. 20),* edited by Nicolaas A. Rupke (London: Wellcome Trust Centre for the History of Medicine, 2000), 3–28; Valencius, *The Health of the Country: How American Settlers Understood Themselves and Their Land* (New York: Basic Books, 2002); Wendy Jepson, "Of Soil, Situation, and Salubrity: Medical Topography and Medical Officers in Early Nineteenth-Century British India," *Historical Geography* 32 (2004); Nash, *Inescapable Ecologies,* 67.

43. Luis Urteaga, "Miseria, miasmas y microbios. Las topografías médicas y el estudio del medio ambiente en el siglo XIX," *GeoCrítica, Cuadernos Críticos de Geografía Humana (Barcelona)* 29 (September 1980): 11.

44. Ibid., 12; Steven Johnson, *The Ghost Map: The Story of London's Most Terrifying Epidemic* (New York: Riverhead Books, 2006).

45. The *Oxford English Dictionary* (Short Version, 1933) gives this as the first definition of "malaria": "The unwholesome atmosphere which results from the exhalations of marshy districts."

46. United States Sanitary Commission, *Report of a Committee of the Associate Medical Members of the United States Sanitary Commission on the Subject of the Nature and Treatment of Miasmatic Fevers* (Washington, DC: United States Sanitary Commission, 1863), 5–6. Cited in Kenneth Thompson, "Insalubrious California: Perception and Reality," *Annals of the Association of American Geographers* 59, no. 1 (1969): 55.

47. M. S. Meade, "The Rise and Demise of Malaria: Some Reflections on Southern Settlement and Landscape," *Southeastern Geographer* 20 (1980): 77–99; Humphreys, *Malaria.*

48. Penna and Barbieri, *El paludismo y su profilaxis en la Argentina,* 9.

49. Cantón figured in a tightly knit network of Tucumán elites, many of whom could be considered part of the national "Generation of 1880" and the province's progressive "Generation of the Centennial" (see chapter 3). Julio Argentino Roca (1843–1914) was born in Tucumán, twice served as president of Argentina, and controlled the provincial and national political oligarchy from the 1880s to his death. The major political figure of his era, he was also a close friend of Cantón. Cantón, Alberto L. de Soldati, Tiburcio Padilla Jr., and Gregorio Aráoz Alfaro all

matriculated from the Colegio Nacional between 1876 and 1885, and all went on to receive their medical degrees at the University of Buenos Aires, which, per Julia Rodriguez, was the major node of the national network of scientist-bureaucrats. Cantón, de Soldati, and Tiburcio Padilla Sr. led the campaign against cholera in Tucumán from 1886 to 1887. As a national congressman, de Soldati sponsored bills that created the Malaria Service and Parque 9 de Julio on reclaimed marshes in Tucumán. The Padillas were important members of the sugar elite and well connected, via Roca, to the national oligarchy. Tiburcio Sr. served at different times as Tucumán's governor and representative in the national senate; Tiburcio III (Tiburcio Jr.'s son) also became a politician and served as secretary general of the DNH from 1931 through 1932; a cousin, Ernesto Padilla, also served as governor of Tucumán. Ernesto Padilla also figured prominently in the movement to revive regional folklore and between 1920 and 1940 "led a powerful clan of sugar industrialists and conservative politicians from the northwest, which had direct control over the Ministry of Education, the National Board of Education, and the University of Tucumán." Aráoz Alfaro served three times as the president of the DNH, founded the Argentine eugenics society, and was a protagonist in the malaria campaign from the 1910s to the 1930s. Luis F. Nougués (Colegio Nacional class of 1888) was the scion of a leading sugar family (the owners of Ingenio San Pablo) and, as governor from 1906 to 1909, lobbied for the establishment of a national malaria service. Juan B. Terán (class of 1895), one of the leaders of the Tucumán's "Generation of the Centennial," founded the University of Tucumán (during the governorship of Ernesto Padilla) and was the first to reach out to the Rockefeller Foundation for their assistance in malaria control in the Northwest (see chapter 3). The botanical institute of the University of Tucumán bears the name of Miguel Lillo (class of 1881), the leading naturalist of his era in the Northwest. Prudencio Santillán Jr. (whose father was a classmate of Alberto L. de Soldati at the Colegio Nacional), graduated from the Colegio Nacional in 1911 and went on to be a leading official in the Malaria Service in the 1930s and 1940s. While it is difficult to discern the substance of the personal, professional, and political connections among these men, there is little doubt that this network of elites shaped the politics of malaria control, and public health more generally, in Tucumán, regionally, and nationally. However, the influence of this network probably waned substantially after the 1930s or so. Provincia de Tucumán, *Album general de la provincia de Tucumán el el primer centenario de la independencia argentina* (Buenos Aires: M. Rodríguez Giles, 1916); Carlos María Gelly y Obes, "La personalidad de Ernesto E. Padilla," in *Asociación Tucumana Ciclo Cultural Año 1956* (Buenos Aires: 1957); Vicente Osvaldo Cutolo, *Nuevo diccionario biográfico argentino (1750–1930)* (Buenos Aires: Editorial ELCHE, 1978); Osvaldo Loudet, "Tres sabios médicos tucumanos. Eliseo Cantón, Gregorio Aráoz Alfaro, Tiburcio Padilla," *La Semana Médica* 159, no. 9 (1981); Carlos Páez de la Torre, *Historia de Tucumán* (Buenos Aires: Plus Ultra, 1987); de la Torre, "Apenas ayer: Un gran médico. Hace cien años nació Tiburcio Padilla," *La Gaceta,* October 23, 1993; Chamosa, "Indigenous or Criollo," 100. See also "Personalidades del Olvido" series in *La Gaceta* (Tucumán), 1965–1969, Archives of *La Gaceta,* Tucumán.

50. Cantón served in the legislature of the province of Tucumán from 1890–1892, as representative of Tucumán in the national congress from 1894 to 1902, and as representative of the city of Buenos Aires in the national congress from 1904 to 1912. Sánchez, *La higiene y los higienistas,* 501–2. On the cohort of medical doctors with public policy influence in Tucumán, including Benjamín Aráoz, Ignacio Colombres, Alberto de Soldati, Tiburcio Padilla, Benigno Vallejo, and Eliseo Cantón, see María Estela Fernández, "Salud y condiciones de vida. Iniciativas estatales y privadas en Tucumán. Fines del siglo XIX y comienzos del XX," in *Historias de enfermedades, salud y medicina,* edited by Adriana Alvarez, Irene Molinari, and Daniel Reynoso (Mar del Plata: Universidad Nacional de Mar del Plata, 2004), 121.

51. Rodriguez, *Civilizing Argentina,* 5.

52. Urteaga, "Miseria, miasmas y microbios"; Jepson, "Of Soil, Situation, and Salubrity"; Paolo Mantegazza, *Cartas médicas sobre la América meridional. Traducción de la edición de Milan (1858–1860), por el Dr. Juan Heller. Prologo por el Dr. Gregorio Araoz Alfaro,* translated by Juan Heller (Buenos Aires: Coni, 1949); J. Amadeo Baldrich, *Las comarcas vírgenes. El Chaco Central norte,* 2nd ed. (Buenos Aires: Impr. de J. Peuser, 1890).

53. Armus, "El descubrimiento de la enfermedad," 513; Rodriguez, *Civilizing Argentina,* 183.

54. Cantón, *El paludismo y su geografía médica,* 74.

55. Ibid., 87.

56. Ibid., 60.

57. See explanation of malaria in the northeastern provinces and territories in the book's introduction (note 46).

58. Cantón, *El paludismo y su geografía médica,* 148.

59. Ibid.

60. Ibid., 149.

61. Eucalyptus trees were introduced to Tucumán in 1877, through a donation of seeds from the National Department of Agriculture. Even then, the provincial government underscored the malaria-fighting properties of the trees and distributed the seeds among one hundred property owners in the city and the country. They became commonplace throughout the province; many, such as those found in and around Monteros, or in the Parque 9 de Julio in Tucumán, were planted as part of sanitation efforts. Carlos Páez de la Torre, "Apenas ayer: Eucalyptus vs. paludismo. En 1877, el gobierno propició la plantación de esos árboles," *La Gaceta,* April 18, 1995. In contemporary California, the planting of eucalyptus was also widely promoted, for similar reasons. Nash, *Inescapable Ecologies,* 72. Indeed, the trees are known to have some of the properties nineteenth-century physicians, foresters, and boosters ascribed to them: they dry out the soil, inhibit the growth of other vegetation, and, in a way, fight disease. An extract of the eucalyptus tree, eucalyptol, is a common ingredient in insect repellents.

62. Cantón, *El paludismo y su geografía médica,* 194.

63. Eliseo Cantón, "Discurso en su recepción académica. Paludismo," *Anales de la Universidad de Buenos Aires* 15 (1899): 157.

64. Cantón, "Profilaxia del paludismo y provisión de aguas corrientes a varias provincias argentinas," *Anales del Círculo Médico Argentino* 16 (1893): 368.

65. Cantón, *El paludismo y su geografía médica,* 282.

66. Ibid., 283; Cantón, "Discurso en su recepción académica. Paludismo," 155.

67. Stepan, *Hour of Eugenics,* 60; Zimmermann, "Racial Ideas and Social Reform"; Zimmermann, *Los liberales reformistas.*

68. Juarez-Dappe, *When Sugar Ruled,* 95, 111.

69. Cantón, *El paludismo y su geografía médica,* 171.

70. Ibid., 283.

71. Jorge Balán, "El origen de la cuestión regional: Las alianzas con las oligarquías provinciales, requisito para el fortalecimiento del Estado nacional," in *El desarrollo rural en el noroeste argentino. Antología,* edited by Mabel Manzanal (Salta: Proyecto Desarrollo Agroforestal en Comunidades Rurales del Noroeste Argentino, 1996); Osvaldo Barsky and Jorge Gelman, *Historia del agro argentino, desde la conquista hasta fines del siglo XX* (Buenos Aires: Mondadori, 2001), 204–15.

72. Guy, *Argentine Sugar Politics.*

73. Campi, "Economía y sociedad en las provincias del Norte," 85.

74. Juarez-Dappe, *When Sugar Ruled,* 98.

75. Páez de la Torre, *Historia de Tucumán;* Carlos Wauters, "Zonas de regadío en Tucumán," *Anales de la S.C.A.* 63 (1907): 185–274.

76. Juarez-Dappe, *When Sugar Ruled,* 133–42.

77. Annual message of Governor Quinteros, September 1889, *Compilación ordenada de leyes, decretos y mensajes del periodo constitucional de la provincia de Tucumán* (hereafter cited as *CO-Tucumán*), 15:395. Quinteros had been installed in office through the heavy-handed intervention of Roca's ally Miguel Juárez Celman.

78. Quinteros, quoted in Ley No. 591, "Autorizando al P.E. para mandar practicar los estudios necesarios a objeto de establecer un sistema general de irrigación en la provincia," I. Mensaje del P.E. Tucumán, December 3, 1888, *CO-Tucumán,* 14:48–50.

79. For example, Ley No. 585, "Autorizando al P.E. para mandar practicar estudios de saneamiento de los terrenos que lo requieran," *CO-Tucumán,* 14 (1889–1890): 22–23; Ley No. 591 (note 78); Ley No. 942, "Sobre desecamiento y drenaje de terrenos insalubres o impropios para la industria," *CO-Tucumán,* 29 (1907): 585–91.

80. Argentina, Congreso, Cámara de Diputados, *Investigación parlamentaria sobre agricultura, ganadería, industrias derivadas y colonización; Ordenada por La H. Cámara de diputados en resolución de 19 de junio de 1896. Anexo G: Tucumán y Santiago del Estero* (Buenos Aires: Tip. de la Penitenciaría Nacional, 1898); Argentina, Comisión Nacional del Censo, *Tercer censo nacional, levantado el 1 de junio de 1914,* 10 vols. (Buenos Aires: Talleres gráficos de L. J. Rosso, 1916–1919), 1:202; Juarez-Dappe, *When Sugar Ruled,* 97–99. As in the rest of Argentina, most European immigrants to Tucumán (as enumerated in the 1914 census) were from Spain and Italy. There was

also a large contingent of different nationalities (e.g., Turkish, Syrian, Lebanese) classified as "Ottoman." Bolivians comprised only about 1 percent of the foreign-born population. Argentina, Comisión Nacional del Censo, *Tercer censo nacional,* 2:302–3.

81. Argentina, Congreso, Cámara de Diputados, *Investigación parlamentaria,* 159–60.

82. Cantón, "Profilaxia del paludismo y provisión de aguas corrientes a varias provincias argentinas," 367.

83. Ley No. 585, "Autorizando al P.E. para mandar practicar estudios de saneamiento de los terrenos que lo requieran," I. Mensaje del P.E. Tucumán, November 23, 1888, *CO-Tucumán,* 14:22–23.

84. Cantón, Address to National Congress, August 2, 1895, reprinted in *CO-Tucumán,* 19:190.

85. Ibid., 19:187.

86. Ibid.

87. Páez de la Torre, *Historia de Tucumán,* 587.

88. *El Orden* (Tucumán), January 22, 1907; Ley No. 912, *CO-Tucumán,* 29 (1907): 55–72; Antenor Alvarez, *Paludismo. Plan de defensa aprobado por el Congreso Médico para la ciudad y centros rurales de la provincia (Santiago del Estero)* (Buenos Aires: J. Peuser, 1902); D.N.H., *Saneamiento de la ciudad de Salta. Informe de la comisión especial (anexo a la memoria del Ministerio del Interior)* (Buenos Aires: La Semana Médica/Spinelli, 1901), 163–83; *Diario de Sesiones de la Cámara de Senadores de la Nación* (hereafter cited as *Diario-Senadores*), September 22, 1906, 1:770–73, 1692; Páez de la Torre, *Historia de Tucumán,* 590; Olga Paterlini de Koch, *Parque 9 de Julio* (Tucumán: Grafica Noroeste, 1992), 34; Jules Huret, *La Argentina de Buenos Aires al Gran Chaco,* translated by E. Gómez Carrillo (Paris: E. Fasquelle, 1913), 253–62.

89. Campi, "Economía y sociedad en las provincias del Norte," 197.

90. Jules Huret, visiting Tucumán in 1912, perceived locals' claims of being "on the same level as Europe" as an expression not so much of overweening pride as one of obsessive admiration and collective anxiety. In some quarters, Huret detected resentment of Buenos Aires: former governor Luis Nougués argued that shiftless Porteños had grown rich from speculation, collecting rents, and the work of immigrants, whereas Tucumán's wealth derived from the labor and industry of "native sons." Huret, *La Argentina,* 262, 73–74.

91. *El Orden* (Tucumán), October 28, 1907. This newspaper editorial supported and expanded on the proposal of Governor Luis Nougués for a law making mandatory the drainage of "unhealthy or waste lands." See also Ley No. 942 (note 79).

92. Rufino Cossio, *La campaña antipalúdica en Tucumán. D.N.H.* (Tucumán: La Gaceta, 1928), 44. By some accounts, this outside perception of the Northwest's unhealthfulness persisted for decades: a retired public health bureaucrat, recalling the view outsiders held of Tucumán in the 1950s, told me, "Tucumán was synonymous with malaria. People were afraid to come to Tucumán." Author's interview with Francisco Sotelo, August 22, 2002, Tucumán, Argentina.

93. Huret, *La Argentina,* 62.

94. D.N.H., *Saneamiento de la ciudad de Salta,* xv.

95. Ibid., 1–3.

96. The city suffered from epidemics of cholera in 1868 and 1886, bubonic plague in 1899 and 1900, measles in 1896, and small pox in 1901 and1902. See Scobie and Baily, *Secondary Cities of Argentina,* 99.

97. G. M. Wrigley, "Salta, an Early Commercial Center of Argentina," *Geographical Review* 2, no. 2 (1916): 117.

98. Scobie and Baily, *Secondary Cities of Argentina,* 99.

99. Wrigley, "Salta, an Early Commercial Center of Argentina," 117–19.

100. Cantón, *El paludismo y su geografía médica,* 26.

101. Ricardo Aráoz, *Introducción al estudio de la Higiene de Salta. Memoria presentada a la Junta de Sanidad por el Dr. Ricardo Aráoz con motivo de la posible invasión del cólera* (Salta: Emilio Sylvester, 1895).

102. Fabio Ovejero, "Consideraciones sobre el saneamiento de la ciudad de Salta" (doctoral thesis, Universidad Nacional de Buenos Aires, 1895), 17.

103. Wrigley, "Salta, an Early Commercial Center of Argentina," 119–20; Scobie and Baily, *Secondary Cities of Argentina.*

104. Aráoz, *Introducción al estudio.*

105. Cantón, *El paludismo y su geografía médica,* 27.

106. Aráoz, *Introducción al estudio,* 110.

107. D.N.H., *Saneamiento de la ciudad de Salta,* xiii.

108. Ovejero, "Consideraciones," 55–56.

109. Aráoz, *Introducción al estudio,* 91.

110. D.N.H., *Saneamiento de la ciudad de Salta,* 238.

111. *El Cívico* (Salta), August 21, 1900; *Tribuna Popular* (Salta), September 14, 1905; D.N.H., *Saneamiento de la ciudad de Salta,* 111, 41.

112. D.N.H., *Saneamiento de la ciudad de Salta,* 142. In 1899, Cantón cited a mortality rate for the city of Salta of 60 per 1,000. Cantón, "Discurso en su recepción académica. Paludismo," 155. The true figure is difficult to determine, but in official documents and public health reports Salta was consistently found to be among the cities with the highest mortality rate in Argentina during the late 1800s into the early 1900s.

113. D.N.H., *Saneamiento de la ciudad de Salta,* 104.

114. Ibid., 38.

115. Cecilio Morón, "Endemias y epidemias en la historia de Salta," in *Los primeros cuatro siglos de Salta, 1582–1982* (Salta: Universidad Nacional de Salta, 1982); D.N.H., *Saneamiento de la ciudad de Salta;* Scobie and Baily, *Secondary Cities of Argentina,* 99.

116. D.N.H., *Saneamiento de la ciudad de Salta.*

117. Aráoz, *Introducción al estudio,* 26, 90.

118. *El Cívico* (Salta), August 4, 1898. Today, of course, yerba maté is the national beverage of Argentina and often celebrated for its healthfulness.

119. On the supposed contrast between Salta's conservative culture and Tucumán's entrepreneurial liberalism, see Huret, *La Argentina,* 329.

120. *La Montaña* (Salta), December 6, 1904.

121. *Tribuna Popular* (Salta), November 19, 1905, February 17, 1907.

122. Ibid., March 31, 1907.

123. D.N.H., *Saneamiento de la ciudad de Salta,* 1.

124. Ley No. 3592, "Autorizando al P.E. a invertir hasta la cantidad de cien mil pesos moneda nacional en los estudios y trabajos más indispensables para el saneamiento de Salta," October 11, 1897, cited in "Saneamiento de la ciudad de Salta," *Anales del D.N.H.* 7 (1897): 517–18.

125. D.N.H., *Saneamiento de la ciudad de Salta.*

126. Ibid., 368–83.

127. Ibid., 104.

128. Ibid.

129. Ley No. 654, "Autorizando la expropiación de tierras y la adquisición de derechos de servidumbre para el saneamiento de la ciudad de Salta," June 19, 1903; Ley No. 659, "Declarando de utilidad pública y sujetos a expropiación," July 28, 1903, in *Recopilación general de leyes de la provincia de Salta,* vol. 7.

130. "Las obras de saneamiento," *Tribuna Popular* (Salta), September 27, 1905.

131. Huret, *La Argentina,* 331.

132. *El Orden* (Tucumán), December 21, 1908. Even as late as 1929, a Salta newspaper complained of "unbearable miasmas" arising from a mix of stagnant water, decomposing garbage, and fecal matter; yet, just days later, the same paper called for the elimination of mosquito-breeding areas in the city. *Nueva Epoca* (Salta), January 4, 1929, January 23, 1929, January 31, 1929.

CHAPTER 2

1. Antenor Alvarez, "La invasión del paludismo a la ciudad del Santiago del Estero y su saneamiento," in *Tercer Congreso Nacional de Medicina: Actas y Trabajos, Tomo I* (Buenos Aires: Las Ciencias, 1926), 685.

2. D.N.H., "El paludismo en la república. Conferencia Nacional de Médicos, Buenos Aires (Mayo 1902)," *Anales del D.N.H.* 9, no. 10 (1902): 467.

3. Alvarez, *Paludismo. Plan de defensa;* Alvarez, "La invasión del paludismo a la ciudad del Santiago del Estero y su saneamiento"; Juan Carlos Delfino, "Epidemiología del paludismo. Su estado en la República Argentina," *Anales del D.N.H.* 11 (1904). This epidemic was subject to sometimes hyperbolic assessments, with some sources even claiming 100 percent incidence in the city, which seems unlikely. See D.N.H., *Guía oficial* (Buenos Aires: D.N.H., 1913), 115.

4. Tom Koch, "The Map as Intent: Variations on the Theme of John Snow," *Cartographica* 39, no. 4 (2004); Johnson, *Ghost Map.*

5. Penna and Barbieri, *El paludismo y su profilaxis en la Argentina;* Nicolás Lozano and Domingo Selva, "Nueva orientación en la lucha antipalúdica," in *Quinto Congreso Nacional de Medicina: Actas y trabajos* (Rosario: Talleres Graficos Pomponio, 1934).

6. Alvarez, *Paludismo. Plan de defensa;* Alvarez, "La invasión del paludismo a la ciudad del Santiago del Estero y su saneamiento"; Alvarez, "El saneamiento antipalúdico de La Dársena," *Cátedra y Clínica* 7 (1940).

7. Packard, *The Making of a Tropical Disease.*

8. For example, *El Cívico* (Salta) reported anxiously on the spreading of the bubonic plague from Paraguay to Rosario to Buenos Aires (January 25, February 5, June 9, 1900); see also Scobie and Baily, *Secondary Cities of Argentina.*

9. Although the national government agency in charge of the malaria campaigns had many different names and administrative alignments over the years, I use the term "Malaria Service" for the sake of consistency. For much of this period, it was known officially as the Dirección General de Paludismo, but it was often simply referred to as "Campaña antipalúdica" or "Defensa antipalúdica."

10. Rodriguez, *Civilizing Argentina,* 40–41.

11. Carter, "State Visions."

12. D.N.H., *Precauciones contra el paludismo* (Buenos Aires: Taller Tipográfico de la Penitenciaría Nacional, 1900). The DNH pamphlet is basically a translation of recommendations for a malaria campaign based on control of the mosquito vector, published by the French National Academy of Medicine in the *Revue d'Hygiene* earlier the same year. While no historical works (that I know of) mention the *Revue d'Hygiene* as a vehicle for dissemination of the mosquito discovery, the hygienists of the DNH were loyal followers of the latest advances from the Parisian medical community.

13. Jaime Carrillo, "El paludismo en Jujuy," *Anales del D.N.H.* 9, no. 3 (1901); Ricardo Aráoz, "El paludismo en Salta," *Anales del D.N.H.* 9, no. 4 (1902); Eleodoro Gallastegui, "El paludismo en los departamentos de Tinogasta y Belén (Catamarca)," *Anales del D.N.H.* 9, no. 12 (1902); Eleodoro R. Giménez, "El paludismo en La Rioja," *Anales del D.N.H.* 9, no. 13 (1902); B. E. Vallejo, "El paludismo en Tucumán," *Anales del D.N.H.* 9, no. 4 (1902). José María Ramos Mejía, while also embracing the view of bacteriologists, strove to make medical geography central to organizing sanitary missions in the provinces and territories. D.N.H., *Guía oficial,* 100.

14. D.N.H., "El paludismo en la república," 449. According to Norma Isabel Sánchez, Malbrán's 1887 thesis on cholera is widely considered the first "complete" work of bacteriology in Argentina. Later, at the University of Buenos Aires, Malbrán led the Department of Bacteriology and directed the DNH bacteriological lab before becoming president of the department. The national bacteriological institute is named in his honor. Sánchez, *La higiene y los higienistas,* 503. Other representatives from the provinces to the commission included Antenor Alvarez, who was leading the campaign against malaria in Santiago del Estero; Ricardo Aráoz, a hygienist from Salta who had played an important role in that city's sanitary reforms; and Alberto de Soldati, a physician, Tucumán aristocrat, and close associate of Eliseo Cantón, who would be the major spokesman for the malaria bill in the national senate.

15. Saul Franco Agudelo, *El paludismo en América Latina* (Guadalajara: Editorial Universidad de Guadalajara, 1990), 87–102.

16. *El Orden,* a Tucumán newspaper, reported frequently on hygiene matters. Often, its editorials linked the malaria problem to the larger problems of wetland reclamation and irrigation improvements. See *El Orden,* October 28, 1907; October

26, 1907; November 19, 1907; November 29, 1907; July 30, 1908; July 31, 1908; August 1, 1908. The problem of high mortality, especially infant mortality, and the associated threat of depopulation also were focal points of discussion. *El Orden,* January 23, 1907; February 14, 1908; April 7, 1908. Reports in Salta newspapers were even more alarmist, and perhaps reasonably so, about the gradual depopulation of the region as a result of disease and unsanitary conditions. "A city that is depopulating" (Una ciudad que se despuebla), *El Cívico,* August 21, 1900; also August 22, 1900.

17. Carlos Malbrán, "El paludismo y su profilaxis. Fundamento la ley de paludismo sobre la transmisión por el Anopheles," *Anales del D.N.H.* 10, no. 10 (1903): 443.

18. In the mid-1800s, when Rawson supposedly made this observation, Palermo was outside of the built-up urban core; but by 1902 it had become the site of large parks and neighborhoods. See D.N.H., "El paludismo en la república," 453.

19. *Diario de Sesiones de la Cámara de Diputados de la Nación* (hereafter cited as *Diario-Diputados*), 1907, 1:1409–1413. The reasoning that malaria was a mobile threat, with potential to reach the littoral, was also applied later on; for example, see the speech by José W. Tobías at the National Sanitary Conference in 1923. José W. Tobías, "Contribución al estudio de la defensa contra el paludismo en la República Argentina," *La Semana Médica* 30 (1923): 406.

20. Malbrán, "El paludismo y su profilaxis," 443, emphasis added.

21. Letter from Soldati to Antonio F. Piñero, *El Diario* (December 1900). Reprinted in Alberto L. de Soldati, *Iniciativas, proyectos y discursos en el parlamento argentino* (Buenos Aires: n.p., 1913), 43.

22. *Diario-Senadores,* September 23, 1905, 1:980.

23. Ibid., September 23, 1905, 1:979. For Piñero, see *Diario-Diputados,* September 25, 1907, 1:1410. Little shame or stigma was attached to malaria sufferers. Indeed, newspaper writers, politicians, or hygienists rarely remarked on the individual sufferers of malaria; and if they did, the attitude toward them was usually one of pity. This somewhat neutral attitude toward malaria sufferers contrasts strongly with the contemporary moralizing tones of Argentina's hygienists toward carriers of tuberculosis. See Armus, "Salud y anarquismo"; Reber, "Blood, Coughs, and Fever."

24. Malbrán, "El paludismo y su profilaxis," 441–44.

25. Ibid., 441.

26. From the 1910s until the 1940s, there would be numerous proposals, originating from various political sectors, seeking to strengthen the power of the DNH or create more vigorous and effective institutions in its place. See Ramacciotti, *La política sanitaria del peronismo,* 21–41. Yet Law 5195 has not really been portrayed in Argentine historiography as a major step toward centralization. Law 5195 was only the second national law to address a specific disease, after the 1904 law on smallpox vaccination, and was the most comprehensive extension of national authority over public health to date, according to the D.N.H., *Guía oficial,* and Alberto Domínguez, *Policía sanitaria: Doctrina, legislación nacional y provincial* (Buenos Aires: Editorial Depalma, 1946). Many historians have ignored how early these centralizing proposals appeared. Julio A. Roca, who led the government during the debates over malaria

control and was perhaps the one individual most responsible for consolidating the power of the national state in the late 1800s, also advocated centralizing matters of sanitation and hygiene within a single national authority, an extension of his "unitary" political ideology and emulative of the legislation of large, progressive countries. Message from Julio A. Roca to the National Congress, accompanying a proposal for a national malaria law, September 16, 1903, in Malbrán, "El paludismo y su profilaxis," 452–53. See also, Romero, *Las ideas políticas en Argentina,* 193.

27. For Tucumán see, for example, *El Orden,* July 26, 1895 ("Board of hygiene. Its ineffectiveness and inertia"); March 2, 1907 ("The state of sanitation: Dreadful conditions"); March 7, 1907 ("Hygiene: Complete neglect"); March 19, 1907; January 21, 1908 ("Public health. A delicate situation. The action of the authorities. Unspeakable abandonment."); January 21, 1908; April 21, 1908; December 14, 1908. In Salta, the criticisms were, perhaps, even harsher; see *Tribuna Popular,* September 13, 1905 ("Health law. What the Republic needs"); September 19, 1905; September 21, 1905; February 17, 1907 ("What does this Board of Hygiene do?").

28. *Tribuna Popular* (Salta), March 31, 1907.

29. *El Cívico* (Salta), August 27, 1908.

30. Quoted in *El Orden* (Tucumán), November 29, 1907.

31. Antonio Restagnio, "Resultado de la misión a la región palúdica," *Anales del D.N.H.* 18, no. 5 (1911); Restagnio, "Campaña antipalúdica. La acción profiláctica concurrente de la Ingeniería Sanitaria," *Anales del D.N.H.* 19, no. 3 (1912).

32. Denis Cosgrove, "Measures of America," in *Geography and Vision* (London: I. B. Tauris, 2008), 159.

33. Mark S. Monmonier, *How to Lie with Maps,* 2nd ed. (Chicago: University of Chicago Press, 1996); Denis Wood, "Every Map Shows This . . . But Not That," in *The Power of Maps* (New York: Guilford Press, 1992).

34. Here, I am drawing on the work of geographers, sociologists, and other social scientists who have interrogated the spatial projects of modern states. See, in particular, Andermann, *Optic of the State;* Ferguson, *The Anti-politics Machine;* Maria Kaika, *City of Flows: Modernity, Nature, and the City* (New York: Routledge, 2005); Mitchell, *Rule of Experts: Egypt, Techno-Politics, Modernity;* Benjamin S. Orlove, "Mapping Reeds and Reading Maps: The Politics of Representation in Lake Titicaca," *American Ethnologist* 18, no. 1 (1991); Scott, *Seeing like a State;* Peter Vandergeest and Nancy Lee Peluso, "Empires of Forestry: Professional Forestry and State Power in Southeast Asia, Part 1," *Environment and History* 12 (2006).

35. Restagnio, "Campaña antipalúdica," 364–75.

36. Antonio M. Correa, "El paludismo en Tucumán. Datos informativos," *Anales del D.N.H.* 19, no. 2 (1912).

37. Restagnio, "Resultado de la misión a la región palúdica," 11.

38. Ribot, "A History of Fear." For an elaboration of my point here, see Carter, "State Visions."

39. In fairness to Anschütz and Restagnio, railroad-based surveys also took them through the most densely inhabited parts of the region, so they may have cap-

tured the environmental conditions most relevant to a *majority* of the people in the Northwest.

40. José Penna, "Plan de profilaxis antipalúdica. Texto de una comunicación al H. Consejo Consultivo, por el Dr. José Penna," *Anales del D.N.H* 18, no. 4 (1911): 11.

41. The national scope of the campaign was portrayed in the official maps of the DNH, which represented the malarious zone as a dark stain on the national map—the whole country, down to Tierra del Fuego, was included. Such maps also implied the presence and control of the national state. See maps supplements in Penna and Barbieri, *El paludismo y su profilaxis en la Argentina*.

42. Penna and Barbieri, *El paludismo y su profilaxis en la Argentina*, 344–46.

43. Antonio Barbieri was born in Córdoba in 1879 and graduated from the Medical School at the University of Buenos Aires in 1908. In addition to occupying the DNH positions described in the text, he led a department mission to Italy to study malariology in 1924 (discussed in chapter 3) and edited the agency's *Annals*. He was a corresponding member of the League of Nations hygiene committee in 1934 and a member of the Sociedad Científica Argentina until 1939. During this time, he continued the clinical practice of ophthalmology, the specialization for which he was most renowned, and published works on color perception. He does not even rate a mention in Norma Isabel Sánchez's exhaustive compendium of biographies of famous hygienists, and no historian of medicine I spoke to had any familiarity with him or his work. Biographical information drawn from Diego A. de Santillán, ed., *Gran Enciclopedia Argentina* (Buenos Aires: Ediar, 1956); *Personalidades de la Argentina. Diccionario Biográfico Contemporaneo*, 3rd ed. (Buenos Aires: Veritas-F. Antonio Rizzuto, 1948).

44. Sánchez, *La higiene y los higienistas*, 94.

45. Dirección Regional de la defensa antipalúdica de Tucumán, *Memoria de la Dirección Regional de la defensa antipalúdica de Tucumán correspondiente al año 1913. Al presidente del D.N.H.* (Tucumán: Tip. Cárcel Penitenciaria, 1914), 15. Jose L. Aráoz was director of the regional office of the Malaria Service in Tucumán and probably drafted most of this report.

46. Rodriguez, *Civilizing Argentina*, 144–45; Otero, *Estadística y nación*. One of the best examples of this effort toward quantification is the publication of *Demographic Annuals* beginning in 1911. These large volumes compiled mortality data from every department (i.e., county) in every Argentine province and territory. The *Annuals* appeared in their original, comprehensive format for six years, but the same budgetary shortfalls that impacted the Malaria Service caused their reduction to summary format starting in 1917. In their geographic and diagnostic detail, the comprehensiveness of these *Annuals* would not be matched for many decades. See Departamento Nacional de Higiene, Oficina de demografía, *Anuario demográfico: Natalidad, nupcialidad y mortalidad* (Buenos Aires: Oficina de Demografía, 1911–1916); D.N.H., *Guía oficial;* Eric D. Carter, "Malaria, Landscape, and Society in Northwest Argentina," *Journal of Latin American Geography* 7, no. 1 (2008). Even before this initiative, Tucumán's government had begun compiling the massively detailed *Anu-*

arios Estadísticos under the direction of Paulino Rodríguez Marquina. These have become invaluable sources for research on public health and historical demography in Tucumán. See Fernández, "Salud y condiciones de vida"; Alfredo S. C. Bolsi and J. Patricia Ortiz de D'Arterio, *Población y azúcar en el Noroeste Argentino: Mortalidad infantil y transición demográfica durante el siglo XX* (Tucumán: Instituto de Estudios Geográficos, Facultad de Filosofía y Letras, Universidad Nacional de Tucumán, 2001).

47. Infection was determined mostly by clinical examinations, conducted inconsistently, drawing on patient histories (e.g., self-reporting of intermittent fevers), visual signs (e.g., wasting, anemia, or jaundice), and diagnoses of enlarged spleens (usually a telltale sign of infection). Only sometimes—yet fairly frequently in some districts, such as Tucumán—were blood examinations carried out.

48. Penna and Barbieri, *El paludismo y su profilaxis en la Argentina,* 233. Some officials acknowledged this statistical problem at the time; see, for example, the remarks of Jose L. Aráoz of the Tucumán office, in Dirección Regional de la defensa antipalúdica de Tucumán, *Memoria de la Dirección Regional,* 11, 15–21.

49. The *P. vivax* parasite produced "tertian" malaria (in Spanish, *malaria terciana*) with a spike of high fever at approximately forty-eight-hour intervals. This was the most prevalent form of the malaria parasite in Argentina and in most subtropical or temperate climate zones. "Quartan" malaria (in Spanish, *malaria cuartana*) was caused by the *P. malariae* parasite and had very regular seventy-two-hour intervals between fevers. *P. falciparum* produced "tropical" malaria, marked by high, constant fever and common, often deadly complications. In Spanish there were several terms associated with this strain, including *trópica, maligna,* and *estivo-otoñal* (the latter term meaning "summer-fall," due to its frequent appearance late in the malaria season). For straightforward yet comprehensive explanations of malaria etiology, see Humphreys, *Malaria,* 8–20; Packard, *The Making of a Tropical Disease,* 19–35.

50. Penna and Barbieri, *El paludismo y su profilaxis en la Argentina,* 68–69; *Anuario estadístico de la provincia de Tucumán,* 1915, 86.

51. Penna and Barbieri, *El paludismo y su profilaxis en la Argentina,* 70–71; Dirección Regional de la defensa antipalúdica de Tucumán, *Memoria de la Dirección Regional.*

52. Dirección Regional de la defensa antipalúdica de Tucumán, *Memoria de la Dirección Regional,* 15–21. During this era, the proportion of malaria sufferers attended at the city of Tucumán's main public hospitals oscillated between 5 and 12 percent. *Anuarios estadísticos de la provincia de Tucumán,* 1905–1915.

53. Dirección Regional de la defensa antipalúdica de Tucumán, *Memoria de la Dirección Regional,* 17.

54. Armus, "El descubrimiento de la enfermedad."

55. The Malaria Service also borrowed photographs of the clinical symptoms of malaria (especially enlarged spleens) from research carried out in Algeria, probably by Edmond and Etienne Sergent. See Penna and Barbieri, *El paludismo y su profilaxis en la Argentina,* 138–39.

56. The active ingredient in quinine is an alkaloid found in the bark of the cinchona plant, which is native to the Andes Mountains. By the end of the nineteenth

century, however, most of the world's supply of cinchona was grown in Dutch and British colonies in South Asia and Southeast Asia, and a handful of European drug companies monopolized quinine manufacturing. Before World War I, the DNH purchased quinine on the international market at a price of 32 to 50 pesos per kilogram, depending on the preparation (powder form, tablets, chocolate bars); Barbieri estimated that in 1914 the department spent 45,000 pesos (roughly US $19,350) on quinine. The leaders of the malaria campaign hoped to establish a domestic supply of quinine by exploiting the natural conditions of the Northwest, believing that the cinchona plant would acclimate favorably to parts of Salta and Jujuy located in the *yungas,* the same physiographic province where the plant thrived in Bolivia. The Reglamentación of Law 5195 (a decree issued by President Sáenz Peña in 1911 to lay out in specific terms the technical and administrative norms of the Malaria Service) also projected the establishment of experimental quinine plantations in the Northwest. Local newspapers even argued that cinchona plantations and quinine manufacturing could give a tremendous boost to the regional economy. These schemes only materialized in 1920, when the national congress offered 15,000 pesos to start an experimental cinchona nursery in Calilegua (Jujuy) after World War I provoked a global shortage in quinine. "El cultivo de la quina. Su ensayo en el norte. Una buena iniciativa," *El Orden* (Tucumán), January 29, 1920; "La escasez de quinina. Una situación inquietante," *El Orden,* April 22, 1920. See also Herbert Michael Gilles, D. A. Warrell, and Leonard Jan Bruce-Chwatt, *Bruce-Chwatt's Essential Malariology,* 3rd ed. (London; Boston: Edward Arnold, 1993), 164–78; William Campbell Steere, "The Cinchona-Bark Industry of South America," *Scientific Monthly* 61, no. 2 (1945); Mark Honigsbaum, *The Fever Trail: In Search of the Cure for Malaria* (New York: Farrar Straus & Giroux, 2002), 215; Antonio Barbieri, "Cultivo y explotación de quinas en la República Argentina," *Anales del D.N.H.* 21, no. 2 (1914), cited in Penna and Barbieri, *El paludismo y su profilaxis en la Argentina,* 235.

57. Penna and Barbieri, *El paludismo y su profilaxis en la Argentina,* 266.

58. Ibid., 249.

59. "Falleció otro niño intoxicado con quinina," *Nueva Epoca* (Salta), January 30, 1929.

60. For example, *El Orden,* December 31, 1908; January 8, 1908; December 22, 1920; *La Montaña* (Salta), February 23, 1904; *La Provincia* (Salta), August 2, 1924. Not surprisingly, these advertisements tended to appear from November to April, the height of the malaria season, or what *El Orden* labeled "the dark months" (*los meses negros*), November 8, 1927.

61. Penna and Barbieri, *El paludismo y su profilaxis en la Argentina,* 304–6.

62. Ibid., 306.

63. Ibid., 308.

64. Ibid., 295–314.

65. Ibid., 311.

66. Ibid., 191.

67. Ibid., 313–17.

68. Armus, "El descubrimiento de la enfermedad"; Zimmermann, *Los liberales reformistas.*

69. Rodriguez, *Civilizing Argentina,* 180.

70. Armus, "El descubrimiento de la enfermedad."

71. Rodriguez, *Civilizing Argentina,* 180; Reber, "Blood, Coughs, and Fever," 89; Sánchez, *La higiene y los higienistas,* 257–63, 483–85. For a local (northwestern) perspective on Coni's work, see "Higiene y salubridad. La sociedad de profilaxis," *Tribuna Popular* (Salta), March 13, 1907. On the Drop of Milk league, the broader "puericulture" movement it represented, and its connection to Argentine eugenics, see Stepan, *Hour of Eugenics,* 76–82; Rodriguez, *Civlizing Argentina,* 117–18.

72. D.N.H., *Guía oficial,* 182.

73. Juarez-Dappe, *When Sugar Ruled,* 136. The significance of the decline in infant mortality is debatable. Juarez-Dappe claims that the infant mortality rate (IMR) declined substantially from 1900 to 1914, yet the province's own statistics from the *Anuarios Estadísticos* show only a slight decline, from 225.45 (per 1,000) to 213.04 (per 1,000) during that timeframe. In any case, IMR was widely variable from year to year, so that IMR was actually higher in 1914 than it was in 1899 (187.15 per 1,000). Comparing five-year averages from 1898–1902 and 1912–1916, we do see a decline from an average of 232.04 to 201.24 per 1,000, a 13 percent drop. Yet from 1918 to 1919, IMR rose to its highest levels in Tucumán since 1902, though possibly as a result of the global influenza pandemic. Whatever decline in infant mortality that Tucumán did experience could be due to a combination of factors, including the Gota de Leche dispensaries, but also to malaria control, which took place simultaneously, and general, slight improvements in living conditions. See Bolsi and Ortiz de D'Arterio, *Población y azúcar en el Noroeste Argentino,* 43–56, 108–9.

74. Founders included the Tucumán oligarchs Alberto Rougés, Rufino Cossio Jr., and Juan B. Terán. See "La Liag [*sic*] sanitaria del Norte. Una patriótica iniciativa," *El Orden,* May 28, 1919. The name of this organization may also have been an allusion to the historical Liga del Norte, an alliance of northern provinces led by the Tucumano Marco Avellaneda, in opposition to Juan Manuel de Rosas in the 1840s. This short-lived effort, and Avellaneda's martyrdom for the cause, featured prominently in a historical narrative of loss, redemption, and federalist autonomy in the Northwest.

75. "Ecos del día. El problema sanitario," *El Orden,* May 28, 1919. For similar sentiments, see Penna, "Plan de profilaxis," 6–7.

76. The most famous exposé on miserable working conditions, especially in the provinces, was the "Report on the Status of the Working Class" by Juan Bialet Massé, commissioned by Joaquín V. González, minister of the interior under Roca, and completed in 1904. This work has been cited extensively in social histories of labor and public health, especially for the Northwest, due to its shocking revelations about the sugar industry, and had concrete effects, such as the creation of the National Department of Labor in 1907. See Juan Bialet Massé, *Informe sobre el estado de las clases obreras en el interior de la República Argentina* (1904; repr., Montevideo: Universidad de la República, Facultad de Humanidades y Ciencias, 1966);

Daniel Campi, "Los ingenios del Norte: Un mundo de contrastes," in *Historia de la vida privada en la Argentina: La Argentina plural, 1870–1930,* edited by Fernando Devoto and Marta Madero (Buenos Aires: Taurus, 1999); Campi, "Economía y sociedad en las provincias del Norte"; Fernández, "Salud y condiciones de vida. Iniciativas estatales y privadas en Tucumán," 115–17; Marcelo Lagos, María Silvia Fleitas, and María Teresa Bovi, eds., *A cien años del informe de Bialet Massé* (Jujuy: Unidad de Investigación en Historia Regional, Facultad de Humanidades y Ciencias Sociales, Universidad Nacional de Jujuy, 2004); Rodriguez, *Civilizing Argentina,* 113–14; Sánchez, *La higiene y los higienistas,* 377–87. A few years later, Department of Labor inspectors reported on conditions of Chaco Indians laboring in the *zafra* of Salta and Jujuy; see José E. Nikilson, "Investigación sobre los indios matacos trabajadores," *Boletín del Departamento Nacional del Trabajo* 35 (1917); Lagos, *La cuestión indígena en el Estado y en la sociedad nacional. Gran Chaco, 1870–1920;* Gordillo, *Landscapes of Devils,* 53–69. Although there was considerable overlap between the realms of hygiene and labor, the reports of Bialet Massé and the Department of Labor inspectors were seldom, if ever, mentioned in the Malaria Service's extensive reports. This may reflect the compartmentalized character of the government bureaucracy, political-administrative rivalries, or ideological differences.

77. Armus, "Salud y anarquismo," 95. The "capitalist system" quotation comes from *El Rebelde,* June 22, 1901, a Radical newspaper that Armus cites here.

78. Juarez-Dappe, *When Sugar Ruled,* 106–18.

79. Packard, *The Making of a Tropical Disease,* 117. This was not the case everywhere: in contemporary Italy, according to Snowden, "antimalaria legislation . . . defined malaria as an occupational disease" and the malaria campaign was connected to the expansion of women's rights and the abolition of latifundia and other vestiges of feudal labor relations and property rights. Snowden, *The Conquest of Malaria,* 54. In the 1920s, some leaders of the malaria campaign would become more outspoken and strident in their critiques of social inequality.

80. Penna, "Plan de profilaxis," 14.

81. D.N.H., *Que es el chucho? Como se transmite? Como se combate? Instrucciones populares* (Buenos Aires: Talleres Gráficos de la Penitenciaría Nacional, 1909). The pamphlet must have proved successful, at least from the perspective of DNH, since it was reissued, with few modifications, in 1912, 1921, and 1931.

82. A reproduction of one such poster can be found in Penna and Barbieri, *El paludismo y su profilaxis en la Argentina,* 337.

83. Pedro J. García, "Factores de éxito de la campaña antipalúdica," *Anales del D.N.H.* 18, no. 6 (1911): 16. Margaret Humphreys has pointed out that in the southern United States, during roughly the same era, young children were the primary targets of education to promote malaria control and became among its most fervent promoters. Humphreys, *Malaria,* 133.

84. "Clases sobre el paludismo en los colegios nacionales y escuelas normales," *El Cívico* (Salta), September 7, 1908.

85. María Teresa Bussolatti and Nicolás Lozano, "El paludismo. Conferencia dada por la Srta. María Teresa Bussolatti, alumna del 40. año normal," *Anales del D.N.H.* 18, no. 6 (1911).

86. Universidad de Tucumán, Extensión Popular, *El chucho (malaria, paludismo, etc.). Urgencia y manera de disminuir esta temible enfermedad* (Tucumán: Universidad de Tucumán, 1914).

87. Sánchez, *La higiene y los higienistas,* 98.

88. D.N.H., *Que es el chucho?,* 33–35. It is worth noting that there was a parallel "folk" discourse on the causes of malaria, which could be classified as a discourse on acts and events that "triggered" a malaria infection or recrudescence of symptoms. Mentioned in newspapers and some scientific reports (usually, with great skepticism) was the idea that malaria infection could be triggered by a fright (*susto*) or a cold bath or other exposure to chill. In 1926, one army physician argued that a bout of malaria was often preceded by a fall from a horse or a similarly sudden injury. See Francisco Aráoz Castellano, "El paludismo en la guarnición de Salta," in *Tercer Congreso Nacional de Medicina: Actas y Trabajos, Tomo I* (Buenos Aires: Las Ciencias, 1926), 701.

89. Malbrán, quoted in "El paludismo. Su profilaxis. Reportaje al doctor Malbrán," *El Orden,* August 4, 1908.

90. D.N.H., *Que es el chucho?,* 44.

91. See, for example, "Hay que eliminar de la ciudad los criaderos de mosquitos," *Nueva Epoca* (Salta), January 31, 1929.

92. García, "Factores de éxito de la campaña antipalúdica," 18. Notably, perhaps, the "folk healer" is a *curandera*—female—while the scientists are always portrayed as men.

93. Universidad de Tucumán, Extensión Popular, *El chucho,* 5.

94. Penna and Barbieri, *El paludismo y su profilaxis en la Argentina,* 337.

95. Universidad de Tucumán, Extensión Popular, *El chucho,* 1.

96. Ibid., 11.

97. Bussolatti and Lozano, "El paludismo," 73.

98. Nicolás Lozano, "La higiene pública en la Argentina. Trabajo presentado al V Congreso Médico Latino-Americano y VI Panamericano," *Anales del D.N.H.* 20, no. 5 (1913): 995.

99. Ibid., 1024.

100. Bussolatti and Lozano, "El paludismo," 83.

101. Ibid. On the floor of the national senate in support of the malaria bill, Alberto de Soldati made a similar remark about "maps that circulate profusely in Europe" marked with "red stains" to show emigrants unhealthy areas, such as the Northwest, that are to be avoided. *Diario-Senadores,* September 23, 1905, 1:980.

102. Lozano, "La higiene pública," 1048.

103. Ibid., 1073.

104. Rodriguez, *Civilizing Argentina,* 212–17; Romero, *Las ideas políticas en Argentina,* 189–209.

105. García, "Factores de éxito de la campaña antipalúdica." See also the opinions of Gregorio Aráoz Alfaro on this subject, in Osvaldo Fustinoni, "El académico Gregorio Aráoz Alfaro (conferencia pronunciada por el Académico Osvaldo Fustinoni en el Círculo Médico de Córdoba, 1 Julio 1994)," *Boletín de la Academia Nacional de Medicina de Buenos Aires* 72 (1994): 485–90.

106. Penna, "Plan de profilaxis," 8.

107. Rock, *Argentina, 1516–1987*, 162–63, 172–83.

108. The crisis began with an increase in interest rates in Britain in expectation of war and a resulting decline in foreign capital investment in Argentina. The situation was exacerbated by a failed wheat harvest in 1914, caused by an invasion of locusts; then, with the outbreak of hostilities in Europe, markets for Argentina's agricultural exports dried up, the import of manufactured goods declined precipitously, and, for the first time, emigrants to Europe (principally men returning to serve in the armies of their native countries) outnumbered immigrants to Argentina. Barsky and Gelman, *Historia del agro argentino*, 223–27; Rock, *Argentina, 1516–1987*, 191–99; José Luis Romero, *Breve historia de la Argentina* (1965; repr., Buenos Aires: Fondo de Cultura Económica, 1996), 129–30.

109. Penna and Barbieri, *El paludismo y su profilaxis en la Argentina*, 350–52; Antonio Barbieri, "El problema de saneamiento antimalárico en la Argentina. Consideraciones y antecedentes," *Anales del D.N.H.* 25, no. 2 (1919): 23.

110. Penna and Barbieri, *El paludismo y su profilaxis en la Argentina*, 350.

111. *Anuarios estadísticos de la provincia de Tucumán*, 1915–1919. The number admitted rose from 281 (about 6 percent of all admissions) to 806 (about 11 percent of all admissions).

112. Penna and Barbieri, *El paludismo y su profilaxis en la Argentina*, 348–49. Leopoldo Bard, a politician and social reformer discussed in more detail in the next chapter, would make a similar argument in the 1920s. Leopoldo Bard, *Profilaxis del paludismo e impuesto sanitario. Proyecto de ley presentado por el diputado Dr. Leopoldo Bard a la Cámara de Diputados de la Nación, en la sesión del 25 de Octubre de 1923* (Buenos Aires: Cámara de Diputados, 1923), 34–35.

113. Penna and Barbieri, *El paludismo y su profilaxis en la Argentina*, 356.

114. Lozano, "La higiene pública," 1072–73.

115. Penna, "Plan de profilaxis," 8.

116. Gregorio Aráoz Alfaro, "Profilaxis del paludismo. Plan de campaña del Departamento Nacional de Higiene," *La Semana Médica* 25 (May 23, 1918): 603. Such frustration with the public's inability or unwillingness to take proper courses of quinine was also felt by malaria control officials in Italy and the United States and was one of the major flaws of the quinine therapy strategy, according to mosquito control advocates. See Humphreys, *Malaria*, 76–79; Snowden, *The Conquest of Malaria*, 96–97.

117. Jaime Carrillo, "Informe. Memoria de la profilaxis antipalúdica correspondiente al año 1912," *Anales del D.N.H.* 20 (1913): 860–61.

118. I borrow the phrase "missionaries of science" from Marcos Cueto's book of the same name. Marcos Cueto, ed., *Missionaries of Science: The Rockefeller Foundation and Latin America* (Bloomington: Indiana University Press, 1994).

CHAPTER 3

1. Tobías, "Contribución al estudio," 406; Jeronimo del Barco, "Proyecto de organizacion del Departamento Nacional de Higiene," in *Conferencia Sanitaria Na-*

cional, Buenos Aires 1923:Antecedentes, sesiones y conclusiones (Buenos Aires: D.N.H., 1923), 131; Antonio Barbieri, "La profilaxis del paludismo en la Argentina: Proyecto de modificaciones a la Ley 5195," in *Conferencia Sanitaria Nacional, Buenos Aires 1923:Antecedentes, sesiones y conclusiones* (Buenos Aires: D.N.H., 1923), 255.

2. As Carolina Biernat puts it, in Argentina eugenics influenced sciences such as "medicine, biology, criminology, sociology or psychiatry"; followers came from diverse ideological foundations, including "socialists, anarchists, liberals and conservatives." The common denominator was a "preoccupation with the perfection of the 'race,'" which was broadly construed to include "geographical, biological, climatic, historical and cultural components." Carolina Biernat, "La eugenesia argentina y el debate sobre el crecimiento de la población en los años de entreguerras," *Cuad. Sur, Hist.* 34 (2005), para. 7; see also Zimmermann, "Racial Ideas and Social Reform," 25–28.

3. On the idea of nationalism as a social construction, see, inter alia, Benedict R. O'G. Anderson, *Imagined Communities: Reflections on the Origin and Spread of Nationalism* (London: Verso Editions/NLB, 1983); Craib, *Cartographic Mexico;* Peter C. Perdue, "Where Do Incorrect Political Ideas Come From? Writing the History of the Qing Empire and the Chinese Nation," in *The Teleology of the Modern Nation-State: Japan and China,* edited by Joshua A. Fogel (Philadelphia: University of Pennsylvania Press, 2005); Tilley, *Seeing Indians;* Thongchai Winichakul, *Siam Mapped: A History of the Geo-Body of a Nation* (Honolulu: University of Hawaii Press, 1994).

4. A similar interpretation is offered by Jeane H. DeLaney, "Imagining El Ser Argentino: Cultural Nationalism and Romantic Concepts of Nationhood in Early Twentieth-Century Argentina," *Journal of Latin American Studies* 34, no. 3 (2002): 626–28.

5. Bard, *Profilaxis del paludismo,* 95; Gregorio Aráoz Alfaro, "La formacion de un pueblo fuerte," *Anales del Instituto Popular de Conferencias* 4 (1924): 213; Bunge, *Las industrias del Norte,* 60–90.

6. Bunge was, in many ways, an intellectual forerunner of Peronist social welfare and economic policy in his pro-natalist, statist, and protectionist stances. See Carolina Biernat, *¿Buenos o útiles?: La política inmigratoria del peronismo* (Buenos Aires: Biblos, 2007), 30–31; Otero, *Estadística y nación,* 223–38.

7. Land colonization has a checkered history in Argentina; although liberal mid-nineteenth-century leaders such as Sarmiento or Mitre hoped for widespread homesteading and colonization of government-owned land, in the end private colonization schemes were most successful in the Pampas of Santa Fe and Córdoba and the territory of Misiones. See Mark Jefferson, *Peopling the Argentine Pampas* (New York: AGS, 1926); Robert C. Eidt, *Pioneer Settlement in Northeast Argentina* (Madison: University of Wisconsin Press, 1971).

8. Otero, "La transición demográfica argentina a debate," 88; Carolina Biernat, "Inmigración, natalidad y urbanización. El poblacionismo argentino y sus contradicciones frente a las preguntas por el desarrollo económico (1914–1955)," in *El mosaico argentino: Modelos y representaciones del espacio y de la población, siglos XIX–XX,*

edited by Hernán Otero (Buenos Aires: Siglo Veintiuno de Argentina Editores, 2004), 471.

9. Aráoz Alfaro, "La formacion de un pueblo fuerte," 217. On the idea of the "Latin" race that emerged at different times across the continent and in Argentina, see Aims McGuinness, "Searching for 'Latin America': Race and Sovereignty in the Americas in the 1850s," in *Race and Nation in Modern Latin America,* edited by Nancy P. Appelbaum, Anne S. Macpherson, and Karin Alejandra Rosemblatt (Chapel Hill: University of North Carolina Press, 2003), 97–102; Tilley, *Seeing Indians,* 197; Marilyn G. Miller, *Rise and Fall of the Cosmic Race* (Austin: University of Texas Press, 2004), 81–82.

10. By 1932, Aráoz Alfaro had hardened his eugenicist stance on immigration, arguing that immigrant families in Argentina were comprised of "cripples of every type" including "dwarves," "stunted" people, "alcoholics," "epileptics," "idiots," "criminals," and "psychopaths of every kind." Gregorio Aráoz Alfaro, "Nuestros problemas eugénicos, verdades dolorosas," *El Hospital Argentino* 3, no. 11 (1932): 516–17, cited in Biernat, "La eugenesia argentina."

11. Nancy Leys Stepan suggests that the carnage of World War I produced a disillusionment among many hygienists and other elites with the European modernism and ideals of progress. Particularly in Brazil, but also in other countries, this disenchantment with European "civilization" intensified the focus of eugenists on discovering the core of national identities and perfecting national races. Stepan, *Hour of Eugenics,* 36.

12. Leopoldo Bard, "Fuentes de recursos para la lucha antipalúdica en la República Argentina," in *Tercer Congreso Nacional de Medicina: Actas y Trabajos, Tomo I* (Buenos Aires: Las Ciencias, 1926), 473.

13. Tobías, "Contribución al estudio," 407–8.

14. David N. Livingstone, *The Geographical Tradition: Episodes in the History of a Contested Enterprise* (Oxford, UK; Cambridge, MA: Blackwell Publishers, 1993), 216–59; Mark Harrison, *Climates and Constitutions: Health, Race, Environment and British Imperialism in India* (Delhi; Oxford: Oxford University Press, 1999); Anderson, *Colonial Pathologies,* 73–103.

15. David Rock, *Authoritarian Argentina: The Nationalist Movement, Its History, and Its Impact* (Berkeley: University of California Press, 1992), 14.

16. Levillier, *Orígenes argentinos,* 314–16; Shumway, *The Invention of Argentina,* chapter 10; Stepan, *Hour of Eugenics,* 16–17, 84–95.

17. DeLaney, "Imagining El Ser Argentino," 646; see also Zimmermann, "Racial Ideas and Social Reform," 39–40, 44.

18. Gregorio Aráoz Alfaro, *Para que la patria sea grande y fuerte* (Buenos Aires: Flaiban & Camilloni, 1916), 28.

19. Ibid., 4–9; Quintero, "La interpretación del territorio argentino," 293.

20. Aráoz Alfaro, "La formacion de un pueblo fuerte," 215.

21. Shumway, *The Invention of Argentina;* Chamosa, "Indigenous or Criollo"; DeLaney, "Imagining El Ser Argentino."

22. Chamosa, "Indigenous or Criollo," 71–72.

23. Stepan, *Hour of Eugenics,* 36; Zimmermann, "Racial Ideas and Social Reform," 46.

24. Juan G. Dietsch and Elías Goligorsky, "Cursos de malariología seguidos en Italia por la misión médica argentina," *Anales del D.N.H.* 31 (1925): 191–203.

25. Caprotti, "Malaria and Technological Networks."

26. It is not clear when this phrase was first formulated. According to Kohn Loncarica and his colleagues, Carlos Alberto Alvarado, the Argentine malariologist, was in Italy for field studies when he heard Mussolini refer to the drainage of the Pontine Marshes in these terms. Kohn Loncarica, Agüero, and Sánchez, "Nacionalismo e internacionalismo," 154. My quotation of this slogan is taken from an epigraph in an English translation of Cesare Longobardi's propagandistic book on land reclamation in Italy. Cesare Longobardi, *Land-Reclamation in Italy: Rural Revival in the Building of a Nation,* translated by Olivia Rossetti Agresti (London: P. S. King & Son, Ltd., 1936). Surprisingly, although he does discuss Mussolini's intention to transform the Pontine Marshes into a "racial utopia" through bonifica integrale, Snowden does not use this vivid quotation. Snowden, *The Conquest of Malaria,* 173.

27. Caprotti, "Malaria and Technological Networks," 150.

28. Longobardi, *Land-Reclamation in Italy,* 10.

29. Federico Caprotti, "Destructive Creation: Fascist Urban Planning, Architecture, and New Towns in the Pontine Marshes," *Journal of Historical Geography* 33 (2007), 656–62; Caprotti, "Malaria and Technological Networks," 150–51.

30. Snowden, *The Conquest of Malaria,* 153.

31. Malcolm Watson, "The Geographical Aspects of Malaria," *Geographical Journal* 99, no. 4 (1942): 168, cited in Caprotti, "Malaria and Technological Networks," 152. Watson went on to say, "Perhaps this will be [Mussolini's] greatest, or only, abiding claim to fame."

32. Antonio Barbieri, "El saneamiento antipalúdico del Norte Argentino por la bonifica integral," in *Tercer Congreso Nacional de Medicina: Actas y Trabajos, Tomo I* (Buenos Aires: Las Ciencias, 1926), 459, emphasis in original

33. Barbieri, "Concepto de la lucha antipalúdica y su legislación," *Anales del D.N.H.* 31 (1925): 9–12; Dietsch and Goligorsky, "Cursos de malariología seguidos en Italia," 178–82; Snowden, *The Conquest of Malaria.* The Pontine Marshes were peripheral from the standpoint of social development, but could hardly be called geographically remote, given their location some thirty miles from Rome.

34. One such map, designed by Antonio Restagnio, can be found in the endpapers of Penna and Barbieri, *El paludismo y su profilaxis en la Argentina.*

35. Giuseppe Sanarelli, quoted in Lozano and Selva, "Nueva orientación en la lucha antipalúdica," 777. Sanarelli, though generally a proponent of the *bonifica* strategy, challenged the Fascist government's dominance of malaria control. In particular, he took issue with the Fascists' abandonment of original research in malariology, based on their assumption that a comprehensive solution (*bonifica integrale*) was already in place. Snowden, *The Conquest of Malaria,* 177–78.

36. Gregorio Aráoz Alfaro, *Orientación y estado actual de la lucha antipalúdica. Discurso presentado al Tercer Congreso Nacional de Medicina* (Buenos Aires: La Semana

Médica [E. Spinelli], 1926), 37; "Proyecto de plan de lucha contra el paludismo sancionado por el Tercer Congreso Nacional de Medicina," *La Semana Médica* 33 (1926): 9–12.

37. These locales are as follows: in Catamarca Province, Catamarca (capital), Paclín, Piedra Blanca, and Pomancillo; in Jujuy Province, San Salvador (capital), Ledesma, La Mendieta, Perico del Carmen, and San Pedro; in La Rioja, Tama; in Salta Province, Salta (capital), Güemes, Cerrillos, Campo Santo, El Carril, Chicoana, Guachipas, Metán, Rosario de la Frontera, and Rosario de Lerma; in Santiago del Estero Province, Santiago del Estero (capital), Canal de la Cuarteada, and La Banda; in Tucumán, San Miguel (capital), Aguilares, Concepción, Famaillá, La Corona, Lules, Medinas-Trinidad, Monteros, Simoca, Trancas, Río Colorado, and Villa Alberdi. In some places, especially provincial capitals, sanitation works were carried out at multiple sites and multiple times over the years. See Aráoz Alfaro, *Orientación y estado actual*, 21–29; Antonio Barbieri, *La lucha antimalárica en la Argentina. Campaña contra la anquilostomiasis* (Buenos Aires: D.N.H., 1928), 11–14, 16, 18–20, 35, 38–40, photo appendix; Bard, *Profilaxis del paludismo,* 152–58; Cossio, *La campaña antipalúdica en Tucumán. D.N.H.,* 65–77, 93, 103–9, 23, 30; Nelson C. Davis, Martín M. Lobo, and Félix G. Cabarrou, "Lucha antipalúdica en Medinas (pcia. de Tucumán)," *La Semana Médica* 34 (1927): 5, 12.

38. Alberto Pérez and Rufino Cossio, "Trabajos en Monteros Viejo," *Anales del D.N.H.* 32 (1926).

39. As with Salta, these observations are based on my personal reconnaissance of the area with the able assistance of local experts. In Monteros, local historian Tulio Ottonello (author's interview, August 31, 2002) and I retraced topographic maps of the DNH control works. See Pérez and Cossio, "Trabajos en Monteros Viejo"; Barbieri, *La lucha antimalárica,* 13.

40. "Prolífica labor que realiza el Ingeniero Pickel," *Nueva Epoca* (Salta), March 3, 1927; "Una gira a Laguna de Chartas y al Lazareto," *Nueva Epoca* (Salta), April 30, 1927. This work, carried out by the American sanitary engineer Oscar Pickel under contract with the DNH, is also summarized in Barbieri, *La lucha antimalárica,* 18. Ingeniero Pickel and the Rockefeller Foundation officers stationed in Argentina (N. C. Davis and E. R. Rickard) seem to have crossed paths in the Northwest; and, as we will see later on, they were skeptical of the value of his work.

41. This is based on my personal observation of the area in 2003. My appreciation also to Miguel Angel Cáseres, a local educator and historian who resides in the neighborhood around Plaza Gurruchaga, for explaining in detail the environmental history of the area, especially its changing hydrography.

42. As early as 1902, even before the federal malaria campaign began, the province of Tucumán sent Dr. Carlos A. Vera on an expedition to Italy, where he studied malaria science with Giovanni Battista Grassi and Angelo Celli and witnessed malaria control in action. Carlos A. Vera, *Informe de los estudios practicado en Italia sobre paludismo, comisionado por el Gobierno de la Provincia de Tucumán* (Buenos Aires: Galileo, 1902). Even at this formative stage of malaria control in both countries, Argentine scientists looked for social and environmental analogues between the two

countries. Vera, in a report to the governor of Tucumán, explained the *bonifica agraria* concept and how it might be applied to the province's agricultural landscape, in particular to control wet rice farming in southern Tucumán. Vera, *Informe de los estudios,* 34. After assuming leadership of the DNH in 1918, at the end of World War I, Aráoz Alfaro renewed intellectual exchange with Italy. At his insistence, in 1924 Barbieri and other Malaria Service officials spent five months studying at the Scuola Superiore di Malariologia at the University of Rome. Despite some clashes between the Argentine pupils and their Italian teachers, the lessons of this scientific expedition were related in a special number of the *Annals* of the Department of Hygiene the following year; see D.N.H., *Anales del D.N.H.* 31 (1925).

43. Giulio Alessandrini, "L'organizzazione della lotta antimalarica in Italia (con presentazione di film)," in *Tercer Congreso Nacional de Medicina: Actas y Trabajos, Tomo I* (Buenos Aires: Las Ciencias, 1926); Gustavo Pittaluga, "La habitación humana en la epidemiología del paludismo," in *Tercer Congreso Nacional de Medicina,* 232. Pittaluga was born in Italy and trained under Grassi at the University of Rome. By the time of his visit to Argentina, he was nationalized Spanish and renowned for his leadership in Spain's malaria campaign and in the League of Nations Malaria Commission. See Esteban Rodríguez Ocaña et al., *La acción médico-social contra el paludismo en la España metropolitana y colonial del siglo XX* (Madrid: Consejo Superior de Investigaciones Científicas, 2003). Also present at the 1926 conference were Vittorio Ascoli, also of Italy, and George K. Strode, of the Rockefeller Foundation. Aráoz Alfaro, *Orientación y estado actual,* 10.

44. Pittaluga, "La habitación humana," 232.

45. L. W. Hackett, *Malaria in Europe: An Ecological Study* (London: Oxford University Press, 1937), 19; Snowden, *The Conquest of Malaria,* 142–80.

46. Lozano and Selva, "Nueva orientación en la lucha antipalúdica," 776–78; Rufino Cossio, *Informe sobre el proyecto de ley de profilaxis y lucha antipalúdica. Producido en nombre de la comisión de higiene y asistencia social del H. Senado de la Nación, 3 de Septiembre 1941 (21a. reunión 19a. sesión ordinaria)* (Tucumán: Editorial La Raza, 1941), 9.

47. See, for example, Cossio, *Informe sobre el proyecto de ley;* Palacios, *Pueblos desamparados.* There was also a congressional debate on "Profilaxis and lucha antipalúdica," in *Diario-Senadores,* September 4, 1941. In July 1941, Lewis W. Hackett, of the Rockefeller Foundation (see also chapter 5), was called to testify in the national senate on the proposals of Cossio and Palacios to reorganize the Malaria Service. He characterized Palacios' bill as "very bad indeed" and argued that the legislators' concept of malaria and its control was mired in erroneous comparisons to Italy's malaria situation, which Hackett knew well from years of research there. He advised a focus on vector control and dismissed other rural development programs as useless in the fight against malaria. Lewis W. Hackett's officer's diary (hereafter cited as L. W. Hackett diary), July 24, 1941, RG 12.1, RF Archives, Rockefeller Archive Center, Sleepy Hollow, New York (hereafter cited as RAC).

48. Marcos Cueto, *Excelencia científica en la periferia: Actividades científicas e investigación biomédica en el Perú, 1890–1950* (Lima: GRADE, 1989).

49. Sandra Sánchez de Maldonado, "Creación y evolución de la Universidad

de Tucumán (1914–1921)," in *La cultura en Tucumán y en el Noroeste Argentino en la primera mitad del siglo XX* (Tucumán: Fundación Miguel Lillo y Centro Cultural Alberto Rougés, 1997), 46.

50. Juan B. Terán, *Una nueva universidad* (Tucumán: Prebisch y Violetto, 1917).

51. This was prior to the university reforms of 1919, which diminished elite privilege in the University of Buenos Aires. Ricardo Rojas was one of the prime movers and major beneficiaries of these reforms.

52. From Terán's May 1914 speech inaugurating the University of Tucumán, published in Terán, *Una nueva universidad,* 41.

53. A. J. Defant de Bravo and A. M. Orce de Llobeta, "Reflectura y reflexiones sobre el pensamiento educativo de Juan B. Terán," in *La 'Generación del Centenario' y su proyección en el Noroeste Argentino (1900–1950). Actas de las IV Jornadas realizadas en San Miguel de Tucumán del 3 al 5 de octubre de 2001,* edited by Florencia Aráoz de Isas (Tucumán: Fundación Miguel Lillo, Centro Cultural Alberto Rougés, 2002), 133.

54. For a good overview of Rojas's brand of nationalism, see Fernando Devoto, *Nacionalismo, fascismo y tradicionalismo en la Argentina moderna: Una historia* (Buenos Aires: Siglo Veintiuno, 2002), 54–77. As further proof of the tight connections among Tucumán's Generation of the Centennial and their somewhat mystical view of regional culture, see Ricardo Rojas's tribute to his friend Gregorio Aráoz Alfaro at his retirement from the Facultad de Medicina in 1929. Ricardo Rojas, "Gregorio Aráoz Alfaro," in *Libro de Oro en Homenaje al Dr. Gregorio Aráoz Alfaro* (Buenos Aires: Imprenta de la Universidad, 1929), v–xvi.

55. Ricardo Rojas, *La Universidad de Tucumán. Tres conferencias* (Buenos Aires: Librería Argentina de Enrique García, 1915), 95.

56. Soledad Terán, "La biblioteca de la Fundación Miguel Lillo y sus aportes al desarrollo geológico," in *La cultura en Tucumán y en el Noroeste Argentino,* 117–21; Silvia Eugenia Formoso, "Padilla, Rougés y la cultura folklórica," in *La 'Generación del Centenario' y su proyección en el Noroeste Argentino,* 171–81; Chamosa, "Indigenous or Criollo," 100–102.

57. Universidad de Tucumán, Extensión Popular, *El chucho.* The university also attempted to establish an institute of regional medicine, as Gregorio Aráoz Alfaro proposed in a speech at the university in 1915. See Gregorio Aráoz Alfaro, "La acción social de la universidad," in *Dos conferencias en la Universidad de Tucumán, Julio 1915* (Buenos Aires: Imprenta de Coni Hermanos, 1915), 35.

58. Benjamín Villafañe, *Nuestros males y sus causas* (Buenos Aires: Juan Perrotti, 1919), 44.

59. Mario C. Nascimbene, *El nacionalismo liberal y tradicionalista y la Argentina inmigratoria: Benjamín Villafañe (h.), 1916–1944* (Buenos Aires: Editorial Biblos, 1997), 41.

60. Ibid., 56.

61. Benjamin Villafañe, ed., *El atraso del interior: Documentos oficiales del gobierno de Jujuy pidiendo amparo para las industrias del Norte. Apendice a la conferencia leída en la Reunión de Gobernadores en Salta* (Jujuy: B. Buttazzoni, 1926), 147.

62. See Bunge, *Las industrias del Norte,* 42–44, 177–89. Although this "dis-

equilibrium" between the littoral and the national periphery is now an obvious theme of Argentine history, Bunge was one of the first economists to point out the severe regional disparities in Argentina's economic development; see Jose Luis de Imaz, "Alejandro E. Bunge, economista y sociólogo (1880–1943)," *Desarrollo Económico* 14, no. 55 (1974); Jimena Caravaca and Mariano Plotkin, "Crisis, ciencias sociales y elites estatales: La constitución del campo de los economistas estatales en la Argentina, 1910–1935," *Desarrollo Económico* 47, no. 187 (2007). It would not be a stretch to call Bunge the "godfather" of dependency theory, since Raúl Prebisch, a Tucumano and future leader at ECLA (Economic Commission on Latin America), was one of his pupils, and important features of dependency theory— such as the core-periphery dynamic and the need for government subsidies for industrialization—figure prominently in Bunge's analyses.

63. Biographical details on Paterson, Mazza, and Alvarado owe a great deal to the work of Dr. Jobino Pedro Sierra Iglesias, also of San Pedro (Jujuy), who in the 1980s and 1990s wrote biographies of each. These works, while not merely hagiographies, resist any criticism of these men and, generally, offer little in the way of broader historical context. In a way, the books themselves are an extension of the celebratory mode of regionalism that began with Terán, Villafañe, and others. Nevertheless, they are indispensable because of their amazing detail and the author's access to primary sources and interview subjects (many now deceased) that were inaccessible to me. Jobino Pedro Sierra Iglesias, *Salvador Mazza: Su vida, su obra* (San Salvador de Jujuy: Universidad Nacional de Jujuy, 1990); Sierra Iglesias, *Carlos Alberto Alvarado;* Jobino Pedro Sierra Iglesias, *Vida y obra del Doctor Guillermo Cleland Paterson* (San Salvador de Jujuy: Universidad Nacional de Jujuy, 1996).

64. Guillermo C. Paterson, "Las fiebres palúdicas en Jujuy," *Anales del D.N.H.* 18 (1911): 31–57. See chapter 4 for a more extensive discussion of Paterson's findings and how they were integrated into malaria control planning.

65. Sierra Iglesias, *Vida y obra del Doctor Guillermo Cleland Paterson,* 70–77. He also taught the subjects of bacteriology and chemistry. His early resignation from these positions, mainly for financial reasons, probably delayed Tucumán's progress in establishing a real curriculum in medicine, hygiene, and microbiology.

66. According to one biographer, Mazza's rural upbringing shaped his outlook; in the small provincial town of Rauch, Mazza witnessed the "neglect" of public health in a community of poor immigrants and organized a vaccination service in the town even before he entered medical school. See Jonathan Leonard, "Investigaciones en el interior de la Argentina: La búsqueda de la salud emprendida por Salvador Mazza," *Boletín de la Oficina Sanitaria Panamericana* 113, no. 4 (1992): 256–57.

67. For example, the guest list at his bachelor party in 1914 included Carlos Malbrán, José Penna, and Gregorio Aráoz Alfaro, all presidents of the National Department of Hygiene; Nicolás Lozano and Antonio Restagnio, important officials in the Malaria Service; and Bernardo Houssay, future Nobel laureate in physiology. Sierra Iglesias, *Salvador Mazza,* 19.

68. Leonard, "Investigaciones en el interior," 259. Nicolle was awarded the Nobel Prize for his research on the lice-borne transmission of typhus in 1928. See

Kim Pelis, *Charles Nicolle, Pasteur's Imperial Missionary: Typhus and Tunisia* (Rochester, NY: University of Rochester Press, 2006).

69. Leonard, "Investigaciones en el interior," 259.

70. Ricardo Alvarado was uncle to Carlos Alvarado, who would succeed him as director of the Jujuy office of the Malaria Service and go on to become the key figure in the eradication of malaria in the country.

71. Sierra Iglesias, *Salvador Mazza,* 62.

72. Andrés Cornejo, "La universidad de Buenos Aires y los médicos del norte argentino," *Cátedra y Clínica* 7 (1940).

73. Sierra Iglesias, *Salvador Mazza,* 527.

74. Ibid., 86.

75. Ibid., 93–94. Sierra Iglesias writes that the *huaco* represented in the logo belonged to the collection of Dr. Napoleón Alvarez Soto, one of Mazza's close colleagues, and was unearthed by the Austrian archaeologist Carlos Schuel. The ceramic piece was itself a representation of a funerary rite of many pre-Columbian cultures of the Andes, wherein the remains of a person (especially dignitaries) were wrapped inside the hide of a llama (or guanaco) with its head still attached. Prepared in such a way, the llama, a sacred animal, was something like the "attendant" or "porter" of the soul in the afterlife.

76. Andrés Cornejo, *Atlas de Enfermedades Regionales del Norte Argentino* (Salta: Ministerio de Bienestar Social de la Provincia, 1980), 51.

77. Personal interview with Dr. Rodolfo U. Carcavallo, Buenos Aires, July 17, 2002.

78. Leonard, "Investigaciones en el interior."

79. Cornejo, *Atlas de Enfermedades Regionales del Norte Argentino,* 51–52.

80. Sierra Iglesias, *Salvador Mazza,* 97–98.

81. Salvador Mazza and E. R. Rickard, "Investigación sobre las relaciones entre paludismo y cultivo de arroz en la provincia de Tucumán," in *Cuarta reunión de la Sociedad Argentina de patología regional del norte: Santiago del Estero, 7, 8 y 9 de mayo de 1928* (Buenos Aires: Imprenta La Universidad, 1928); Mazza and Rickard, "Relación del cultivo de arroz con la difusión del paludismo en la provincia de Tucumán," in *Quinta reunión de la Sociedad Argentina de patología regional del norte: Jujuy del 7 al 10 de octubre de 1929* (Buenos Aires: Imprenta La Universidad, 1929).

82. Simone Petraglia Kropf, Nara Azevedo, and Luiz Otávio Ferreira, "Biomedical Research and Public Health in Brazil: The Case of Chagas' Disease (1909–1950)," *Social History of Medicine* 16, no. 1 (2003): 120–21; Sánchez, *La higiene y los higienistas,* 44–49.

83. Leonard, "Investigaciones en el interior," 259–263.

84. Personal interview with Rodolfo U. Carcavallo, Buenos Aires, July 17, 2002.

85. L. W. Hackett diary, July 10, 1941, RG 12.1, RF Archives, RAC.

86. The Rockefeller Foundation constituted the International Health Commission in 1913 with the objective of extending its hookworm eradication campaign from the U.S. South to other countries where the disease was a problem. Ettling, *Germ of Laziness;* Cueto, *Missionaries of Science,* x. The commission later became the board and, subsequently, the division. Since this agency was called the International

Health Board through the period of the foundation's most intensive activities in Argentina, this is the name used here, abbreviated IHB.

87. This phrase is borrowed from Marcos Cueto's edited volume of the same name. Cueto, *Missionaries of Science.*

88. J. Farley, "Mosquitoes or Malaria? Rockefeller Campaigns in the American South and Sardinia," *Parassitologia* 36 (1994): 165–73: Darwin H. Stapleton, "Lessons of History? Anti-malaria Strategies of the International Health Board and the Rockefeller Foundation from the 1920s to the Era of DDT," *Public Health Reports* 119 (2004): 206–15.

89. Armus, "Disease in the Historiography," 10. The literature on the Rockefeller Foundation's activity in Latin America is vast; in addition to *Missionaries of Science,* see, for example, Christian Brannstrom, "Polluted Soils, Polluted Souls: The Rockefeller Hookworm Eradication Campaign in São Paulo, Brazil, 1917–1926," *Historical Geography* 25 (1997); Cueto, *El regreso de las epidemias,* chapter 2; Steven Palmer, "Central American Encounters with Rockefeller Public Health, 1914–1921," in *Close Encounters of Empire: Writing the Cultural History of U.S.–Latin American Relations,* edited by Gilbert M. Joseph, Catherine C. LeGrand, and Ricardo D. Salvatore (Durham: Duke University Press, 1998).

90. The RF's first cooperative demonstrations for malaria control outside of the United States began only in 1924, in Brazil. However, the RF had been conducting malaria control operations in the southern United States since the mid-1910s. Research and control work for other infectious diseases, such as hookworm, tuberculosis, and yellow fever, had begun earlier (TB work exclusively in France, only to 1924). Warwick Anderson cites malaria control work starting in the Philippines in 1922, but IHB budget reports show malaria control demonstration projects starting there only in 1926. Rockefeller Foundation, *Annual Report* (New York: Rockefeller Foundation, 1925–1927), 1925, 290–301, 1927, 204–5; Anderson, *Colonial Pathologies,* 217.

91. The overseer may have taken this step on the advice of Alois Bachmann, a close friend of Yrigoyen's. Apparently, Yrigoyen had installed Bachmann as the director of the DNH bacteriological laboratory, replacing Dr. Kraus, who had been Mazza's mentor there. This would seem to reflect Yrigoyen's well-known penchant for using patronage to maintain political support. Bachmann (for unknown reasons, but presumably rooted in some professional rivalry) chose to disdain the IHB. This account is, unfortunately, hearsay: it was told to L. W. Hackett in 1941, during his directorship of the RF's office in Buenos Aires, by William A. Cross, the director of the Agricultural Experiment Station in Tucumán. L. W. Hackett diary, October 8, 1941, RG 12.1, RF Archives, RAC. Mieldazis is not a well-known figure in the history of malaria control; however, this sanitary engineer worked in Rockefeller-sponsored malaria control projects in British Palestine and in the Philippines in the 1920s. Anderson, *Colonial Pathologies,* 218; Sufian, *Healing the Land and the Nation,* 206–7.

92. The "representatives" of the Argentine government were unnamed, but pre-

sumably involved with the DNH; Terán's support was persistent throughout. Wickliffe Rose Officer's Diary, March 10, 1921, 111, RG 12.1, RF Archives, RAC.

93. H. A. Taylor, "Preliminary Malaria Survey. Tucuman District, Argentine," 1921, Folder 57, Box 5, Series 301, RG 1.1, RF Archives, RAC.

94. Taylor, "Preliminary Malaria Survey."

95. Ettling, *Germ of Laziness;* Humphreys, *Malaria,* 49–68.

96. Rockefeller Foundation, *Annual Report,* 1925, 298–301.

97. Shannon was technically "on loan" from the "National Museum" (probably meaning the Smithsonian) in the United States to the DNH bacteriology laboratory for most of 1926 and 1927, but worked closely with Davis and Argentine collaborators, especially Eduardo Del Ponte and Martin M. Lobo, on the distribution, feeding habits, and breeding conditions of anopheles mosquitoes. "Annual Report of the Argentina Malaria Service, 1927," 66–67, Folder 1375, Box 105, Series 300I, RG 5.3, RF Archives, RAC. See also Nelson C. Davis and Raymond C. Shannon, "The Habits of Anopheles Rondini in the Argentine Republic," *American Journal of Hygiene* 8, no. 2 (1928): 448–56; Raymond C. Shannon and Nelson C. Davis, "Condiciones de reproducción de A. pseudopunctipennis en la provincia de Tucumán durante la estación seca," *Revista del Instituto Bacteriológico del D.N.H.* 4, no. 7 (1927): 662–77; R. C. Shannon, N. C. Davis, and E. Del Ponte, "La distribución del Anopheles pseudopunctipennis y su relación con el paludismo, en la Argentina," *Revista del Instituto Bacteriológico del D.N.H.* 4, no. 7 (1927): 679–705.

98. Randall M. Packard and Paulo Gadelha, "A Land Filled with Mosquitoes: Fred L. Soper, the Rockefeller Foundation, and the *Anopheles gambiae* invasion of Brazil," *Parassitologia* 36 (1994); Malcolm Gladwell, "The Mosquito Killer," *New Yorker,* July 2, 2001.

99. Most of the letters and reports by Soper relating to the Argentina malaria control operation can be found in the Rockefeller Archive Center, while his extremely detailed and often droll diary is in the Fred L. Soper Papers at the National Library of Medicine in Bethesda, Maryland (hereafter cited as Fred L. Soper Papers).

100. "Argentina—Malaria Control—Annual Report—1925—Narrative and Statistical" ("Report on the Work of the International Health Board in Brazil, Argentina and Paraguay," 235–71), Folder 1371, Box 105, Series 300I, RG 5.3, RF Archives, RAC.

101. Nelson C. Davis's response to a questionnaire on malaria control, sent to him by Claudio Fermi (Hygiene Institute, University of Sassari, Sardinia, Italy). Davis's response is attached to letter from Davis to Fermi, Bahia, Brazil, August 13, 1928, Folder 3, Box 1, Nelson C. Davis Papers, RF Archives, RAC.

102. Letter from Davis to F. F. Russell, October 23, 1927, Folder 59, Box 5, Series 301, RG 1.1 Projects, RF Archives, RAC.

103. "Argentina—Malaria Control—Annual Report—1925—Narrative and Statistical," 250; Argentina Malaria Service Report, 2nd Quarter, 1926, 64–66, Folder 1371, Box 105, Series 300I, RG 5.3, RF Archives, RAC.

104. Photo #18965, "Laguna 'La Paludica' before draining. Situated in Lower

Course of Arroyo" [Medinas]; and Photo #18966, "Site of 'La Paludica' after drain-ing" [Medinas], included in "Preliminary Report, One Year in Medinas," 1926 (Folder 1371, Box 105, Series 3, RG5), but photographs themselves are found in RG RF Photographs. Photo #20095R, "XXII-One of series of small ponds near Calle San Martin, Concepción. Prolific focus for *A. pseudopunctipennis*"; and photo #20095S, "XXIII-Same locality as XXII after ponds have been drained by canal 'E9.' Land now used for agriculture," 1927 Annual Malaria Service Report, 39, Folder 1375, Box 105, Series 300I, RG 5.3. All in RF Archives, RAC.

105. Indeed, many of these DNH photographs could have been used in this book to illustrate the same point, if not for their very poor quality. The original, reproduction-quality photographs are presumed lost. For series of before-and-after saneamiento images published by the DNH, see Penna and Barbieri, *El paludismo y su profilaxis en la Argentina;* Barbieri, *La lucha antimalárica.*

106. Letter from Strode to Russell, September 11, 1925, Folder 58, Box 5, Series 301, RG 1.1, RF Archives, RAC.

107. Soper's exact assessment of Barbieri's entomological knowhow: "the bi-onomics of various mosquito genera are not clearly differentiated in his mind." Soper's diary, December 7, 1928, Box 7, Folder 8, Fred L. Soper Papers.

108. See Pedro Mühlens et al., "Estudios sobre paludismo y hematología en el Norte Argentino," *Revista del Instituto Bacteriológico del D.N.H.* 4, no. 3 (1925). The RF also had a coincidental connection to this expedition; during the tour, the staff entomologist at the DNH Bacteriological Institute, Juana Petrocchi, died sud-denly of appendicitis, and Raymond Shannon, the American entomologist who also worked for the RF, replaced her. Peter Mühlens (his name was Hispanicized as "Pedro") was affiliated with the Tropical Diseases Institute in Hamburg, Germany, and he also carried out malaria control work in Palestine in 1912 and 1913. Sufian, *Healing the Land and the Nation,* 187.

109. "Annual Report of the Argentina Malaria Service, 1926," 201; "Annual Report of the Argentina Malaria Service, 1927," 63, Folder 1375, Box 105, Series 300I, RG 5.3, RF Archives, RAC; Raymond C. Shannon, "Summary of Investiga-tions on Anopheles in Argentina, 1926–1927," *Rockefeller Foundation Quarterly Bul-letin* 1, no. 4 (1928).

110. "Argentina—Malaria Control—Annual Report—1925—Narrative and Statistical," 256–57, Folder 1371, Box 105, Series 300I, RG 5.3, RF Archives, RAC.

111. Mazza and Rickard, "Investigación sobre las relaciones"; Mazza and Rick-ard, "Relación del cultivo de arroz"; "Report on the Work of International Health Division in Argentina from January 1st to December 31st, 1928," Folder 1379, Box 105, Series 3, RG 5, RF Archives, RAC.

112. E. R. Rickard, "Estudios sobre el alcance de vuelo del Anopheles pseudo-punctipennis en el norte argentino," in *Cuarta reunión de la Sociedad Argentina de patología regional del norte: Santiago del Estero, 7, 8 y 9 de mayo de 1928* (Buenos Aires: Imprenta La Universidad, 1928); "Annual Report of the Argentina Malaria Ser-vice, 1927," 64; Letter from Soper to Russell (No. 485), Río de Janeiro, February 6, 1928, Folder 59, Box 5, Series 301, RG 1.1, RF Archives, RAC.

113. "Annual Report of the Argentina Malaria Service, 1927," 64.

114. Letter from Rickard to Davis, Tucumán, June 20, 1928, Folder 3, Box 1, Nelson C. Davis Papers, RF Archives, RAC.

115. Barbieri, *La lucha antimalárica,* 18.

116. Romero, *Breve historia de la Argentina,* 137; Rock, *Authoritarian Argentina,* 88–90.

117. Gregorio Aráoz Alfaro advised Soper, months prior to the election, that Yrigoyen was opposed to the activities of the RF in Argentina, although he did not specify why. See Soper diary, July 28, 1927, and December 6, 1927, Box 7, Folder 8, Fred L. Soper Papers.

118. Letter from Soper to Russell (#1338), June 5, 1929, Folder 59, Box 5, Series 301, RG 1.1, RF Archives, RAC.

119. Letter from Rickard to Soper, May 28, 1929, attached to letter from Soper to Russell (#1338), June 5, 1929, Folder 59, Box 5, Series 301, RG 1.1, RF Archives, RAC.

120. "Report on the Work of the International Health Division in Argentina, for the Quarter Ending June 30th, 1929," Folder 1381, Box 105, Series 3, RG 5, RF Archives, RAC.

121. Soper's diary, December 6–10, 1928, Box 7, Folder 8, Fred L. Soper Papers.

122. Robert A. Potash, *The Army and Politics in Argentina* (Stanford, CA: Stanford University Press, 1969), 52–53.

123. Frederick A. Hollander, "Oligarchy and the Politics of Petroleum in Argentina: The Case of the Salta Oligarchy and Standard Oil, 1918–1933" (PhD diss., University of California, 1976); Nicholas L. Biddle, "Oil and Democracy in Argentina, 1916–1930" (PhD diss., Duke University, 1991).

124. L. W. Hackett diary, October 8, 1941, RG 12.1, RF Archives, RAC.

125. Letter from Soper to Russell (#1507), September 12, 1929, Folder 59, Box 5, Series 301, RG 1.1, RF Archives, RAC.

126. On this point, see also Adriana Alvarez, "Malaria and the Emergence of Rural Health," 155–56.

CHAPTER 4

1. This chapter includes fragments from Eric D. Carter, "Development Narratives and the Uses of Ecology: Malaria Control in Northwest Argentina, 1890–1940," *Journal of Historical Geography* 33, no. 3 (2007): 619–50.

2. Although Tucumán remained the undisputed center of sugar production, with the output of its ingenios exceeding that of all other provinces combined, the production of sugar in Salta and Jujuy was growing at a much faster rate. Between 1920 and 1930, the sugarcane processed (by weight) increased by 41 percent in Tucumán, by 101 percent in Jujuy, and 525 percent in Salta. See statistical tables in E. J. Schleh, *La industria azucarera* (Buenos Aires: Centro Azucarero Argentino, 1935).

3. See Carter, "Malaria, Landscape, and Society," 15. According to my analysis, the population of "malarious" or "very malarious" departments (i.e.,

counties) of the Northwest grew by 52.4 percent between 1895 and 1914, while the region as a whole grew by 42.8 percent. For the subsequent intercensal period, 1914–1947, population continued to grow faster in the malaria zone, though some of the fastest growing departments, such as San Antonio de los Cobres, a mining center in the highlands, were not malarious at all. As far as internal migration goes, data for this era are generally sparse, but we can infer the magnitude of these movements from census data. In the province of Jujuy, for example, in 1895 only 3.4 percent of the native-born Argentine population had been born in another province or territory. By 1914, 25.8 percent of native-born Argentines had been born outside of Jujuy, and by 1947, it was 27.2 percent. Between 1914 and 1947 the province's population would more than double, from 76,631 to 166,700. Given the small number of foreign immigrants, most of this growth came from natural increase and internal migration. Argentina, Dirección Nacional de Estadística y Censos, *Cuarto censo general de la nación, 1947* (Buenos Aires: Dirección Nacional de Estadística y Censos, 1951), 1:254. See also Juarez-Dappe, *When Sugar Ruled,* 92–93; Kirchner, *Sugar and Seasonal Labor Migration.*

4. Rock, *Authoritarian Argentina,* 90.

5. Romero, *Las ideas políticas en Argentina,* 240–43.

6. Rock, *Argentina, 1516–1987,* 234–37.

7. Sussini was a surgeon from Corrientes Province who served in the national congress (Chamber of Deputies) from 1924 to 1928. A member of the Radical Party, Sussini took the side of the *antipersonalistas,* that faction of the party aligned against Hipólito Yrigoyen. According to Soper, Mazza and Sussini were not allies either. Soper's diary, August 26, 1932, Series I, Box 8, Folder 5, Fred L. Soper Papers. See also Sánchez, *La higiene y los higienistas,* 527; Enrique Pereira, "Miguel Sussini," in *Diccionario Biográfico Nacional de la Unión Cívica Radical* (2009), http://diccionarioradical.blogspot.com/search/label/Corrientes. Accessed September 12, 2009.

8. Personal interview with Pedro "Peter" Alvarado, Jujuy, March 24, 2003.

9. Houssay earned the Nobel Prize particularly for his work in endocrinology. See his Nobel Institute biography, http://nobelprize.org/medicine/laureates/1947/houssay-bio.html. Accessed September 12, 2009.

10. Sierra Iglesias, *Carlos Alberto Alvarado,* 7–8.

11. This recollection was supplied by Lewis W. Hackett, a major leader in the Rockefeller Foundation's malaria programs at the time, according to Sierra Iglesias, *Carlos Alberto Alvarado,* 8. It's not clear if Alvarado met Hackett in Italy, where he was stationed with the RF at the time, or not until later. In 1940, Hackett recalled meeting Alvarado two years earlier at a conference on tropical medicine in Amsterdam. L. W. Hackett diary, October 9, 1940, RAC.

12. Personal interview with Pedro "Peter" Alvarado, Jujuy, March 24, 2003.

13. Salvador Mazza was intensely involved, in Bolivia and Argentina, with the study of this epidemic. Writing years later, Lewis W. Hackett reported that Mazza was deeply offended by Alvarado's having been appointed over him to supervise yellow fever control, and afterward the two were no longer on speaking terms. L. W. Hackett diary, October 12, 1941, RAC.

14. In Jujuy, soon after the inception of the Malaria Service, Jaime Carrillo had executed a few intensive saneamiento works on the banks of the Río Grande (see chapter 3), but after 1916 no work was done for about a decade, due to budgetary problems. Starting up again in 1924, Ricardo Alvarado directed various works similar to those in Monteros, that is, based on a model of *piccola bonifica*. The 1928 DNH report on progress against malaria proudly proclaimed the advances in saneamiento in Jujuy. According to the report, malaria indices had declined from 40.11 percent in 1913 to an average of 26.00 percent in 1927 (the late-season or "epidemic" index). Starting in 1928, E. R. Rickard collaborated with Ricardo Alvarado in a study of the malaria problem in Jujuy. This study included a thorough census of San Salvador and its suburbs; the highest malaria incidence (blood index) of any neighborhood was 33.6 percent, and the low was 2.8 percent. Rickard was unable to continue research in Jujuy because of the RF's sudden departure. Letter from Rickard to Davis, Tucumán, June 20, 1928, Nelson C. Davis Papers, Folder 3, Box 1, RF Archives, RAC; Barbieri, *La lucha antimalárica*, 19.

15. E. R. Rickard, "Report upon Eleven Months of Study of the Malaria Problem," 1929, unpublished report, Folder 62, Box 5, Series 301, RG 1.1, RF Archives, RAC.

16. Miguel Sussini, "El paludismo en la Argentina. Contribución al conocimiento de la biologia del Anofeles pseudopunctipennis. Nuevos métodos de lucha antipalúdica. Estudio presentado en la Novena Conferencia Panamericana, Buenos Aires, 12–22/XI/1934," *Anales del D.N.H.* 36, no. 1 (1935): 12.

17. Rickard, "Report upon Eleven Months of Study."

18. Sussini, "El paludismo en la Argentina," 16.

19. Antonio Barbieri, "Resultados alcanzados en la lucha contra el paludismo en la última década," *La Prensa Médica Argentina* 20 (1933): 379.

20. Ibid., 381.

21. Lozano and Selva, "Nueva orientación en la lucha antipalúdica," 776–78.

22. This meeting and the Second Panamerican Conference on Eugenics and Homiculture were held back-to-back since they involved many of the same public health professionals. Although public health and eugenics had many common interests, the panels on malaria at the sanitary conference mostly avoided reference to eugenics and race, unlike the proceedings of the 1926 National Medical Conference or the 1923 National Sanitary Conference, discussed in the previous chapter. See *Actas generales de la Novena Conferencia Sanitaria Panamericana* (Buenos Aires: n.p., 1934); *Actas de la Segunda Conferencia Panamericana de Eugenesia y Homicultura de las Repúblicas Americanas, Celebrada en Buenos Aires desde el 23 hasta el 25 de Noviembre de 1934* (Buenos Aires: Imp. Frascoli y Bindi, 1934); Stepan, *Hour of Eugenics.* See also various articles in *La Prensa* (Buenos Aires), November 12–26, 1934; Soper's diary, November 10–23, 1934, Fred L. Soper Papers.

23. Paterson, "Las fiebres palúdicas en Jujuy," 31–57.

24. Sierra Iglesias, *Vida y obra del Doctor Guillermo Cleland Paterson,* 36–39.

25. Emphasis mine.

26. Paterson, "Las fiebres palúdicas en Jujuy," 48, emphasis mine.

27. Ibid.

28. Juana Petrocchi, *Mosquitos trasmisores: Guía para su clasificación. D.N.H.* (Buenos Aires: R.A.C.P., 1924), 22. Emphasis on "springs" (*vertientes*) and "lama" retained from the original text. I have retained *lama* without translation because its multivalent meanings are part of the crux of the problem of understanding malarious wetland environments and because Petrocchi defines it so carefully in the text. Petrocchi participated in a research expedition in 1924 led by Peter Mühlens, where she expanded on her research on anopheles mosquitoes of the region, but died before the study was published. See Mühlens et al., "Estudios sobre paludismo y hematología," esp. 251–70.

29. Alois Bachmann, "Programa de lucha para llevarse a cabo en Famaillá contra los anófeles y sus larvas," *Anales del D.N.H.* 27, no. 3 (1921): 117–37.

30. Bachmann, "Programa de lucha," cited in Sussini, "El paludismo en la Argentina," 13; emphasis mine. I have translated the word *lama* from the original text to "mat of algae," but Driever and Espejo-Saavedra's Spanish-English geographical dictionary also includes "slime," "mud," "silt," "ooze," "alga found in pools of water or in a mire," and "layer of cryptogamic (nonflowering) plants (algae, ferns, etc.) that grow in fresh water" as definitions. Steven L. Driever and Rafael Espejo-Saavedra, *Spanish/English Dictionary of Human and Physical Geography* (Westport, CT: Greenwood Press, 1994).

31. Barbieri, *La lucha antimalárica,* 14.

32. Compare Barbieri, *La lucha antimalárica,* 14–15, with Bachmann, "Programa de lucha," 117–37.

33. Davis, Rickard, and Shannon seemed to be aware of Paterson's research, yet did not always give him due credit. On his initial visit to Jujuy, Davis (in the company of George K. Strode) met with Paterson, who shared his idea that *A. pseudo* was the only important vector for malaria in the region. A few months later, Davis recorded notes from Paterson's 1911 article in his field notebook. However, in his report on control work in Argentina, published as part of the *Annual Report* of the RF for 1926, Davis seems to take credit for the "establishment of *A. pseudopunctipennis* as the chief vector of malaria in Tucumán," but without acknowledging Paterson. Similarly, in a 1927 article published in *La Semana Médica,* Davis, along with Martín Lobo and Félix Cabarrou, implied that their discovery of the intense anthropophilia of *A. pseudo* was independent, again neglecting to mention Paterson. In at least one publication, in a 1927 piece on the distribution of *A. pseudo* in Argentina, in the *Revista del Instituto Bacteriológico,* the RF scientists do cite Paterson's 1911 article. My interpretation is that Davis and his colleagues felt that Paterson's hypothesis was plausible and worth investigating, but that Paterson himself had not done sufficient research to prove it convincingly. Therefore they regarded their own findings as original. Letter from Strode to Russell, September 12, 1925, Folder 58, Box 5, Series 301, RG 1.1, RF Archives, RAC; Nelson C. Davis field notebook, January 1926, Folder 64, Box 9, Nelson C. Davis Papers, RF Archives, RAC; Rockefeller Foundation, *Annual Report,* 1926, 212–14; Davis, Lobo, and Cabarrou, "Lucha antipalúdica en Medinas," 12; Shannon, Davis, and Del Ponte, "La distribución del Anopheles pseudopunctipennis," 680.

34. Shannon, "Summary of Investigations on Anopheles in Argentina 1926–1927," 277; Rickard, "Estudios sobre el alcance de vuelo," 131.

35. Rickard, "Estudios sobre el alcance de vuelo," 138. Sussini and others later exaggerated these results to conclude that the mosquito's flight range was four to six kilometers, but in Rickard's original experiment he characterized four kilometers as the "normal maximum" flight range.

36. Nelson C. Davis and E. R. Rickard, "Plan de lucha contra la malaria urbana en el norte argentino," in *Cuarta reunión de la Sociedad Argentina de patología regional del norte: Santiago del Estero, 7, 8 y 9 de mayo de 1928* (Buenos Aires: Imprenta La Universidad, 1928), 120.

37. Shannon, "Summary of Investigations on Anopheles in Argentina 1926–1927," 275–76. More recent entomological research led by María Julia Dantur Juri in the Argentine Yungas generally confirms Shannon's assessment of the ecology and geographical distribution of *A. pseudo* and discovers, in line with Alvarado, that this mosquito prefers disturbed environments, described as edge habitats between forests and cultivated land. See Maria Julia Dantur Juri, Mario Zaidenberg, and Walter Almiron, "Distribución espacial de Anopheles pseudopunctipennis en las Yungas de Salta, Argentina," *Rev. Saúde Pública* 39, no. 4 (2005): 565–70.

38. Shannon, Davis, and Del Ponte, "La distribución del Anopheles pseudopunctipennis," 693–95.

39. The *Nyssorhynchus* group is a subgenus of anopheles that includes *A. albitarsis, A. argyritarsis,* and *A. darlingi.* Mosquitoes of this group, however, are not necessarily harmless: *A. darlingi* is the major vector of malaria in the Brazilian Amazon and Northeast Argentina. Michael E. Faran and Kenneth J. Linthicum, "A Handbook of the Amazonian Species of Anopheles (Nyssorhynchus) (Diptera: Culicidae)," *Mosquito Systematics* 13, no. 1 (1981): 1–81; E. L. Peyton, Richard C. Wilkerson, and Ralph E. Harbach, "Comparative Analysis of the Subegenera Kerteszia and Nyssorhynchus of Anopheles (Diptera: Culicidae)," *Mosquito Systematics* 24, no. 1 (1992): 51–62.

40. Davis and Rickard, "Plan de lucha contra la malaria urbana," 127.

41. This is hearsay: Sr. Díaz Quieta, who assisted Davis, reported this to Sussini ("El paludismo en la Argentina," 15). However, in an article Davis and Rickard stated, "It was hoped that drainage (commonly known as saneamiento) would resolve the problem. Only in rare places would that happen. In most places, on the other hand, expensive drainage operations not only do not improve the situation but rather could make it worse." Davis and Rickard, "Plan de lucha contra la malaria urbana," 127. Davis and Rickard were clearly ambivalent about drainage for mosquito control, since in the same article they called it "the best means of extinguishing larvae" where it was "practicable" to do so (see note 36).

42. The public health hazards of rice farming had been debated for some time in the Northwest, especially in Tucumán. Some politicians, agronomists, and others believed that Tucumán needed to diversify its agricultural economy, moving away from a reliance on sugarcane into crops like rice, whose demand in Argentina was met by imports. In November of 1914, a bill was proposed in the Tucumán leg-

islature to create a fund to stimulate the production of rice. Legislators who opposed the bill (perhaps representatives of the sugar interests, but that is hard to say for sure) utilized the threat of malaria in an attempt to defeat the law; in their view, the standing water of rice paddies created ideal foci for mosquito breeding. A Japanese agronomist serving as consultant to the legislature on rice cultivation affirmed that the cultivation of rice did not present any malaria risk and suggested that the opposition used the threat of malaria to attempt to defeat a law that went against their own economic interests. The bill passed anyway, but for years to follow the DNH would recommend the prohibition of rice farming in the malarious zone. Even Davis, after the first year of RF control work in Medinas, suspected rice fields west of the town as prime sites of anopheles production (see discussion in chapter 3). *El Orden,* October 26, 1914, D.N.H., "El cultivo de arroz en las zonas palúdicas," *Boletín Sanitario del D.N.H.* 4 (1940): 488; Rockefeller Foundation, *Annual Report,* 1925, 256.

43. Mazza and Rickard, "Relación del cultivo de arroz," 707–11; Mazza and Rickard, "Investigación sobre las relaciones," 175–80.

44. For his part, Alvarado was not convinced that rice cultivation was so innocuous. In the late 1930s, he commissioned epidemiological studies in rice-cultivating areas in southern Tucumán and the Salta lowlands and found that some irrigation techniques promoted *A. pseudo* breeding. But Hackett, testifying on malaria legislation in the Argentine senate in 1941, argued that there was no evidence that rice farming increased incidence of malaria in the Northwest. See Alvarado, "Arrozales y paludismo," *La Prensa* (Buenos Aires), October 2–3, 1941; L. W. Hackett diary, July 24, 1941, RAC; *Memoria de la Dirección General de Paludismo 1939* (1940), 35; *Memoria de la Dirección General de Paludismo 1941* (1942), 31. These *Memorias* (reports) of the Malaria Service were published on a yearly basis from 1938 to 1946. All of them were authored by Carlos Alvarado, drawing on data reported by other agency officials. Hereafter, I will cite this publication simply as *Memoria,* followed by the year of coverage, and the year of publication in parentheses. Prior to 1943, the report was published by the DNH, and after that by the new DNSP (Dirección Nacional de Salud Pública).

45. Sussini, "El paludismo en la Argentina," 17.

46. Carlos A. Alvarado, "La lucha contra el paludismo en el país," *Boletín Sanitario del D.N.H.* 2, no. 5 (1938): 5. Perhaps Alvarado was being charitable, since the impact of saneamiento on agricultural development was also dubious. I have translated *lodazales* from the original text as "quagmires," though it could also mean "any place full of mud (mudhole, quagmire)" according to Driever and Espejo-Saavedra, *Spanish/English Dictionary.*

47. Miguel Sussini and Carlos Alberto Alvarado, "Paludismo," *Monitor de Enfermedades Sociales y Endémicas* 2, no. 1 (1936): 27.

48. For a somewhat different interpretation, in which malaria control strategy in Argentina changes in response to continuous advances in entomology, within an atmosphere of perfect information-sharing among experts of diverse national origins, free of the political machinations I have described in the last two chapters, see Alvarez, "Malaria and the Emergence of Rural Health," 151–54.

49. It should be noted that Antonio Barbieri defended the Malaria Service's approach and accomplishments during his tenure. Perhaps sensing the self-serving nature of Alvarado's storytelling, Barbieri disputed the notion that foci patrol was radically different from saneamiento. Antonio Barbieri, "Los procedimientos de la lucha antipalúdica en la Argentina. Resultados hasta 1936," *La Prensa Médica Argentina* 24, no. 48 (1937): 2297.

50. Personal interview with Pedro "Peter" Alvarado, Jujuy, March 24, 2003.

51. D. J. Bradley, "Watson, Swellengrebel and Species Sanitation: Environmental and Ecological Aspects," *Parassitologia* 36 (1994): 137–47; Packard, *The Making of a Tropical Disease,* 136–40; Sufian, *Healing the Land and the Nation,* 204.

52. Bradley, "Watson, Swellengrebel and Species Sanitation," 137–47; Hughes Evans, "European Malaria Policy in the 1920s and 1930s: The Epidemiology of Minutiae," *Isis* 80, no. 1 (1989): 40–59; Hackett, *Malaria in Europe.*

53. Bradley, "Watson, Swellengrebel and Species Sanitation," 144.

54. Ibid., 138.

55. Ibid.; Stapleton, "Lessons of History?," 206–15.

56. Evans, "European Malaria Policy," 59. Evans writes, "The social-disease proponents [e.g., *bonifica* advocates] could not disentangle the disease process from its concomitant social ills; the entomological malariologist saw disentanglement as a necessary first step in conquering malaria."

57. Evans, "European Malaria Policy," 40–59; Paul F. Russell, *Man's Mastery of Malaria* (London: Oxford University Press, 1955), 207.

58. Due to the leading role of RF scientists such as Soper and Hackett, species sanitation became known as the "American" solution, while the social development approach of the League of Nations was labeled as "European." Coincidentally, Raymond Shannon, whose entomological research in Argentina inspired Alvarado, also discovered the first *A. gambiae* mosquitoes in Brazil in 1930. Fred L. Soper and John Duffy, *Ventures in World Health: The Memoirs of Fred Lowe Soper* (Washington, DC: Pan American Health Organization, 1977), 202.

59. Sierra Iglesias, *Carlos Alberto Alvarado,* 7–8.

60. Evans, "European Malaria Policy," 44–45.

61. As Hackett saw it, Fascist politics undermined the integrity and progress of malaria science in Italy. See Snowden, *The Conquest of Malaria,* 178–80.

62. *Register of Students,* 11: 97, Archives of the London School of Hygiene and Tropical Medicine, London, England (hereafter cited as LSHTM Archives).

63. The national ecological society in Argentina (Asociación Argentina de Ecología) was not founded until 1972. José Babini's comprehensive tome on the history of science in Argentina, published in 1954, offers no mention of ecology. See José Babini, *La evolución del pensamiento científico en la Argentina* (Buenos Aires: Ediciones La Fragua, 1954).

64. Lucy J. Howland, "A Four Years' Investigation of a Hertfordshire Pond," *New Phytologist* 30, no. 4 (1931): 221–65.

65. P. A. Buxton, "Applied Entomology of Palestine, Being a Report to the Palestine Government," *Bulletin of Entomological Research* 24 (1924): 289–340. See also Sufian, *Healing the Land and the Nation,* 145–46. In British Mandate Palestine,

Buxton conducted malaria work with Jerome Mieldazis, the sanitary engineer who accompanied H. A. Taylor on the first RF survey of Northwest Argentina in 1921. Buxton was also acquainted with L. W. Hackett, the RF's outstanding medical entomologist and malariologist, and traveled with him to Algeria, Tunis, and Sardinia in 1930. Letter from P. A. Buxton to Andrew Balfour (director, LSHTM), March 10, 1930, Patrick A. Buxton papers, part 1, LSHTM Archives. Buxton also played a role in some of the first testing of DDT against insects (lice, in this case), during World War II. V. B. Wigglesworth, "Patrick Alfred Buxton, 1892–1955," *Biographical Memoirs of Fellows of the Royal Society* 2 (1956): 75.

66. P. A. Buxton, "Seasonal Changes in Vegetation in the North of Nigeria," *Journal of Ecology* 23, no. 1 (1935): 134–39; Buxton, *The Natural History of Tsetse Flies; An Account of the Biology of the Genus Glossina (Diptera)* (London: H. K. Lewis, 1955).

67. F. E. Fritsch, "Some Aspects of the Ecology of Fresh-Water Algae (with Special Reference to Static Waters)," *Journal of Ecology* 19, no. 2 (1931): 233–72.

68. Lucy J. Howland, "Bionomical Investigation of English Mosquito Larvae with Special Reference to Their Algal Food," *Journal of Ecology* 18, no. 1 (1930): 81–125; Mary V. F. Beattie, "Physico-Chemical Factors in Relation to Mosquito Prevalence in Ponds," *Journal of Ecology* 18, no. 1 (1930): 67–80.

69. For further explanation of their collaborative research on mosquito-algae associations, see Mary V. F. Beattie and Lucy J. Howland, "The Bionomics of Some Tree-Hole Mosquitoes," *Bulletin of Entomological Research* 20, no. 1 (1929): 45–56.

70. Shannon, Davis, and Del Ponte had said as much in a 1927 article published in the *Annals* of the Institute of Bacteriology of the DNH. They also pointed out that the habits of *A. pseudo* differed in other countries (it was found from California, almost continuously in the foothills and valleys of mountain chains, through Mexico, Central America, and the Andes). In some places, depending in part on conditions of competition with other mosquitoes, it could be found in more "swampy" areas. See Shannon, Davis, and Del Ponte, "La distribución del Anopheles pseudopunctipennis," 67.

71. Donald Worster, *Nature's Economy: A History of Ecological Ideas,* 2nd ed. (Cambridge: Cambridge University Press, 1994), 207.

72. Alvarado, "La lucha contra el paludismo en el país," 7.

73. Carlos A. Alvarado, *Por la formación de una conciencia sanitaria en el país* (Tucumán: Ventriglia, 1938), 17. All italics in original, except "sine qua non," where I added italics. Original phrase for "see and record" is *ver y registrar.*

74. Sussini, "El paludismo en la Argentina," 20.

75. Alvarado, "La lucha contra el paludismo en el país," 15.

76. Paul F. Russell, "A Classification of Measures of Malaria Prophylaxis and Mosquito Control," *American Journal of Tropical Medicine and Hygiene* s1–21, no. 5 (1941): 681–87.

77. Prudencio Santillán, "Appendix: El paludismo en la República Argentina," in *Manual de control del paludismo,* edited by R. Svensson (Buenos Aires: Editorial Shell, 1945), 154–56. For a thorough classification of "natural," "chemical," and

"mechanical" methods of larval mosquito control (before DDT obviated the need for most of them), see Russell, "A Classification of Measures of Malaria Prophylaxis and Mosquito Control," 681–87.

78. In his comments on a 1942 congressional bill to reorganize the Malaria Service, Alvarado questioned the legislation's very specific language regarding control methods, even though it basically conformed to the foci patrol strategy. Alvarado argued that "any procedure recognized as effective" should be used in malaria control. It seems, first, that Alvarado wished to keep strategic decisions the prerogative of the Malaria Service, rather than having them codified in legislation. Second, this demonstrates again that he was not convinced that foci patrol was the best technique for malaria control—just the best available one. See, Carlos Alberto Alvarado, "Comentarios a los proyectos de nueva ley de profilaxis y lucha antipalúdica," *La Semana Médica* 49, no. 28 (1942): 82.

79. D.N.H., "Memoria del D.N.H. correspondiente al año 1935. Buenos Aires, 10 Marzo 1936," *Boletín Sanitario del D.N.H.* Supl. No. 1 (1937): 100. The use of prison laborers in the earliest stages of this work was exceptional, since by necessity they worked in teams under the supervision of guards. See Sierra Iglesias, *Carlos Alberto Alvarado,* 59.

80. Sierra Iglesias, *Carlos Alberto Alvarado,* 49.

81. C. A. Alvarado, "Métodos de lucha antipalúdica en la República Argentina. Informe presentado a la Décima Conferencia Sanitaria Panamericana por el Dr. Miguel Sussini, presidente del Departamento Nacional de Higiene," *Boletín Sanitario del D.N.H.* 3 (1938): 14. For a version of one of these malaria control zone maps (for Ledesma), see Sierra Iglesias, *Carlos Alberto Alvarado,* 163.

82. *Memoria 1944* (1945), 7. Alvarado and other Malaria Service scientists hypothesized that *A. pseudo* could also hibernate in egg state, but never discovered any conclusive evidence. In Ledesma and points north (e.g., Orán, Tartagal) *A. pseudo* mosquitoes commonly continued breeding, though at a slower rate, through the winter. While larvae of *A. pseudo* could withstand extreme cold better than other mosquito species, harsh winters usually resulted in relatively mild malaria seasons.

83. See, for example, Paul S. Sutter, "Nature's Agents or Agents of Empire? Entomological Workers and Environmental Change during the Construction of the Panama Canal," *Isis* 98 (2007): 738; Packard and Gadelha, "A Land Filled with Mosquitoes," 197–213; Snowden, *The Conquest of Malaria,* 165; Edmund Russell, *War and Nature: Fighting Humans and Insects with Chemicals from World War I to Silent Spring* (Cambridge: Cambridge University Press, 2001), 112–18.

84. Alvarado, *Por la formación de una conciencia sanitaria,* 17.

85. Personal interview with Pedro "Peter" Alvarado, Jujuy, March 24, 2003.

86. Alvarado, "La lucha contra el paludismo en el país," 3.

87. Sussini and Alvarado, "Paludismo," 28.

88. Personal interview with Pedro "Peter" Alvarado, Jujuy, March 24, 2003.

89. Ibid.

90. Alvarado, "La lucha contra el paludismo en el país," 7.

91. Alvarado, "Métodos de lucha antipalúdica," 14.

92. Alvarado, *Por la formación de una conciencia sanitaria,* 11.

93. The blood surveys conducted by Mühlens et al. ("Estudios sobre paludismo y hematología"), Malaria Service surveys in Monteros, and the RF-sponsored activity in Concepción and Medinas were among the few instances where baseline epidemiological surveys (e.g., blood or spleen indices) were conducted before Alvarado took over.

94. Barbieri, *La lucha antimalárica.* This document *does* feature some blood and spleen indices, but almost all relate to locales where the RF experiments were being carried out; other statistics, such as number of malaria cases (even differentiated by parasite type) are aggregated to such a broad spatial scale (province or, at best, Malaria Service district) as to be useless for assessing the effectiveness of control works.

95. Alvarado, "La lucha contra el paludismo en el país," 13.

96. Ibid. For reference, in 1938 one US dollar was worth about 3.86 pesos. Gerardo Della Paolera and Alan M. Taylor, *Straining at the Anchor: The Argentine Currency Board and the Search for Macroeconomic Stability, 1880–1935* (Chicago: University of Chicago Press, 2001), 191. But, without knowing much about relative costs (i.e., purchasing power of the currencies) it is hard to assess the accuracy of Alvarado's estimates.

97. Alvarado, "La lucha contra el paludismo en el país," 13; exclamation point in the original text.

98. By 1939, the total budget for the Servicios de Saneamiento, including labor and supplies, was 426,000 pesos, equivalent to 3.55 pesos per square kilometer covered by the services, or about 0.50 pesos per inhabitant of the area served by the Malaria Service. *Memoria 1939* (1940), 17.

99. *Memoria 1937* (1938), 4; Sierra Iglesias, *Carlos Alberto Alvarado,* 91.

100. *Memoria 1937* (1938), 3; Sierra Iglesias, *Carlos Alberto Alvarado,* 90.

101. These were Jujuy and Ledesma (Jujuy); Salta and Tártagal (Salta); Monteros, Famaillá, Concepción, and Aguilares (Tucumán); Catamarca (capital); and Río Hondo (Santiago del Estero). For reasons that are unclear, the Monteros office pertained to the Escuela de Oficiales Sanitarios (Sanitary Officers' School), which answered directly to Alvarado; this office used Monteros for field experiments and handled sanitation work in other locales in southern Tucumán Province. Sierra Iglesias, *Carlos Alberto Alvarado,* 95.

102. *Memoria 1945* (1946), 54. Outside contributions to the Malaria Service budget increased from around 45,000 pesos in 1940 to about 130,000 pesos in 1945.

103. Hollander, "Oligarchy and the Politics of Petroleum"; *Memoria 1943* (1944), 7; *Memoria 1939* (1940), 39–40. L. W. Hackett diary, August 23–31, 1944, RAC. On the industrialization of the Northwest in the 1930s, see Jorge Schvarzer, "Los avatares de la industria nacional," in *Lo mejor de Todo es Historia,* edited by Félix Luna (Buenos Aires: Taurus, 2002), 451.

104. *Memoria 1943* (1944), 37.

105. *Memoria 1942* (1943), 26.

106. Alvarado, *Por la formación de una conciencia sanitaria.*

107. Ibid., 5.

108. Dirección General de Paludismo, *Almanaque Sanitario* (Tucumán: Dirección General de Paludismo, 1939); Sierra Iglesias, *Carlos Alberto Alvarado,* 201–4.

109. *Memoria 1943* (1944), 34.

110. Páez de la Torre, *Historia de Tucumán,* 633–34; Eduardo Rosenzvaig, *Historia social de Tucumán y del azúcar* (Tucumán: UNT, 1986), 227.

111. Centro Azucarero Argentino, *Asistencia social en la industria azucarera,* edited by Emilio Schleh (Buenos Aires: Ferrari Hnos., 1943), 143.

112. Bolsi and Ortiz de D'Arterio, *Población y azúcar en el Noroeste Argentino,* 33–41; Campi, "Los ingenios del Norte: Un mundo de contrastes," 208; Emilio J. Schleh, *La industria azucarera en su primer centenario, 1821–1921; consideraciones sobre su desarrollo y estado actual* (Buenos Aires: Establecimiento Grafico Ferrari Hnos., 1921), 264; Palacios, *El dolor argentino;* Palacios, *Pueblos desamparados.*

113. The yearly reports, published from 1938 to 1946, were in themselves a manifestation of the organizational maturity, autonomy, and professionalization of the Malaria Service.

114. *Memoria 1942* (1943), 6.

115. See data tables in *Memorias* of the Malaria Service, 1940–1945.

116. *Anuario estadístico de la provincia de Tucumán,* 1905–1943; see also Carter, "Malaria, Landscape, and Society," 12–15.

117. Humphreys, *Malaria,* 149; Meade, "The Rise and Demise of Malaria," 77–99.

118. Julia Patricia Ortiz de D'Arterio, "Azúcar y mortalidad. Un análisis evolutivo de la mortalidad infantil y de menores de 15 años en el área cañera de la provincia de Tucumán," in *El complejo azucarero en Tucumán: Dinámica y articulaciones* (CD-ROM), edited by Alfredo S. C. Bolsi (Tucumán: Instituto de Estudios Geográficos, Universidad Nacional de Tucumán, 2002), 6–7.

119. Asociación de Profesionales de la Salud de Salta, Central de Trabajadores Argentinos, and Asociación Trabajadores del Estado, *El paludismo en la Argentina,* 3.

120. Curto de Casas, "Geografía de los complejos patógenos"; Martine and Jorge, "Se acabó el chucho," 70–88; Sierra Iglesias, *Carlos Alberto Alvarado;* Kohn Loncarica, Agüero, and Sánchez, "Nacionalismo e internacionalismo," 147–63; Alvarez, "Malaria and the Emergence of Rural Health," 137–60.

121. Antonio Elio Brailovsky and Dina Foguelman, *Memoria verde: Historia ecológica de la Argentina* (Buenos Aires: Editorial Sudamericana, 1991), 292–93; italics mine.

122. Ibid., 294; italics mine.

123. See, for example, James Stevens Simmons, "The Transmission of Malaria by the Anopheles Mosquitoes of North America," in *A Symposium on Human Malaria with Special Reference to North America and the Caribbean Region,* edited by Forest Ray Moulton (Washington, DC: AAAS, 1941), 121.

124. Petrocchi, *Mosquitos trasmisores;* "Juana Petrocchi," *Revista del Instituto Bacteriológico del D.N.H.* 4, no. 2 (1925); Susana V. Garcia, "Ni solas ni resignadas: La participación femenina en las actividades científico-académicas de la Argentina en los inicios del siglo XX," *Cadernos Pagu* 27 (2006): 162–64.

125. Indeed, this lack of expertise in entomology would even afflict the malaria campaign under Alvarado. The need for better entomological foundations for malaria control work in Latin America was pointed out at meetings of the Pan American Sanitary Bureau. During his tenure in Argentina, Hackett sometimes advised the DNH leadership and, perhaps not surprisingly, given his background, urged the agency to hire a full-time entomologist. Eduardo Del Ponte did part-time entomological work for the DNH, mainly on anopheles mosquitoes, and consulted frequently with Hackett. See L. W. Hackett diary, October 10, 1940, December 20, 1940, RAC.

CHAPTER 5

1. This chapter is a slightly revised version of Eric D. Carter, "'God Bless General Perón': DDT and the Endgame of Malaria Eradication in Argentina in the 1940s," *Journal of the History of Medicine and Allied Sciences* 64 (2009): 78–122.

2. Ramacciotti, *La política sanitaria del peronismo,* 169–71.

3. "Thoughts on South America," memorandum from IAL, November 22, 1937, and "An RF Program in Latin America," memorandum, December 10, 1937, Folder 1097, Box 148, Series 301, RG 2, RF Archives, RAC.

4. Marcos Cueto, "Laboratory Styles in Argentine Physiology," *Isis* 85 (1994): 228–46.

5. Marcos Cueto, "The Rockefeller Foundation's Medical Policy and Scientific Research in Latin America: The Case of Physiology," in *Missionaries of Science: The Rockefeller Foundation and Latin America,* edited by Marcos Cueto (Bloomington: Indiana University Press, 1994).

6. Ibid.

7. L. W. Hackett diary (see chapter 3, note 47).

8. Russell, *War and Nature.*

9. Cueto, *Cold War, Deadly Fevers.*

10. Oficina Sanitaria Panamericana, "Llamamiento regional a las armas, 1946–1958," *Boletín de la Oficina Sanitaria Panamericana* 113 (1992): 396–405; Cueto, *The Value of Health.* The PASB is presently known as the PAHO, Pan American Health Organization, with headquarters in Washington, DC.

11. Stepan, *Hour of Eugenics;* Karina Inés Ramacciotti, "Las huellas eugénicas en la política sanitaria argentina (1946–1955)," in *Darwinismo social y eugenesia en el mundo latino,* edited by Marisa Miranda and Gustavo Vallejo (Buenos Aires: Siglo XXI de Argentina Editores, 2005). For a discussion of Perón co-opting leftist social policy, see Donald Clark Hodges, *Argentina, 1943–1987: The National Revolution and Resistance* (Albuquerque: University of New Mexico Press, 1988), 24. Other scholars have challenged interpretations of Peronism as "top-down" political centralization and co-opting of class-based interests, instead emphasizing the agency of the labor movement in its affiliation with Perón; see, for example, Daniel James, *Resistance and Integration: Peronism and the Argentine Working Class* (Cambridge: Cambridge University Press, 1988). However, such interpretations seem less relevant to

the case of malaria control, negotiations of which took place within a relatively in-sular political arena of national government bureaucracy.

12. For details of Carrillo's biography and the diverse intellectual ingredients of his social policy, see Ramacciotti, "Las huellas eugénicas," 311–50; Ramacciotti, *La política sanitaria,* 45–52.

13. R. F. Alzugaray, "Ramon Carrillo o la salud pública," *Todo es Historia* 117 (1977): 10; Ramón Carrillo, "Hace veinticinco años cuando escribí la *Glosa de los Humildes,*" in *Contribuciones Al Conocimiento Sanitario, Obras Completas* (Buenos Aires: Editorial Universitaria de Buenos Aires, 1974), 2:278.

14. Alzugaray, "Ramon Carrillo o la salud pública," 12; Ramacciotti, *La política sanitaria,* 38.

15. Romero, *Breve historia de la Argentina,* 149–51; Rock, *Authoritarian Argentina,* 125–31.

16. Rock, *Authoritarian Argentina,* 125–31; Cueto, "Laboratory Styles in Argentine Physiology."

17. Romero, *Breve historia de la Argentina,* 153.

18. Hodges, *Argentina, 1943–1987,* 24; Romero, *Breve historia de la Argentina,* 156; Félix Luna, *Perón y su tiempo* (Buenos Aires: Editorial Sudamericana, 1984), 1:29.

19. Paul H. Lewis, "Was Peron a Fascist? An Inquiry into the Nature of Fascism," *Journal of Politics* 42, no. 1 (1980); Alberto Spektorowski, "The Ideological Origins of Right and Left Nationalism in Argentina, 1930–43," *Journal of Contemporary History* 29, no. 1 (1994): 169.

20. The iconography of Peronist propaganda was inspired not only by fascism, but also by Roosevelt's New Deal and Soviet Communism; see Marcela M. Gené, *Un mundo feliz: Imágenes de los trabajadores en el primer peronismo, 1946–1955* (Victoria, Buenos Aires: Universidad de San Andrés, 2005).

21. Romero, *Breve historia de la Argentina,* 159.

22. Ramacciotti, *La política sanitaria,* 49.

23. Alzugaray, "Ramon Carrillo o la salud pública," 17.

24. In fact, there was a short period under the pre-Perón military government when a new entity, the National Directorate of Public Health, subsumed the National Department of Hygiene (1943–1946). Technically, the Secretariat of Public Health replaced the National Directorate of Public Health in May 1946, and the Secretariat became the Ministry of Public Health in 1949. Ramacciotti, *La política sanitaria,* 32–38; Sánchez, *La higiene y los higienistas,* 107.

25. Carrillo, *Contribuciones al conocimiento sanitario,* 22, cited in Karina Inés Ramacciotti, "La política sanitaria argentina entre 1946–1954: Las propuestas de Ramón Carrillo," *Taller* 6 (2001): 52.

26. Carrillo, *Política sanitaria argentina* (Buenos Aires: Ministerio de Salud Pública de la Nación, 1949), 1:271; emphasis mine.

27. Ibid., 1:255.

28. Ibid., 1:292.

29. Hodges, *Argentina, 1943–1987,* 31; Hugo E. Ratier, *El Cabecita Negra* (Buenos Aires: Centro Editor de América Latina, 1972); Luna, *Perón y su tiempo,*

1:29; Rock, *Argentina 1516–1987,* 235. Figures from the 1947 national census validate this trend. In 1914, only 18.1 percent of native-born Argentines had been born outside of Capital Federal, but in 1947, 43.0 percent of native-born Argentines in the district originated from elsewhere in the country. For the province of Buenos Aires, analogous figures for 1914 and 1947 were 9.6 percent and 27.6 percent, respectively. Argentina, Dirección Nacional de Estadística y Censos, *Cuarto censo general de la nación, 1947,* 1:lxvi.

30. Carrillo, *Política sanitaria argentina,* 1:102.

31. Ibid., 1:168.

32. The moral critique of inequalities in health and social welfare that Carrillo and Perón developed drew on a long tradition in Argentine social thought. In fact, it followed a long line of writing on sanitation and public welfare going back to the parliamentary debates over the establishment of the national Malaria Service, the case for which was built, in part, on the severe inequality between the Northwest and Buenos Aires. The desire to resolve inter-regional imbalances in health had prompted many proposals to create a centralized national sanitary or public health authority, such as that proposed by the socialist legislator Leopoldo Bard in 1923. There was also a long line of muckraking journalism, often written by politicians and/or commissioned by the government, meant to expose the appalling conditions of the working class in the interior and particularly the Northwest. This tradition included Juan Bialet Massé's "Report on the State of the Working Classes in the Interior of the Republic" (1904); Alfredo Palacios's *The Pain of Argentina* (1938) and *Forgotten Peoples* (1944); and Juan Solari's *Argentine Pariahs: Exploitation and Misery of the Workers of the North* (1940). See Bard, *Profilaxis del paludismo;* Juan Bialet Massé, *Informe sobre el estado;* Palacios, *El dolor argentino;* Palacios, *Pueblos desamparados;* Juan Antonio Solari, *Parias argentinos: Explotación y miseria de los trabajadores en el norte del país* (Buenos Aires: La Vanguardia, 1940). See also Lagos, Fleitas, and Bovi, eds., *A cien años del informe de Bialet Massé;* Ramacciotti, *La política sanitaria,* 21–41.

33. Ramacciotti, *La política sanitaria,* 27, 31–39, 65.

34. Ibid., 46–52.

35. Museo Social Argentino, *Primer Congreso de la Población,* 1941, 377–78, cited in Ramacciotti, "Las huellas eugénicas."

36. Carrillo, *Política sanitaria argentina,* 1:167.

37. Ramón Carrillo, "Conferencia inaugural del Sr. Secretario de salud pública con motivo de la iniciación de los cursos de la Escuela de Biotipología y Ciencias afines," *Archivos de la Secretaría de Salud Pública,* April 1947; Carrillo, *Plan esquemático de salud pública (1952–1958)* (Buenos Aires: Eudeba, 1974), 4:100. Both are cited in Ramacciotti, "Las huellas eugénicas."

38. Karina Inés Ramacciotti, "Ramón Carrillo," in *Dictionary of Medical Biography,* edited by W. F. Bynum and Helen Bynum (Westport, CT: Greenwood Press, 2007), 308–10.

39. Susana Belmartino and Carlos Bloch, "Estado, clases sociales y salud," *Social Science and Medicine* 28 (1989): 501.

40. In an interview with Martine and Jorge in the early 1980s, Alvarado remarked that he took pride in *never* singing the Peronist anthem at public events—he only mouthed the words. Nevertheless, he and Perón appear to have gotten along well. Martine and Jorge, "Se acabó el chucho," 80–82.

41. Manuel A. Viera was one of Carrillo's predecessors, before the Secretariat of Public Health was formed in 1946. L. W. Hackett diary, May 2, 1945, RAC.

42. Later, it would become clear that the organizers of the conference had little political influence themselves, and most reputable physicians (in the eyes of Hackett) and many in the Peronist faction (such as Carrillo) also boycotted the conference. L. W. Hackett diary, September 25, 1945, RAC.

43. L. W. Hackett diary, September 25, 1945.

44. Ibid., September 23, 1945; *Memoria 1945* (1946).

45. L. W. Hackett diary, October 24, 1945.

46. Ibid., May 30, 1947.

47. Ramacciotti, *La política sanitaria,* 76.

48. Alzugaray, "Ramon Carrillo o la salud pública," 21.

49. Martine and Jorge, "Se acabó el chucho."

50. Ramón Carrillo, *Plan analítico de salud pública* (Buenos Aires: n.p., 1947), 2:785–830.

51. Ibid., 2:785; emphasis mine. Historian Karina Ramacciotti (pers. comm.) points out that Carrillo let subordinates compose most of the sections of the enormous *Analytical Plan,* so Alvarado was likely responsible for the section on malaria.

52. Carrillo, *Plan analítico de salud pública,* 2:810. It is noteworthy, however, that these improvements did not include outright swamp drainage, the classic saneamiento technique.

53. Harrison, *Mosquitoes, Malaria, and Man,* 218.

54. Ibid., 222.

55. Ibid.; Humphreys, *Malaria,* 140–54; Franco Agudelo, *El paludismo en América Latina,* 130–31.

56. Russell, *War and Nature,* 165–83.

57. For his part, Alvarado maintained a well-appointed library at the Malaria Service office in Tucumán, which received journals from Brazil, Great Britain, Italy, France, and the United States, among others. According to Sierra Iglesias, in 1944 the library had 2,301 books and pamphlets and 285 journals. See Sierra Iglesias, *Carlos Alberto Alvarado,* 105. When I visited this now-abandoned but mostly intact library (which resides in what is known as the Federal Sanitary Delegation to Tucumán), I discovered a ledger accounting for all of the library's loans. In 1946, to take one year as an example, Alvarado checked out well over one hundred articles, from such journals as the *Bulletin of the Panamerican Health Office, Bulletin of the U.S. Army Medical Department, Tropical Disease Bulletin, Transactions of the Royal Society of Tropical Medicine and Hygiene,* and the *Journal of the National Malaria Society* (US). Many of these articles focused on the use of DDT in malaria control.

58. Sierra Iglesias, *Carlos Alberto Alvarado,* 194.

59. Daniel Campi, "Los Ingenios del Norte," 186–221.

60. Letter from Carlos Alvarado to Hermino Arrieta, July 27, 1946, mimeograph in author's possession.

61. Sierra Iglesias, *Carlos Alberto Alvarado,* 274.

62. Carlos A. Alvarado and Héctor A. Coll, "Organización y resultados de la campaña antipalúdica que realiza la Dirección General de Paludismo y Enfermedades Tropicales del Ministerio de Salud Pública de la Nación," in *Primera Reunión Panamericana sobre Enfermedad de Chagas, Primera Reunión Conjunta de la Sociedad Argentina de Patología Infecciosa y Epidemiología de Buenos Aires, y la Sociedad Argentina de Patología y Epidemiología de las Enfermedades Transmisibles del Norte Argentino, Tucumán, July 10–16, 1949* (Tucumán: UNT, 1949), 6; emphasis mine.

63. L. W. Hackett diary, June 15, 1947, RAC. Later, Fred L. Soper recounted this incident, which may well be apocryphal: Alvarado, to make a point about "shutting the door on the past," literally conducted a "public burial" of the tools employed in the larvicidal phase of the campaign. J. Austin Kerr, ed., *Building the Health Bridge: Selections from the Works of Fred L. Soper* (Bloomington: Indiana University Press, 1970), 490, originally published as Fred L. Soper, "Nationwide Malaria-Eradication Projects in the Americas. V. General Principles of the Eradication Programs in the Western Hemisphere," *Journal of the National Malaria Society* 10 (1951).

64. Personal interview with Pedro "Peter" Alvarado, Jujuy, March 24, 2003.

65. Martine and Jorge, "Se acabó el chucho," 80. The original quote: "A este muchacho ud. le da lo que le pida."

66. L. W. Hackett diary, July 26, 1947, RAC. Hackett frequently took a jaundiced view of Argentine politics, and the relationship between his office and Perón was "sour and tense" even before Perón rose to power (Marcos Cueto, pers. comm., November 12, 2006). The relationship really deteriorated after Houssay and other RF-supported scientists were ousted from public universities for taking an anti-Peronist stance. Cueto, "Laboratory Styles in Argentine Physiology."

67. Karina Inés Ramacciotti, "Las sombras de la política sanitaria durante el peronismo: Los brotes epidémicos en Buenos Aires," *Asclepio* 58, no. 2 (2006). Ramacciotti, *La política sanitaria,* 127–29.

68. Carrillo, *Política sanitaria argentina,* 1:165.

69. Ramacciotti, "Las sombras."

70. Spektorowski has argued that Peron's "productionist" impulse was just as strong as his "social justice" philosophy. Spektorowski, "The Ideological Origins of Right and Left Nationalism." For more on the intrigues of an expatriate Austrian scientist developing Argentina's atomic capacity, see Mario A. J. Mariscotti, *El secreto atómico de Humuel. Crónica del origen de la energía atómica en la Argentina* (Buenos Aires: Estudio Sigma S.R.L., 1996).

71. Ramacciotti, "Las sombras."

72. Carrillo, *Contribuciones al conocimiento sanitario,* cited in Martine and Jorge, "Se acabó el chucho," 83.

73. Alvarado, *Por la formación de una conciencia sanitaria en el país* (Tucumán: Ventriglia, 1938), 17.

74. Alvarado, "Conceptos sobre el nuevo plan de lucha antipalúdica de la Secretaría de Salud Pública de la Nación," in *Anuario 1947–1948* (Tucumán: Universidad Nacional de Tucumán, Instituto y Escuela de Higiene, 1948), 21. This was a transcript of a radio broadcast on Radio Tucumán, November 12, 1947.

75. Sierra Iglesias, *Carlos Alberto Alvarado,* 204. Moisés Aizenberg, a doctor and amateur artist from Rosario, drew these cartoons around 1948. In using such imagery, Alvarado (and Aizenberg) may have been imitating the use of cartoon characters for malaria education in U.S. Army propaganda posters and film shorts during World War II. This included the use of the popular character "Private Snafu" in the short "Private Snafu vs. Malaria Mike." See Christopher Dow, "Private Snafu's Hidden War," *Bright Lights Film Journal* 42 (November 2003), http://www.brightlightsfilm.com/42/snafu.htm#4. Accessed February 12, 2006.

76. Russell, *War and Nature.*

77. This connection was made explicit in other Peronist public health propaganda. For example, a poster displayed at the First Argentine Exposition of Public Health in Buenos Aires, starting July 1948, entitled "La salud de la Patagonia," shows an army surplus truck emblazoned with a Red Cross symbol, cartoonishly out of scale, driving over the map of Argentina toward the country's southernmost territories. The headlights of the truck appear to symbolize the "light" of health being made to shine in the dark and forgotten corners of the nation's interior. See also Karina Inés Ramacciotti and Adriana María Valobra, "'Plasmar la raza fuerte.' Relaciones de género en la campaña sanitaria de la Secretaría de Salud Pública de la Argentina (1946–1949)," in *Generando el peronismo. Estudios de cultura, política y género (1946–1955),* edited by Ramacciotti and Valobra (Buenos Aires: Proyecto Editorial, 2004), 19–64.

78. L. W. Hackett diary, June 15, 1947, RAC.

79. *El Laborista* (Buenos Aires), May 29, 1947; personal interview with Pedro "Peter" Alvarado, March 24, 2003; Alzugaray, "Ramon Carrillo o la salud pública"; Angel Jankilevich, "Testimonio De Adolfo Alzugaray," *Hospital y Comunidad* 4, no. 4 (2001), 433.

80. Personal interview with Pedro "Peter" Alvarado, March 24, 2003.

81. *La Gaceta* (Tucumán), June 13, 1947.

82. L. W. Hackett diary, June 15, 1947, RAC. Details about the manufacture of DDT for Argentina's malaria campaign are scarce or ambiguous. It may be that Hackett was mistaken about the domestic manufacture of DDT in Argentina, as Sierra Iglesias states that there were multiple foreign firms from which Alvarado acquired DDT (in addition to Geigy of Switzerland, there were Dupont and Monsanto of the United States and Imperial Chemical of Britain). Only in 1955, again according to Sierra Iglesias, was "technical grade" DDT manufactured in Argentina, at a factory in Río Tercero (Córdoba) under license of Geigy. Sierra Iglesias, *Carlos Alberto Alvarado,* 197.

83. Alvarado, "La lucha contra el paludismo en el país," *Boletín Sanitario del D.N.H.* 2 (1938): 7.

84. Franco Agudelo, *El paludismo en América Latina;* Harrison, *Mosquitoes, Ma-*

laria, and Man; Andrew Spielman and Michael D'Antonio, *Mosquito: A Natural History of Our Most Persistent and Deadly Foe* (New York: Hyperion, 2001).

85. Alvarado and Coll, "Organización y resultados," 6.

86. Ibid.

87. *Noticias Gráficas* (Buenos Aires), September 27, 1947.

88. Alvarado and Coll, "Organización y resultados," 6.

89. Luis A. Silvetti Peña, "Desarrollo y método de la actual lucha antipalúdica en la República Argentina," *Asociación Interamericana de Ingeniería Sanitaria* 1 (1948): 9–20; Sierra Iglesias, *Carlos Alberto Alvarado,* 553. Alvarado might have been inspired by the modern efficiency ideas of Frederick Winslow Taylor; Ramón Carrillo certainly integrated Taylor's ideas into public health planning. See Ramacciotti, *La política sanitaria,* 69.

90. *Noticias Gráficas* (Buenos Aires), September 27, 1947.

91. Alvarado and Coll, "Organización y resultados," 9.

92. Sierra Iglesias, *Carlos Alberto Alvarado,* 196. This is similar to the amount of DDT employed in other countries at the time.

93. The more impervious surface, the longer the residual effect lasts, even for as much as one year. On permeable surfaces such as adobe, the effect is much shorter lived. See Gilles, Warrell, and Bruce-Chwatt, *Bruce-Chwatt's Essential Malariology,* 220–21.

94. Alvarado and Coll, "Organización y resultados," 8; National Pesticide Telecommunications Network, "DDT Fact Sheet," http://npic.orst.edu/factsheets/ddtgen.pdf. Accessed March 25, 2005.

95. Alvarado and Coll, "Organización y resultados," 8.

96. Harrison, *Mosquitoes, Malaria, and Man,* 227.

97. Sierra Iglesias, *Carlos Alberto Alvarado,* 287.

98. Ibid.; Silvetti Peña, "Desarrollo y método."

99. Alvarado and Coll, "Organización y resultados," 10.

100. Ibid; Alvarado, H. A. Coll, and S. F. Laguzzi, "El programa de erradicación del paludismo en la República Argentina. Las fallas de la campaña de dedetización y la organización del Servicio de Vigilancia," *Boletín de la Oficina Sanitaria Panamericana* 29 (1950): 1–6.

101. Silvetti Peña, "Desarrollo y método."

102. Ibid.

103. Carlos Alvarado, "Progresos de la lucha antimalárica en el continente," *Rev. Bras. de Malariol. e D. Trop.* 4 (December 1952): 303; emphasis on "homogeneous unit" mine; on "national," Alvarado's.

104. Ibid., Alvarado and Coll, "Organización y resultados."

105. Franco Agudelo, *El paludismo en América Latina,* 132–34.

106. Since the 1930s, Alvarado and his Malaria Service had engaged in work against other diseases including typhus, yellow fever, small pox, goiter, trachoma, and hookworm. With the dissolution of the old Malaria Service and the creation of the new agency Digesnorte, the responsibilities of his office widened even further.

107. Personal interview with Tulio Ottonello, Monteros, August 31, 2002.

108. Luna, *Perón y su tiempo,* 1:403.

109. Personal interview with Tulio Ottonello, Monteros, August 31, 2002.

110. These DDT-based products were advertised in Tucumán newspapers as early as 1947. According to the advertisements, "Pestroy" was distributed by Sherwin Williams Argentina and had a concentration of 6 percent DDT, more than the solution used by the Malaria Service. The J. R. Geigy Company of Switzerland marketed "Hormiguicida GEIGY" as an ant killer. Philips Argentina S. A. distributed the US-manufactured "Nebulair." *La Gaceta* (Tucumán), October 5, 1947, and October 12, 1947.

111. It is hard to accept this anecdote completely at face value. Alvarado told this story, as part of a speech on the role of Perón's social justice doctrine in public health, to a class at the University of the Littoral, in Santa Fe. According to Sierra Iglesias, Alvarado, who was not a Peronist, tried to avoid giving such a speech but eventually relented. In the speech, Alvarado may have sarcastically overstated his admiration for Perón. But if the story contains at least a grain of truth, it speaks volumes about the way that Perón was able to deliver his political message through "great works" carried out by a powerful state, which had the ability to reach into the remotest corners of the country. Carlos Alberto Alvarado, "Justicialismo en el saneamiento urbano y rural," paper presented at Universidad Nacional del Litoral, 1950, cited in Sierra Iglesias, *Carlos Alberto Alvarado,* 520–21.

112. See Cueto, *El regreso de las epidemias;* Cueto, "Appropriation and Resistance: Local Responses to Malaria Eradication in Mexico, 1955–1970," *Journal of Latin American Studies* 37 (2005): 533–59; Cueto, *Cold War, Deadly Fevers.*

113. Carrillo, *Contribuciones al conocimiento sanitario,* 376.

114. Sierra Iglesias, *Carlos Alberto Alvarado,* 549.

115. Carrillo, *Contribuciones al conocimiento sanitario,* 377. More recently, malaria scientists have admitted that these calculations of economic "savings" through malaria control are frequently exaggerated. See Gilles, Warrell, and Bruce-Chwatt, *Bruce-Chwatt's Essential Malariology,* 266.

116. Luis Guillermo Bähler, ed., *La nación argentina: Justa, libre, soberana* (Buenos Aires: Control de Estado de la Presidencia de la Nación, 1950).

117. Luna, *Perón y su tiempo,* 1:404.

118. Interview with Dr. Serafín Fernando Vera, August 22, 2002, Tucumán; interview with Dr. Néstor Taranto, November 5, 2002, Orán.

119. Decreto No. 16700, July 19, 1949; reprinted in Sierra Iglesias, *Carlos Alberto Alvarado,* 555–56. Karina Ramacciotti suggests another reason why it was fortunate that malaria was eradicated so quickly: in the first few years of his presidency, Perón gave Carrillo considerable latitude to carry out bold experiments in public health planning. After 1950, Carrillo was increasingly marginalized within the government, and control over public health policy was usurped by Eva Perón, who channeled government largesse through her eponymous foundation. Carrillo lacked the political clout to follow through on most of his initiatives in the 1950s. Ramacciotti, *La política sanitaria,* 167–71.

120. Natalio Gruer, Julio H. Ousset, and Carlos E. López Mañan, "Problemas

especiales en la campaña de erradicación del paludismo en la Argentina," *Anales del Instituto Nacional de Microbiologia* 1 (1962): 127–31; Juan F. R. Bejarano, "Paludismo en la cuenca del Plata y su erradicación," in *Segundas Jornadas Entomoepidemiológicas Argentinas* (Buenos Aires: n.p., 1971), 3:261–88; Organización Panamericana de la Salud, *La malaria en las Américas. Bosquejo de la batalla que libra el hemisferio para terminar con un viejo enemigo* (Washington, DC: Organización Panamericana de la Salud, 1963).

121. Alzugaray, "Ramon Carrillo o la salud pública."

122. Ramacciotti, "Ramon Carrillo."

123. Fred L. Soper diary, April 2, 1950, Box 12, Folder 2, Fred L. Soper Papers.

124. Sierra Iglesias, *Carlos Alberto Alvarado;* and Martine and Jorge, "Se acabó el chucho."

125. See letters from Alvarado to Soper, September 27, 1959, and October 19, 1959, Box 14, Folder 3, Fred L. Soper Papers.

126. See Bolsi and Ortiz de D'Arterio, *Población y azúcar en el Noroeste Argentino;* Carter, "Malaria, Landscape, and Society"; Sawers, *The Other Argentina.*

CONCLUSION

1. Jeffrey Sachs and Pia Malaney, "The Economic and Social Burden of Malaria," *Nature* 415 (2002): 680–85; Packard, *The Making of a Tropical Disease,* 216.

2. D. Bagster Wilson, "Malaria in the African," *Central African Journal of Medicine* 4, no. 2 (1958): 73; cited in Webb, *Humanity's Burden,* viii.

3. Peet and Watts, "Liberation Ecology," 15–16.

4. Carter, "State Visions," 279.

5. Craib, *Cartographic Mexico;* Mitchell, *Rule of Experts;* Scott, *Seeing Like a State;* P. Vandergeest, "Mapping Nature: Territorialization of Forest Rights in Thailand," *Society and Natural Resources* 9 (1996); Vandergeest and Peluso, "Empires of Forestry."

6. Brennan and Pianetto, *Region and Nation;* Juarez-Dappe, *When Sugar Ruled,* 6, n. 11–12.

7. See, for example, Rodriguez, *Civilizing Argentina.*

8. Daniel B. Botkin, *Discordant Harmonies: A New Ecology for the Twenty-First Century* (New York: Oxford University Press, 1990).

9. Karl Zimmerer, "Ecology as Cornerstone and Chimera in Human Geography," in *Concepts in Human Geography,* edited by Carville Earle, Martin S. Kenzer, and Kent Mathewson (Lanham, MD: Rowman & Littlefield Publishers, 1996), 180. Examples of the former include human ecology (as in the Chicago School of the 1920s and 1930s) and systems ecology, and of the latter, cultural-historical ecology (the Sauerian School) and political ecology. See also Worster, *Nature's Economy;* Gregg Mitman, *The State of Nature: Ecology, Community, and American Social Thought, 1900–1950* (Chicago: University of Chicago Press, 1992); Warwick Anderson, "Natural Histories of Infectious Disease: Ecological Vision in Twentieth-Century Biomedical Science," *Osiris* 19 (2004), 39–61.

10. Packard, *The Making of a Tropical Disease,* 10–11.

11. Anthony J. McMichael, "Environmental and Social Influences on Emerging Infectious Diseases: Past, Present and Future," *Philosophical Transactions of the Royal Society of London Series B-Biological Sciences* 359, no. 1447 (2004): 1057.

EPILOGUE

1. The discussion in this concluding section is based mainly on field observations and interviews conducted in northern Salta Province in November 2002 and March 2003. I spent most of that time in and around Orán, mainly traveling with personnel of the Malaria Service, with a shorter stay in Tartagal, where I also observed the Malaria Service in action (mainly conducting its newer dengue fever control work). At this time the Malaria Service was known as the Programa Nacional de Paludismo (National Malaria Program, often referred to as "La Palúdica" for simplicity's sake), a dependency of the Ministry of Public Health and Social Welfare, which also has a related agency, the Programa Nacional de Control de Vectores (National Vector Control Program). Statements from Malaria Service personnel and others in the area are taken either from transcripts of recorded interviews or my own field notes.

2. "Paludismo: Confirmaron el brote en El Cadillal," *La Gaceta* (Tucumán), January 8, 1979; Curto de Casas, "Geografía de los complejos patógenos en el territorio argentino," 138.

3. "Indice de láminas positivas, gestion 1995–2001 distrito V Bermejo," unpublished report, Programa Nacional de Paludismo (Argentina), 2002; author's interview with Nestor Taranto, Orán, November 5, 2002.

4. Recent research by the entomologist Maria Julia Dantur Juri, done with the cooperation of the Malaria Service, has begun to update and improve understanding of anopheles ecology in the Northwest. See Maria Julia Dantur Juri, W. R. Almirón, and G. L. Claps, "Population Fluctuation of Anopheles (Diptera: Culicidae) in Forest and Forest Edge Habitats in Tucumán Province, Argentina," *Journal of Vector Ecology* 35 (2010): 28–34.

5. Juan J. Burgos et al., "Global Climate Change Influence in the Distribution of Some Pathogenic Complexes (Malaria and Chagas' Disease) in Argentina," *Entomología y Vectores* 1, no. 2 (1994); S. I. Curto de Casas et al., "Environmental Risk Factors for Diseases Transmitted by Vectors: A Case Study in North-Argentina," *GeoJournal* 44 (1998); Yola Verhasselt et al., "Geografía de la salud. Algunos factores ambientales de riesgo para enfermedades transmitidas por mosquitos (Salvador Mazza, Salta, Argentina)," *GAEA, Anales de la Sociedad Argentina de Estudios Geográficos* 20 (1996): 288–97.

6. Noemí R. Aparicio, Miguel A. Sánchez, and Marcelo G. Cornejo, *Leishmaniasis: El mal del norte Argentino, Enfoque laboral sobre una patología rural* (Tartagal: self-published, 2002); O. Daniel Salomon et al., "American Cutaneous Leishmaniasis Outbreak, Tartagal City, Province of Salta, Argentina, 1993," *Rev. Inst. Med. Trop. S. Paulo* 43 (2001), 105–8.

7. On the relationship between climate and malaria incidence in El Oculto, see Dantur Juri et al., "Malaria Transmission in Two Localities in North-Western Argentina," 18.

8. Jan A. Rozendaal, "Vector Control: Methods for Use by Individuals and Communities," (Geneva: World Health Organization, 1997), chapter 9.

9. Ministerio de Bienestar Social de Jujuy, "Taller de Control de Foco para Prevención de Dengue," Microsoft PowerPoint presentation for public health workshop on control of dengue fever, Jujuy, January 2002.

10. Ramy Wurgat, "Viaje al corazón de la epidemia de dengue de Argentina," April 22, 2009, http://tejiendoelmundo.wordpress.com/2009/04/22/viaje-al-corazon-de-la-epidemia-de-dengue-de-argentina/. Accessed July 25, 2010.

11. Daniel Muchnik, "Dengue y otras pestes," April 4, 2009, http://weblogs.clarin.com/detrasdeltelon/archives/2009/04/dengue_y_otras_pestes.html. Accessed July 25, 2010.

Glossary

anopheles: Genus of mosquitoes, comprised of approximately four hundred species, that are the only vectors of malaria.

Anopheles albitarsis: Anopheline species commonly found in the Northwest, but ultimately harmless as a malaria vector.

Anopheles argyritarsis: Anopheline species commonly found in the Northwest, but ultimately harmless as a malaria vector.

Anopheles darlingi: A major vector of malaria in tropical South America, especially Brazil, and also found in Northeast Argentina.

Anopheles gambiae: The main vector for malaria in tropical Africa.

Anopheles pseudopunctipennis: The principal mosquito vector for malaria in Northwest Argentina; also found throughout the Andean countries and in Central America.

anthropophilia: Propensity of a female mosquito to take blood meals from humans.

arroyo: Creek or stream.

berro: Watercress.

bonifica: Italian term that was roughly equivalent in usage to the Argentine *saneamiento,* meaning "sanitation" and "beautification." *Bonifica umana* referred to treating or preventing malaria infections through the timely prescription of quinine. *Piccola bonifica* encompassed a suite of strategies aimed at mosquitoes in their adult and larval stages. *Grande bonifica,* which translated into Spanish as *gran saneamiento, saneamiento agrario,* or *saneamiento hidráulico,* consisted of massive drainage and land reclamation projects, at the landscape scale: river valleys, marshlands, and so forth.

brigada: Brigade.

Cámara de Diputados: Chamber of Deputies, the lower house of the Argentine national congress.

Cámara de Senadores: Chamber of Senators, the upper house of the Argentine national congress.

caudillos: In the politics of nineteenth-century Argentina, regional strongmen who controlled their subjects through patronage relations.

chucho: Commonplace vernacular term for malaria in Argentina's Northwest; derived from Quechua *chúhchu;* still a common term for "shivers" or "chills."

ciénaga: Swamp.

cinchona: A genus of trees (*Cinchona* spp.) from which quinine is derived; these trees are native to the eastern flank of the Andes Mountains and foothills.

Chagas disease: A parasitic disease spread by insects (*Triatoma* spp., or *vinchucas*) in South America.

criadero: Mosquito breeding or nursery area.

criollo: Creole or Hispanic; in Argentina, the meaning of this term has been subject to much debate but usually refers to the racial admixture of European, indigenous, and, to a lesser extent, African, that was characteristic of Argentine society before the great migrations of the late nineteenth century. See also chapter 1, note 13.

croquis: Sketch map.

culex: Genus of mosquitoes, comprised of common and generally harmless species.

curandero/a: Folk healer.

dedetización: Literally, DDT-ization, a strategy of house spraying for anopheles mosquitoes with DDT.

descamisados: Shirtless ones, a name given to (and cherished by) Juan D. Perón's followers from the lower classes.

encargado de sección: Section manager, designation used in place of "peon" in Carlos Alvarado's foci patrol model.

foci patrol: See *policía de focos.*

gaucho: The peasant or cowboy of the Pampas, a central figure in the mythology of Argentina's national identity.

higiene: Hygiene.

higienista: Proponent of public hygiene, circa 1880–1940, in Argentina.

ingenio: Sugar mill.

interventor: Federal overseer, appointed by Argentine presidents to govern provinces by decree under *intervención federal* process.

jornal: Workday, the unit of pay for a *jornalero,* or "day laborer."

justicialismo: Social justice ideology of Juan D. Perón's political party, the Partido Justicialista.

laguna: Lagoon or pond.

lama: Roughly, a mat of algae in a pond or stream.

lampazo: Burdock.

latifundio: A large estate, typical of the agrarian structure of Italy and South America into the 1900s (and after).

Law 5195: Federal law passed in 1907 that created Argentina's Malaria Service.

leishmaniasis: A disease, transmitted by sand flies (*Phlebotomus* spp.), that causes a disfiguring and rotting of the flesh; also known as American cutaneous or mucocutaneous leishmaniasis.

littoral: Literally, near the sea; in Argentina, the region comprised of Buenos Aires and other provinces of the lower Río de la Plata Basin. Though its boundaries are ambiguous, historically it is the country's core economic region and the counterpart of the interior.

lucha: Fight or campaign, as in *lucha antipalúdica* (campaign against malaria).

mixed infection: Infection with two or more species of plasmodium parasites simultaneously.

monte: Thick or scrubby vegetation; disused or waste land.

Nyssorhynchus: Subgenus of anopheles mosquitoes that includes *A. albitarsis, A. argyritarsis, A. darlingi, A. tarsimaculatus,* but not *A. pseudopunctipennis.*

paludismo: One Spanish term for malaria, derived from Latin word for swamp (*palus*); in Argentina, more than in other South American countries, malaria is called "paludismo" instead of "malaria."

pantano: Marsh.

patria: Fatherland or country.

peón: Peon or manual laborer.

piccola bonifica: See *bonifica.*

plasmodium: Genus of parasite that causes malaria in humans and animals.

Plasmodium falciparum: The most deadly species of malaria parasite, producing "malignant" or "tropical" malaria.

Plasmodium malariae: A species of malaria parasite, producing "quartan" malaria.

Plasmodium ovale: Rarest of human malaria parasite species, found only in tropical Africa.

Plasmodium vivax: A widespread species of malaria parasite, producing "benign" or "tercian" malaria.

policía de focos: Foci patrol, a malaria control strategy created by Carlos Alberto Alvarado in the 1930s.

Porteño: A native or resident of the city of Buenos Aires.

profilaxis interna: Internal prophylaxis, referring to malaria prevention and treatment efforts focused on the human patient (i.e., quinine medication).

quebrada: A narrow canyon, common in the Andean foothills.

quinine: An alkaloid derived from Cinchona bark, the oldest effective medication against malaria (as a curative and prophylactic).

ranchos: Rural shanties or shacks.

raza: Race, breed, or nationality.

Salteño: A resident or native of Salta.

saneamiento: Roughly, environmental sanitation, the generally preferred approach for malaria control in Argentina until the 1930s. The term can also signify "sanitation," "drainage of land," "reparation," "cleaning up," "reorganization," and "rationalization." Saneamiento encompassed a wide range of malaria control tools, from the personal level of preventive or curative medication (*saneamiento individual*) to agricultural drainage and irrigation works (*saneamiento agrario*) to broader schemes of rural social reform (*saneamiento integral*). Generally, however, saneamiento referred to landscape-

based techniques. Campaign officials also used "saneamiento" as a translation of the Italian term *bonífica*.

saneamiento agrario: See *saneamiento*.

saneamiento del suelo: Sanitation of the land, or sanitation of the soil, roughly
equivalent to environmental sanitation; see *saneamiento*.

saneamiento integral: See *saneamiento*.

spirogyra: A kind of filamentous algae associated with *A. pseudopunctipennis*
breeding sites.

subterráneo biológico: Literally, biological tunnel, a malaria control technique that
involves shading mosquito breeding areas, such as canals, with branches or
leaves.

tierra palustre: Malarious land or swampy land.

Tucumano: A native or resident of Tucumán.

vagón sanitario: Railroad car, equipped with a microbiology lab and medical
clinic, used by the MEPRA.

valle: Valley.

vertiente: Spring or spring-fed stream.

Yungas: A physiographic province of seasonally moist sub-tropical and tropical
foothills along the eastern flank of the Andes in Argentina and Bolivia.

zafra: Sugar harvest, which in Northwest Argentina usually lasted from May to
October.

zafrero: Worker in the *zafra,* or "sugar harvest."

zancudo: Vernacular term in Argentina for mosquito.

zanja: Drainage ditch or canal.

zona azucarera: Sugar-growing zone.

zoophilia: Propensity of a female mosquito to take blood meals from animals.

Note on Sources

This book depends mainly on primary sources that are often difficult to find, whether published or not. Most of the documentary evidence used in this book is found in Argentina, but there are also a few important archives in the United States and England worthy of mention. As an aid to scholars interested in retracing my steps or developing their own research projects, this discussion proceeds geographically, that is, by the physical location of the collections.

In Argentina, I conducted archival research in Buenos Aires, Tucumán, Salta, and Orán. In Buenos Aires, the single most important collection on public health and medicine is found in the general library of the Facultad de Medicina of the University of Buenos Aires. Most of the articles in scientific, medical, and public health journals that I have cited, including those published by the Departamento Nacional de Higiene (DNH), can be found in this library. The library of the Academia Nacional de Historia houses a complete run of the proceedings of the national congress (*Diario de Sesiones de la Cámara de Diputados* and *Diario de Sesiones de la Cámara de Senadores*), key reference materials, and historical monographs and journals. The Biblioteca Tornquist, housed inside one of the buildings of the Banco Central de la Nación, contains good sources related to the political economy of the Northwest, especially the sugar industry. The Archivo General de la Nación has an extensive collection of archival photographs. I also consulted libraries at the Academia Nacional de Medicina, the Asociación Médica Argentina, the Biblioteca Nacional (mainly, the *hemeroteca,* or "periodical room"), the Instituto Geográfico Militar (map library), INDEC (Instituto Nacional de Estadística y Censos), and the Sociedad Científica Argentina.

In Tucumán, the Archivo Histórico de la Provincia was my main source for local historical newspapers, particularly *El Orden,* the city's major newspaper of the late nineteenth and early twentieth centuries. The Biblioteca de la Legislatura houses the *Compilación ordenada de leyes, decretos y mensajes del periodo constitucional de la provincia de Tucumán,* a compendium of provincial legislative proceedings. The library of the Instituto de Estudios Geográficos (IEG) at the Facultad de Filosofía y Letras of the Universidad Nacional de Tucumán has a complete run of the *Anuario estadístico de la provincia de Tucumán,* initially compiled by the demographer Paulino Rodríguez Marquina. These annual volumes represent an invaluable source of information on all quantifiable aspects of Tucumán society from 1897 to 1943. Some of these statistical series, for example, on infant mortality and agriculture, have been compiled in digital spreadsheet format and are available from the IEG. With the help of a research assistant, I compiled data on hospital admissions, classified by cause of illness, which serve as the basis for statistical analysis of malaria incidence. The collection in the derelict library of the Delegación Sanitaria Federal was first developed by Carlos Alvarado himself, when it was the library of the Malaria Service (Dirección General de Paludismo). Having been abandoned, the collection is difficult to access but mostly well preserved; at the same time, it does not feature many unpublished or internal agency documents, which were presumably transferred and then destroyed at the national Ministry of Public Health in Buenos Aires. The archives of *La Gaceta,* the city's major newspaper, include archival photographs, organized by subject. In Tucumán I also consulted libraries at the Universidad Nacional de Tucumán (central library and Miguel Lillo Institute), the Casa Histórica de la Independencia, and the Sociedad Sarmiento.

Most archival research in Salta was conducted at provincial libraries. The Archivo y Biblioteca Históricos de la Provincia houses some historical newspapers, the *Recopilación* (compendium) of provincial laws, and an interesting collection of original registry logs for El Milagro hospital for the early 1900s. I compiled a sampling of hospital registrations to analyze temporal, spatial, and social patterns of malaria; little of this analysis made it into this book, but related results can be found in my 2008 article, "Malaria, Landscape, and Society in Northwest Argentina," in the *Journal of Latin American Geography.* Other Salta newspapers can be found in the hemeroteca of the Biblioteca Provincial Dr. Victorino de la Plaza. Gregorio Caro Figueroa generously granted me access to his private library in nearby Cerrillos, which includes a wide variety of holdings, mainly on the history of Argentina and the Northwest. While in Salta, I also consulted the Biblioteca Dr. Atilio Cornejo and the library of the local office of the Ministerio de Salud Pública. In Orán, Salta Province, at the base of operations for the Programa Nacional de Control de Vectores (today's incarnation of the Malaria Service), I compiled data from original epidemiological reports that detailed the circumstances of each and every case of malaria in the region from the 1970s onward; however, this data ultimately did not make it into the book, falling outside of its temporal scope.

In Argentina, I also received historical documents (originals or copies) from other historical researchers, including Susana Curto, Karina Ramacciotti, and Jobino Pedro Sierra Iglesias. For the most part, these were previously published documents, and I've tried to limit the use of unpublished documents I received from them, given the difficulty other researchers would have in retracing them. I also conducted interviews with people involved in Argentina's malaria campaign or other aspects of public health, and they are identified in the book's acknowledgments.

Generally, in Argentina I lacked access to internal reports, memoranda, correspondence, and other documents that shed light on the everyday politics and social relationships inside the malaria campaign. For example, the personal collection of Carlos Alberto Alvarado, which Jobino Pedro Sierra Iglesias accessed for his research in the 1980s, was said to be too damaged for me to use. Fortunately, and perhaps unexpectedly, two archives in the United States helped fill some of these gaps. The Rockefeller Archive Center (Sleepy Hollow, New York) maintains an extremely well-organized collection of documents related to the International Health Board's action in Argentina from 1925 to 1929, including internal memoranda, photographs, and correspondence, along with the diaries of two important Rockefeller Foundation officers, Nelson C. Davis and Lewis W. Hackett. The latter proved especially useful for understanding the internal politics of public health during the 1940s, when Hackett was stationed in Buenos Aires. In Bethesda, Maryland, at the National Library of Medicine, History of Medicine Division, I had access to the Fred L. Soper Papers, which include his typescript diary. Though Soper is usually not identified with Argentina, during his tenure with the Rockefeller Foundation and, later, with the Pan American Sanitary Bureau, Soper had frequent contact with Argentine public health officials, such as Carlos Alvarado. While Davis, Hackett, Soper, and other Americans were candid about their Argentine counterparts, their testimony must be taken with a grain of salt, since they were outsiders to Argentine culture and politics.

Finally, in England I briefly consulted the archives of the London School of Hygiene and Tropical Medicine for any documentation related to Carlos Alvarado's post-medical school education there, including information on the curriculum in tropical medicine and research by his colleagues and instructors.

Bibliography

PRIMARY SOURCES

Government Documents

Argentina

Cámara de Diputados de la Nación. *Investigación parlamentaria sobre agricultura, ganadería, industrias derivadas y colonización; Ordenada por La H. Cámara de diputados en resolución de 19 de junio de 1896. Anexo G: Tucumán y Santiago del Estero.* Buenos Aires: Tip. de la Penitenciaría Nacional, 1898.

Comisión Directiva del Censo. *Segundo censo de la República Argentina, levantado el 10 de mayo de 1895.* 3 vols. Buenos Aires: Taller Tipográfico de la Penitenciaría Nacional, 1898.

Comisión Nacional del Censo. *Tercer censo nacional, levantado el 1 de junio de 1914.* 10 vols. Buenos Aires: Talleres gráficos de L. J. Rosso, 1916–1919.

Departamento Nacional de Higiene (D.N.H.). *Anales del D.N.H.* 31 (1925): 1–205.

———. "El cultivo de arroz en las zonas palúdicas." *Boletín Sanitario del D.N.H.* 4 (1940): 488.

———. "El paludismo en la república. Conferencia Nacional de Médicos, Buenos Aires (Mayo 1902)." *Anales del D.N.H.* 9, no. 10 (1902): 449–524.

———. *Guía oficial.* Buenos Aires: D.N.H., 1913.

———. "Memoria del D.N.H. correspondiente al año 1935. Buenos Aires, 10 Marzo 1936." *Boletín Sanitario del D.N.H.* Supl. No. 1 (1937): 94–139.

———. *Precauciones contra el paludismo.* Buenos Aires: Taller Tipográfico de la Penitenciaría Nacional, 1900.

———. *Que es el chucho? Como se transmite? Como se combate? Instrucciones populares.* Buenos Aires: Talleres Gráficos de la Penitenciaría Nacional, 1909.

———. *Saneamiento de la ciudad de Salta. Informe de la comisión especial (anexo a la memoria del Ministerio del Interior).* Buenos Aires: La Semana Médica/Spinelli, 1901.

———. "Saneamiento de la ciudad de Salta." *Anales del D.N.H.* 7 (1897): 517–18.

Departamento Nacional de Higiene. Oficina de demografía. *Anuario demográfico: Natalidad, nupcialidad y mortalidad.* Buenos Aires: Oficina de Demografía, 1911–1916.

Diario de Sesiones de la Cámara de Diputados de la Nación, 1895–1949.

Diario de Sesiones de la Cámara de Senadores de la Nación, 1895–1949.

Dirección General de Estadística. *La población y el movimiento demográfico de la República Argentina en el periodo 1910–1925.* Demografía Serie D. No. 1. Buenos Aires: Gmo. Kraft Ltda., 1926.

Dirección General de Paludismo. *Almanaque Sanitario.* Tucumán: Dirección General de Paludismo, 1939.

———. *Memoria de la Dirección General de Paludismo.* Buenos Aires: DNH/DNSP, 1938–1946. (Cited as *Memoria* in the notes.)

Dirección Nacional de Estadística y Censos. *Cuarto censo general de la nación, 1947.* Buenos Aires: Dirección Nacional de Estadística y Censos, 1951.

Dirección Regional de la defensa antipalúdica de Tucumán. *Memoria de la Dirección Regional de la defensa antipalúdica de Tucumán correspondiente al año 1913. Al presidente del D.N.H.* Tucumán: Tip. Cárcel Penitenciaria, 1914.

Programa Nacional de Paludismo (Argentina). "Indice de láminas positivas, gestion 1995–2001 distrito V Bermejo." Unpublished report, 2002.

Jujuy

Ministerio de Bienestar Social de Jujuy. "Taller de control de foco para prevención de dengue." Microsoft PowerPoint presentation. Jujuy, January 2002.

Salta

Recopilación general de leyes de la provincia de Salta. Edited by Gavino Ojeda, 1937.

Tucumán

Album general de la provincia de Tucumán el el primer centenario de la independencia argentina. Buenos Aires: M. Rodríguez Giles, 1916.

Anuario estadistico de la provincia de Tucumán, 1897–1943.

Compilación ordenada de leyes, decretos y mensajes del periodo constitucional de la provincia de Tucumán, 1885–1909. (Cited as *CO-Tucumán* in the notes.)

Newspapers

El Cívico (Salta), 1895–1900, 1908.

El Laborista (Buenos Aires), 1947.

El Orden (Tucumán), 1895–1930.

La Gaceta (Tucumán), 1947–1995.

La Montaña (Salta), 1904.

La Prensa (Buenos Aires), 1934–1947.

La Provincia (Salta), 1924.

Noticias Gráficas (Buenos Aires), 1947.

Nueva Epoca (Salta), 1925–1933.

Tribuna Popular (Salta), 1905–1907.

OTHER PRIMARY SOURCES

Actas de la Segunda Conferencia Panamericana de Eugenesia y Homicultura de las Repúblicas Americanas, Celebrada en Buenos Aires desde el 23 hasta el 25 de Noviembre de 1934. Buenos Aires: Imp. Frascoli y Bindi, 1934.

Actas generales de la Novena Conferencia Sanitaria Panamericana. Buenos Aires: n.p., 1934.

Alberdi, Juan B. *Bases y puntos de partida para la organización política de la República Argentina.* 1852. Reprint, Buenos Aires: Editorial Sudamericana, 1969.

Alessandrini, Giulio. "L'Organizzazione della lotta antimalarica in Italia (con presentazione di film)." In *Tercer Congreso Nacional de Medicina: Actas y Trabajos, Tomo I,* 327–31. Buenos Aires: Las Ciencias, 1926.

Alvarado, Carlos Alberto. "Arrozales y paludismo." *La Prensa* (Buenos Aires), October 2–3, 1941.

———. "Comentarios a los proyectos de nueva ley de profilaxis y lucha antipalúdica." *La Semana Médica* 49, no. 28 (1942): 76–83.

———. "Conceptos sobre el nuevo plan de lucha antipalúdica de la Secretaría de Salud Pública de la Nación." In *Anuario 1947–1948.* Tucumán: Universidad Nacional de Tucumán, Instituto y Escuela de Higiene, 1948.

———. "Justicialismo en el saneamiento urbano y rural." Paper presented at Universidad Nacional del Litoral, 1950.

———. "La lucha antimosquito en la América tropical." In *Proceedings of the Fourth International Congresses on Tropical Medicine and Malaria,* 1577–1585. Washington, DC: US Department of State, 1948.

———. "La lucha contra el paludismo en el país." *Boletín Sanitario del D.N.H.* 2, no. 5 (1938): 451.

———. "Métodos de lucha antipalúdica en la República Argentina. Informe presentado a la Décima Conferencia Sanitaria Panamericana por el Dr. Miguel Sussini, presidente del Departamento Nacional de Higiene." *Boletín Sanitario del D.N.H.* 3 (1938): 891–904.

———. *Por la formación de una conciencia sanitaria en el país.* Tucumán: Ventriglia, 1938.

———. "Progresos de la lucha antimalárica en el continente." *Rev. Bras. de Malariol. e D. Trop.* 4 (1952): 301–5.

Alvarado, Carlos Alberto, and Héctor A. Coll. "Organización y resultados de la campaña antipalúdica que realiza la Dirección General de Paludismo y Enfermedades Tropicales del Ministerio de Salud Pública de la Nación." In *Primera Reunión Panamericana sobre Enfermedad de Chagas, Primera Reunión Conjunta de la Sociedad Argentina de Patología Infecciosa y Epidemiología de Buenos Aires, y la Sociedad Argentina de Patología y Epidemiología de las Enfermedades Transmisibles del Norte Argentino, Tucumán, July 10–16 1949.* Tucumán: UNT, 1949.

Alvarado, Carlos Alberto, Hector A. Coll, and Segundo F. Laguzzi. "El programa de erradicación del paludismo en la República Argentina. Las fallas de la campaña de dedetización y la organización del Servicio de Vigilancia." *Boletín de la Oficina Sanitaria Panamericana* 29 (1950): 1–6.

Alvarez, Antenor. "El saneamiento antipalúdico de La Dársena." *Cátedra y Clínica* 7 (1940): 353.

———. "La invasión del paludismo a la ciudad del Santiago del Estero y su saneamiento." In *Tercer Congreso Nacional de Medicina: Actas y Trabajos, Tomo I,* 685–99. Buenos Aires: Las Ciencias, 1926.

———. *Paludismo. Plan de defensa aprobado por el Congreso Médico para la ciudad y centros rurales de la provincia (Santiago del Estero).* Buenos Aires: J. Peuser, 1902.

Aráoz Alfaro, Gregorio. "La acción social de la universidad." In *Dos conferencias en la Universidad de Tucumán, Julio 1915.* Buenos Aires: Imprenta de Coni Hermanos, 1915.

———. "La formacion de un pueblo fuerte." *Anales del Instituto Popular de Conferencias* 4 (1924): 209–35.

———. "Nuestros problemas eugénicos, verdades dolorosas." *El Hospital Argentino* 3, no. 11 (1932): 516–17.

———. *Orientación y estado actual de la lucha antipalúdica. Discurso presentado al Tercer Congreso Nacional de Medicina.* Buenos Aires: La Semana Médica (E. Spinelli), 1926.

———. *Para que la patria sea grande y fuerte.* Buenos Aires: Flaiban & Camilloni, 1916.

———. "Profilaxis del paludismo. Plan de campaña del Departamento Nacional de Higiene." *La Semana Médica* 25 (May 23, 1918): 602–4.

Aráoz Castellano, Francisco. "El paludismo en la guarnición de Salta." In *Tercer Congreso Nacional de Medicina: Actas y Trabajos, Tomo I,* 700–706. Buenos Aires: Las Ciencias, 1926.

Aráoz, Ricardo. "El paludismo en Salta." *Anales del D.N.H.* 9, no. 4 (1902): 162–64.

———. *Introducción al estudio de la Higiene de Salta. Memoria presentada a la Junta de Sanidad por el Dr. Ricardo Aráoz con motivo de la posible invasión del cólera.* Salta: Emilio Sylvester, 1895.

Bachmann, Alois. "Programa de lucha para llevarse a cabo en Famaillá contra los anófeles y sus larvas." *Anales del D.N.H.* 27, no. 3 (1921): 117–37.

Bähler, Luis Guillermo, ed. *La nación argentina: Justa, libre, soberana.* Buenos Aires: Control de Estado de la Presidencia de la Nación, 1950.

Baldrich, J. Amadeo. *Las comarcas vírgenes. El Chaco Central norte.* 2nd ed. Buenos Aires: Impr. de J. Peuser, 1890.

Barbieri, Antonio. "Concepto de la lucha antipalúdica y su legislación." *Anales del D.N.H.* 31 (1925): 7–44.

———. "Cultivo y explotación de quinas en la República Argentina." *Anales del D.N.H.* 21, no. 2 (1914).

———. "El problema de saneamiento antimalárico en la Argentina. Consideraciones y antecedentes." *Anales del D.N.H.* 25, no. 2 (1919): 21–37.

———. "El saneamiento antipalúdico del Norte Argentino por la bonifica integral." In *Tercer Congreso Nacional de Medicina: Actas y Trabajos, Tomo I,* 455–70. Buenos Aires: Las Ciencias, 1926.

———. *La lucha antimalárica en la Argentina. Campaña contra la anquilostomiasis.* Buenos Aires: D.N.H., 1928.

——. "La profilaxis del paludismo en la Argentina: Proyecto de modificaciones a la Ley 5195." In *Conferencia Sanitaria Nacional, Buenos Aires 1923: Antecedentes, sesiones y conclusiones*. Buenos Aires: D.N.H., 1923.

——. "Los procedimientos de la lucha antipalúdica en la Argentina. Resultados hasta 1936." *La Prensa Médica Argentina* 24, no. 48 (1937): 2297.

——. "Resultados alcanzados en la lucha contra el paludismo en la última década." *La Prensa Médica Argentina* 20 (1933): 375.

Bard, Leopoldo. "Fuentes de recursos para la lucha antipalúdica en la República Argentina." In *Tercer Congreso Nacional de Medicina: Actas y Trabajos, Tomo I*, 471–75. Buenos Aires: Las Ciencias, 1926.

——. *Profilaxis del paludismo e impuesto sanitario. Proyecto de ley presentado por el diputado Dr. Leopoldo Bard a la Cámara de Diputados de la Nación, en la sesión del 25 de Octubre de 1923*. Buenos Aires: Cámara de Diputados, 1923.

Beattie, Mary V. F. "Physico-Chemical Factors in Relation to Mosquito Prevalence in Ponds." *Journal of Ecology* 18, no. 1 (1930): 67–80.

Beattie, Mary V. F., and Lucy J. Howland. "The Bionomics of Some Tree-Hole Mosquitoes." *Bulletin of Entomological Research* 20, no. 1 (1929): 45–56.

Bejarano, J.F.R. "Areas palúdicas de la República Argentina." In *Primeras Jornadas Entomoepidemiológicas Argentinas*, 275–304. Buenos Aires: n.p., 1959.

Bejarano, Juan F. R. "Paludismo en la cuenca del Plata y su erradicación." In *Segundas Jornadas Entomoepidemiológicas Argentinas*, 3:261–88. Buenos Aires: n.p., 1971.

Bialet Massé, Juan. *Informe sobre el estado de las clases obreras en el interior de la República Argentina*. 1904. Reprint, Montevideo: Universidad de la República Facultad de Humanidades y Ciencias, 1966.

Bunge, Alejandro E. *Las industrias del Norte. Contribución al estudio de una nueva política económica argentina*. Buenos Aires: n.p., 1922.

Bussolatti, María Teresa, and Nicolás Lozano. "El paludismo. Conferencia dada por la Srta. María Teresa Bussolatti, alumna del 40. año normal." *Anales del D.N.H.* 18, no. 6 (1911): 71–85.

Buxton, Patrick A. "Applied Entomology of Palestine, Being a Report to the Palestine Government." *Bulletin of Entomological Research* 24 (1924): 289–340.

——. *The Natural History of Tsetse Flies; An Account of the Biology of the Genus Glossina (Diptera)*. London: H. K. Lewis, 1955.

——. "Seasonal Changes in Vegetation in the North of Nigeria." *Journal of Ecology* 23, no. 1 (1935): 134–39.

Cantón, Eliseo. "Discurso en su recepción académica. Paludismo." *Anales de la Universidad de Buenos Aires* 15 (1899): 151–59.

——. *El paludismo y su geografía médica en la República Argentina*. Buenos Aires: Imp. La Universidad, 1891.

——. "Profilaxia del paludismo y provisión de aguas corrientes a varias provincias argentinas." *Anales del Círculo Médico Argentino* 16 (1893): 365.

Carrillo, Jaime. "El paludismo en Jujuy." *Anales del D.N.H.* 9, no. 3 (1901): 97–104.

———. "Informe. Memoria de la profilaxis antipalúdica correspondiente al año 1912." *Anales del D.N.H.* 20 (1913): 859–73.

Carrillo, Ramón. "Conferencia inaugural del Sr. Secretario de salud pública con motivo de la iniciación de los cursos de la Escuela de Biotipología y Ciencias afines." *Archivos de la Secretaría de Salud Pública,* April 1947.

———. *Contribuciones al conocimiento sanitario, obras completas.* Buenos Aires: Editorial Universitaria de Buenos Aires, 1974.

———. *Plan analítico de salud pública.* Buenos Aires: n.p., 1947.

———. *Plan esquemático de salud pública (1952–1958).* Buenos Aires: Eudeba, 1974.

———. *Política Sanitaria Argentina.* 2 vols. Buenos Aires: Ministerio de Salud Pública de la Nación, 1949.

Centro Azucarero Argentino. *Asistencia social en la industria azucarera,* edited by Emilio Schleh. Buenos Aires: Ferrari Hnos., 1943.

Cornejo, Andrés. *Atlas de enfermedades regionales del Norte Argentino.* Salta: Ministerio de Bienestar Social de la Provincia, 1980.

———. "La universidad de Buenos Aires y los médicos del norte argentino." *Cátedra y Clínica* 7 (1940): 365.

Correa, Antonio M. "El paludismo en Tucumán. Datos informativos." *Anales del D.N.H.* 19, no. 2 (1912): 189–207.

Cossio, Rufino. *Informe sobre el proyecto de ley de profilaxis y lucha antipalúdica. Producido en nombre de la comisión de higiene y asistencia social del H. Senado de la Nación, 3 de Septiembre 1941 (21a. reunión 19a. sesión ordinaria).* Tucumán: Editorial La Raza, 1941.

———. *La campaña antipalúdica en Tucumán. D.N.H.* Tucumán: La Gaceta, 1928.

Davis, Nelson C., Martín M. Lobo, and Félix G. Cabarrou. "Lucha antipalúdica en Medinas (pcia. de Tucumán)." *La Semana Médica* 34 (1927).

Davis, Nelson C., and E. R. Rickard. "Plan de lucha contra la malaria urbana en el norte argentino." In *Cuarta reunión de la Sociedad Argentina de patología regional del norte: Santiago del Estero, 7, 8 y 9 de mayo de 1928,* 119–30. Buenos Aires: Imprenta La Universidad, 1928.

Davis, Nelson C., and Raymond C. Shannon. "The Habits of Anopheles Rondini in the Argentine Republic." *American Journal of Hygiene* 8, no. 2 (1928): 448–56.

del Barco, Jeronimo. "Proyecto de organizacion del Departamento Nacional de Higiene." In *Conferencia Sanitaria Nacional, Buenos Aires 1923: Antecedentes, sesiones y conclusiones,* 129–35. Buenos Aires: D.N.H., 1923.

Delfino, Juan Carlos. "Epidemiología del paludismo. Su estado en la República Argentina." *Anales del D.N.H.* 11 (1904): 272–81.

Dietsch, Juan G., and Elías Goligorsky. "Cursos de malariología seguidos en Italia por la misión médica argentina." *Anales del D.N.H.* 31 (1925): 178–203.

Domínguez, Alberto. *Policía sanitaria: Doctrina, legislación nacional y provincial.* Buenos Aires: Editorial Depalma, 1946.

Franck, Harry Alverson. *Working North from Patagonia; Being the Narrative of a Journey, Earned on the Way, through Southern and Eastern South America.* New York: Century Co., 1921.

Fritsch, F. E. "Some Aspects of the Ecology of Fresh-Water Algae (with Special Reference to Static Waters)." *Journal of Ecology* 19, no. 2 (1931): 233–72.

Gallastegui, Eleodoro. "El paludismo en los departamentos de Tinogasta y Belén (Catamarca)." *Anales del D.N.H.* 9, no. 12 (1902): 661–65.

García, Pedro J. "Factores de éxito de la campaña antipalúdica." *Anales del D.N.H.* 18, no. 6 (1911): 15–19.

Gelly y Obes, Carlos María. "La personalidad de Ernesto E. Padilla." In *Asociación Tucumana Ciclo Cultural Año 1956.* Buenos Aires, 1957.

Giménez, Eleodoro R. "El paludismo en La Rioja." *Anales del D.N.H.* 9, no. 13 (1902): 702–7.

Gruer, Natalio, Julio H. Ousset, and Carlos E. López Mañan. "Problemas especiales en la campaña de erradicación del paludismo en la Argentina." *Anales del Instituto Nacional de Microbiologia* 1 (1962): 127–31.

Hackett, L. W. *Malaria in Europe: An Ecological Study.* London: Oxford University Press, 1937.

Howland, Lucy J. "Bionomical Investigation of English Mosquito Larvae with Special Reference to Their Algal Food." *Journal of Ecology* 18, no. 1 (1930): 81–125.

———. "A Four Years' Investigation of a Hertfordshire Pond." *New Phytologist* 30, no. 4 (1931): 221–65.

Huret, Jules. *La Argentina de Buenos Aires al Gran Chaco.* Translated by E. Gómez Carrillo. Paris: E. Fasquelle, 1913.

Jefferson, Mark. *Peopling the Argentine Pampas.* New York: AGS, 1926.

"Juana Petrocchi." *Revista del Instituto Bacteriológico del D.N.H.* 4, no. 2 (1925): 95.

"La campaña contra el paludismo." *Caras y Caretas,* December 23, 1911.

Levillier, Roberto. *Orígenes argentinos: La formación de un gran pueblo.* Paris, Buenos Aires: E. Fasquelle, 1912.

Lozano, Nicolás. "La higiene pública en la Argentina. Trabajo presentado al V Congreso Médico Latino-Americano y VI Panamericano." *Anales del D.N.H.* 20, no. 5 (1913): 991–1079.

Lozano, Nicolás, and Domingo Selva. "Nueva orientación en la lucha antipalúdica." In *Quinto Congreso Nacional de Medicina: Actas y trabajos,* 776–78. Rosario: Talleres Graficos Pomponio, 1934.

Malbrán, Carlos. "El paludismo y su profilaxis. Fundamento la ley de paludismo sobre la transmisión por el Anopheles." *Anales del D.N.H.* 10, no. 10 (1903): 441–53.

Mantegazza, Paolo. *Cartas médicas sobre la América meridional. Traducción de la edición de Milan (1858–1860), por el Dr. Juan Heller. Prologo por el Dr. Gregorio Araoz Alfaro.* Translated by Juan Heller. Buenos Aires: Coni, 1949.

Mazza, Salvador, and F. Calera Vital. "Consideraciones sobre un caso autóctono de paludismo a 3442 metros de altura." In *Quinta reunión de la Sociedad Argentina de patología regional del norte: Jujuy del 7 al 10 de octubre de 1929,* 718–23. Buenos Aires: Imprenta La Universidad, 1929.

Mazza, Salvador, and E. R. Rickard. "Investigación sobre las relaciones entre paludismo y cultivo de arroz en la provincia de Tucumán." In *Cuarta reunión de la Sociedad Argentina de patología regional del norte: Santiago del Estero, 7, 8 y 9 de mayo de 1928,* 175–80. Buenos Aires: Imprenta La Universidad, 1928.

———. "Relación del cultivo de arroz con la difusión del paludismo en la provincia de Tucumán." In *Quinta reunión de la Sociedad Argentina de patología regional del norte: Jujuy del 7 al 10 de octubre de 1929,* 707–11. Buenos Aires: Imprenta La Universidad, 1929.

Mühlens, Pedro, Roberto L. Dios, Juana Petrocchi, and A. Zuccarini. "Estudios sobre paludismo y hematología en el Norte Argentino." *Revista del Instituto Bacteriológico del D.N.H.* 4, no. 3 (1925): 251.

Museo Social Argentino. *Primer Congreso de la Población.* Buenos Aires: Museo Social Argentino, 1941.

Nikilson, José E. "Investigación sobre los indios matacos trabajadores." *Boletín del Departamento Nacional del Trabajo* 35 (1917).

Organización Panamericana de la Salud. *La malaria en las Américas. Bosquejo de la batalla que libra el hemisferio para terminar con un viejo enemigo.* Washington, DC: Organización Panamericana de la Salud, 1963.

Ovejero, Fabio. "Consideraciones sobre el saneamiento de la ciudad de Salta." Doctoral thesis, Universidad Nacional de Buenos Aires, 1895.

Palacios, Alfredo L. *El dolor argentino.* Buenos Aires: Editorial Claridad, 1938.

———. *Pueblos desamparados: Solución de los problemas del Noroeste Argentino.* Buenos Aires: Editorial Kraft, 1944.

Paterson, Guillermo C. "Las fiebres palúdicas en Jujuy." *Anales del D.N.H.* 18 (1911): 31–57.

Penna, José. "Plan de profilaxis antipalúdica. Texto de una comunicación al H. Consejo Consultivo, por el Dr. José Penna." *Anales del D.N.H* 18, no. 4 (1911): 5–17.

Penna, José, and Antonio Barbieri. *El paludismo y su profilaxis en la Argentina.* Buenos Aires: D.N.H., 1916.

Pérez, Alberto, and Rufino Cossio. "Trabajos en Monteros Viejo." *Anales del D.N.H.* 32 (1926): 36–48.

Petrocchi, Juana. *Mosquitos trasmisores: Guía para su clasificación. D.N.H.* Buenos Aires: R.A.C.P., 1924.

Pittaluga, Gustavo. "La habitación humana en la epidemiología del paludismo." In *Tercer Congreso Nacional de Medicina: Actas y Trabajos, Tomo I,* 217–32. Buenos Aires: Las Ciencias, 1926.

"Proyecto de plan de lucha contra el paludismo sancionado por el Tercer Congreso Nacional de Medicina." *La Semana Médica* 33 (1926): 501.

Restagnio, Antonio. "Campaña antipalúdica. La acción profiláctica concurrente de la Ingeniería Sanitaria." *Anales del D.N.H.* 19, no. 3 (1912): 315–414.

———. "Resultado de la misión a la región palúdica." *Anales del D.N.H.* 18, no. 5 (1911): 5–13.

Rickard, E. R. "Estudios sobre el alcance de vuelo del Anopheles pseudopunctipennis en el norte argentino." In *Cuarta reunión de la Sociedad Argentina de patología regional del norte: Santiago del Estero, 7, 8 y 9 de mayo de 1928,* 131–42. Buenos Aires: Imprenta La Universidad, 1928.

Rockefeller Foundation. *Annual Report*. New York: Rockefeller Foundation, 1925–1927.

Rojas, Ricardo. "Gregorio Aráoz Alfaro." In *Libro de Oro en Homenaje al Dr. Gregorio Aráoz Alfaro,* v–xvi. Buenos Aires: Imprenta de la Universidad, 1929.

———. *La Universidad de Tucumán. Tres conferencias.* Buenos Aires: Librería Argentina de Enrique García, 1915.

Russell, Paul F. "A Classification of Measures of Malaria Prophylaxis and Mosquito Control." *American Journal of Tropical Medicine and Hygiene* s1–21, no. 5 (1941): 681–87.

———. *Man's Mastery of Malaria.* London: Oxford University Press, 1955.

Santillán, Prudencio. "Appendix: El paludismo en la República Argentina." In *Manual de control del paludismo,* edited by R. Svensson, 145–69. Buenos Aires: Editorial Shell, 1945.

Sarmiento, Domingo Faustino. *Civilización y barbarie: Vida de Juan Facundo Quiroga.* 1845. Reprint, Mexico City: Editorial Porrúa, 1977.

Schleh, Emilio J. *La industria azucarera.* Buenos Aires: Centro Azucarero Argentino, 1935.

———. *La industria azucarera en su primer centenario, 1821–1921; consideraciones sobre su desarrollo y estado actual.* Buenos Aires: Establecimiento Grafico Ferrari Hnos., 1921.

Shannon, Raymond C. "Summary of Investigations on Anopheles in Argentina 1926–1927." *Rockefeller Foundation Quarterly Bulletin* 1, no. 4 (1928): 271–83.

Shannon, Raymond C., and Nelson C. Davis. "Condiciones de reproducción de A. pseudopunctipennis en la provincia de Tucumán durante la estación seca." *Revista del Instituto Bacteriológico del D.N.H.* 4, no. 7 (1927): 662–77.

Shannon, Raymond C., Nelson C. Davis, and Eduardo Del Ponte. "La distribución del Anopheles pseudopunctipennis y su relación con el paludismo, en la Argentina." *Revista del Instituto Bacteriológico del D.N.H.* 4, no. 7 (1927): 679–705.

Silvetti Peña, Luis A. "Desarrollo y método de la actual lucha antipalúdica en la República Argentina." *Asociación Interaméricana de Ingeniería Sanitaria* 1 (1948): 9–20.

Simmons, James Stevens. "The Transmission of Malaria by the Anopheles Mosquitoes of North America." In *A Symposium on Human Malaria with Special Reference to North America and the Caribbean Region,* edited by Forest Ray Moulton, 113–30. Washington, DC: AAAS, 1941.

Solari, Juan Antonio. *Parias argentinos: Explotación y miseria de los trabajadores en el norte del país.* Buenos Aires: La Vanguardia, 1940.

Soldati, Alberto L. de. *Iniciativas, proyectos y discursos en el parlamento argentino.* Buenos Aires: n.p., 1913.

Soper, Fred L., and John Duffy. *Ventures in World Health: The Memoirs of Fred Lowe Soper.* Washington, DC: Pan American Health Organization, 1977.

Steere, William Campbell. "The Cinchona-Bark Industry of South America." *Scientific Monthly* 61, no. 2 (1945): 114–26.

Sussini, Miguel. "El paludismo en la Argentina. Contribución al conocimiento de la biologia del Anofeles pseudopunctipennis. Nuevos métodos de lucha antipalúdica. Estudio presentado en la Novena Conferencia Panamericana, Buenos Aires, 12–22/XI/1934." *Anales del D.N.H.* 36, no. 1 (1935): 5–22.

Sussini, Miguel, and Carlos Alberto Alvarado. "Paludismo." *Monitor de Enfermedades Sociales y Endémicas* 2, no. 1 (1936): 27–32.

Terán, Juan B. *Una nueva universidad.* Tucumán: Prebisch y Violetto, 1917.

Tobías, José W. "Contribución al estudio de la defensa contra el paludismo en la República Argentina." *La Semana Médica* 30 (1923): 406.

United States Sanitary Commission. *Report of a Committee of the Associate Medical Members of the United States Sanitary Commission on the Subject of the Nature and Treatment of Miasmatic Fevers.* Washington, DC: United States Sanitary Commission, 1863.

Universidad de Tucumán. Extensión Popular. *El chucho (malaria, paludismo, etc.). Urgencia y manera de disminuir esta temible enfermedad.* Tucumán: Universidad de Tucumán, 1914.

Vallejo, B. E. "El paludismo en Tucumán." *Anales del D.N.H.* 9, no. 4 (1902): 168–69.

Vera, Carlos A. *Informe de los estudios practicado en Italia sobre paludismo, comisionado por el Gobierno de la Provincia de Tucumán.* Buenos Aires: Galileo, 1902.

Villafañe, Benjamin, ed. *El atraso del interior: Documentos oficiales del gobierno de Jujuy pidiendo amparo para las industrias del Norte. Apendice a la conferencia leída en la Reunión de Gobernadores en Salta.* Jujuy: B. Buttazzoni, 1926.

———. *Nuestros males y sus causas.* Buenos Aires: Juan Perrotti, 1919.

Watson, Malcolm. "The Geographical Aspects of Malaria " *Geographical Journal* 99, no. 4 (1942): 161–70.

Wauters, Carlos. "Zonas de regadío en Tucumán." *Anales de la S.C.A.* 63 (1907): 185–274.

Wigglesworth, V. B. "Patrick Alfred Buxton, 1892–1955." *Biographical Memoirs of Fellows of the Royal Society* 2 (1956): 69–84.

Wilson, D. Bagster. "Malaria in the African." *Central African Journal of Medicine* 4, no. 2 (1958): 73.

Wrigley, G. M. "Salta, an Early Commercial Center of Argentina." *Geographical Review* 2, no. 2 (1916): 116–33.

SECONDARY SOURCES

Academia Argentina de Letras. *Diccionario del habla de los argentinos.* Buenos Aires: Espasa Calpe, 2003.

Alvarez, Adriana. "Malaria and the Emergence of Rural Health in Argentina: An Analysis from the Perspective of International Interaction and Co-operation." *Canadian Bulletin of the History of Medicine* 25, no. 1 (2008): 137–60.

Alzugaray, R. F. "Ramon Carrillo o la salud pública." *Todo es Historia* 117 (1977): 7–27.

Andermann, Jens. *The Optic of the State: Visuality and Power in Argentina and Brazil.* Pittsburgh: University of Pittsburgh Press, 2007.

Anderson, Benedict R. O'G. *Imagined Communities: Reflections on the Origin and Spread of Nationalism.* London: Verso Editions/NLB, 1983.

Anderson, Warwick. *Colonial Pathologies: American Tropical Medicine, Race, and Hygiene in the Philippines.* Durham: Duke University Press, 2006.

———. "Natural Histories of Infectious Disease: Ecological Vision in Twentieth-Century Biomedical Science." *Osiris* 19 (2004): 39–61.

Aparicio, Noemí R., Miguel A. Sánchez, and Marcelo G. Cornejo. *Leishmaniasis: El mal del norte Argentino, Enfoque laboral sobre una patología rural.* Tartagal: self-published, 2002.

Appelbaum, Nancy P., Anne S. Macpherson, and Karin Alejandra Rosemblatt, eds. *Race and Nation in Modern Latin America.* Chapel Hill: University of North Carolina Press, 2003.

Armus, Diego. "Disease in the Historiography of Modern Latin America." In *Disease in the History of Modern Latin America from Malaria to AIDS,* edited by Diego Armus, 1–24. Durham: Duke University Press, 2003.

———. "El descubrimiento de la enfermedad como problema social." In *Nueva Historia Argentina, Tomo 5: El progreso, la modernización y sus límites (1880–1916),* edited by Mirta Zaida Lobato, 507–52. Buenos Aires: Editorial Sudamericana, 2000.

———. "Salud y anarquismo. La tuberculosis en el discurso libertario argentino, 1890–1940." In *Política, médicos y enfermedades: Lecturas de historia de la salud argentina,* edited by Mirta Zaida Lobato, 91–116. Buenos Aires: Biblos, 1996.

———. "Tango, Gender, and Tuberculosis in Buenos Aires, 1900–1940." In *Disease in the History of Modern Latin America from Malaria to AIDS,* edited by Diego Armus, 101–29. Durham: Duke University Press, 2003.

Asociación de Profesionales de la Salud de Salta, Central de Trabajadores Argentinos, and Asociacion Trabajadores del Estado. *El paludismo en la Argentina.* Salta: Editorial MILOR, 1999.

Babini, José. *La evolución del pensamiento científico en la Argentina.* Buenos Aires: Ediciones La Fragua, 1954.

Balán, Jorge. "El origen de la cuestión regional: Las alianzas con las oligarquías provinciales, requisito para el fortalecimiento del Estado nacional." In *El desarrollo rural en el noroeste argentino. Antología,* edited by Mabel Manzanal, 65–72. Salta: Proyecto Desarrollo Agroforestal en Comunidades Rurales del Noroeste Argentino, 1996.

Barrett, Frank A. *Disease and Geography: The History of an Idea.* Toronto: Atkinson College Dept. of Geography, 2000.

Barsky, Osvaldo, and Jorge Gelman. *Historia del agro argentino, desde la conquista hasta fines del siglo XX.* Buenos Aires: Mondadori, 2001.

Belmartino, Susana, and Carlos Bloch. "Estado, clases sociales y salud." *Social Science and Medicine* 28, no. 5 (1989): 497–514.

Bianchi, A. R., and C. E. Yañez. *Las precipitaciones en el Noroeste Argentino.* 2nd ed. Salta: Instituto Nacional de Tecnología Agropecuaria and Estación Experimental Agropecuaria Salta, 1992.

Biddle, Nicholas L. "Oil and Democracy in Argentina, 1916–1930." PhD thesis, Duke University, 1991.

Biernat, Carolina. *¿Buenos o útiles? La política inmigratoria del peronismo.* Buenos Aires: Biblos, 2007.

———. "Inmigración, natalidad y urbanización. El poblacionismo argentino y sus contradicciones frente a las preguntas por el desarrollo económico (1914–1955)." In *El mosaico argentino: Modelos y representaciones del espacio y de la población, siglos XIX–XX,* edited by Hernán Otero, 471–506. Buenos Aires: Siglo Veintiuno de Argentina Editores, 2004.

———. "La eugenesia argentina y el debate sobre el crecimiento de la población en los años de entreguerras." *Cuad. Sur, Hist.* 34 (2005): 251–73.

Bolsi, Alfredo S. C., and J. Patricia Ortiz de D'Arterio. *Población y azúcar en el Noroeste Argentino: Mortalidad infantil y transición demográfica durante el siglo XX.* Tucumán: Instituto de Estudios Geográficos, Facultad de Filosofía y Letras, Universidad Nacional de Tucumán, 2001.

Bosonetto, Julio C. "Distribución de los ingenios azucareros tucumanos." In *Geographia una et varia: Homenaje al doctor Federico Machatschek con motivo de sus bodas de oro con el doctorado 1899, 5 de noviembre de 1949,* 43–55. Tucumán: Universidad Nacional de Tucumán, 1951.

Botkin, Daniel B. *Discordant Harmonies: A New Ecology for the Twenty-First Century.* New York: Oxford University Press, 1990.

Bradley, D. J. "Watson, Swellengrebel and Species Sanitation: Environmental and Ecological Aspects." *Parassitologia* 36 (1994): 137–47.

Brailovsky, Antonio Elio, and Dina Foguelman. *Memoria verde: Historia ecológica de la Argentina.* Buenos Aires: Editorial Sudamericana, 1991.

Brannstrom, Christian. "Polluted Soils, Polluted Souls: The Rockefeller Hookworm Eradication Campaign in São Paulo, Brazil, 1917–1926." *Historical Geography* 25 (1997): 25–45.

Breeden, James O. "Disease as a Factor in Southern Distinctiveness." In *Disease and Distinctiveness in the American South,* edited by Todd L. Savitt and James Harvey Young, 1–28. Knoxville: University of Tennessee Press, 1988.

Brennan, James P., and Ofelia Pianetto. *Region and Nation: Politics, Economics, and Society in Twentieth-Century Argentina.* 1st ed. New York: St. Martin's Press, 2000.

Briggs, Charles L., and Clara Mantini-Briggs. *Stories in the Time of Cholera: Racial Profiling during a Medical Nightmare.* Berkeley: University of California Press, 2003.

Brown, Alejandro Diego, and Héctor Ricardo Grau. *La naturaleza y el hombre en las selvas de montaña.* Colección Nuestros Ecosistemas. Salta: Proyecto GTZ, 1993.

Burgos, Juan J., Susana I. Curto de Casas, Rodolfo U. Carcavallo, and Itamar

Galíndez Girón. "Global Climate Change Influence in the Distribution of Some Pathogenic Complexes (Malaria and Chagas' Disease) in Argentina." *Entomología y Vectores* 1, no. 2 (1994): 69–78.

Burgos, Juan J., Susana I. Curto de Casas, Rodolfo U. Carcavallo, and Antonio Martínez. "Malaria and Global Climate Change in Argentina." *Entomologia y Vectores* 1, no. 4 (1994): 123–35.

Campi, Daniel. "Economía y sociedad en las provincias del Norte." In *Nueva Historia Argentina, Tomo 5: El progreso, la modernización y sus límites (1880–1916),* edited by Mirta Zaida Lobato, 71–118. Buenos Aires: Editorial Sudamericana, 2000.

———. "Los ingenios del Norte: un mundo de contrastes." In *Historia de la vida privada en la Argentina: La Argentina plural, 1870–1930,* edited by Fernando Devoto and Marta Madero, 186–221. Buenos Aires: Taurus, 1999.

Campi, Daniel, and Marcelo Lagos. "Auge azucarero y mercado de trabajo en el Noroeste Argentino, 1850–1930." *ANDES: Antropología e historia* 6 (1994): 179–208.

Caprotti, Federico. "Destructive Creation: Fascist Urban Planning, Architecture and New Towns in the Pontine Marshes." *Journal of Historical Geography* 33 (2007): 651–79.

———. "Malaria and Technological Networks: Medical Geography in the Pontine Marshes, Italy, in the 1930s." *Geographical Journal* 172, no. 2 (2006): 145–55.

Caravaca, Jimena, and Mariano Plotkin. "Crisis, ciencias sociales y elites estatales: La constitucion del campo de los economistas estatales en la Argentina, 1910–1935." *Desarrollo Económico* 47, no. 187 (2007): 401–28.

Caro Figueroa, Gregorio, and Eduardo M. Ashur. *El NOA como región.* Salta: Centro Unico de Estudiantes de Humanidades, 1974.

Carter, Eric D. "Development Narratives and the Uses of Ecology: Malaria Control in Northwest Argentina, 1890–1940." *Journal of Historical Geography* 33, no. 3 (2007): 619–50.

———. "'God Bless General Perón': DDT and the Endgame of Malaria Eradication in Argentina in the 1940s." *Journal of the History of Medicine and Allied Sciences* 64 (2009): 78–122.

———. "Malaria, Landscape, and Society in Northwest Argentina." *Journal of Latin American Geography* 7, no. 1 (2008): 7–38.

———. "State Visions, Landscape, and Disease: Discovering Malaria in Argentina, 1890–1920." *Geoforum* 39, no. 1 (2008): 278–93.

Chamosa, Oscar. "Indigenous or Criollo: The Myth of White Argentina in Tucumán's Calchaquí Valley." *Hispanic American Historical Review* 88, no. 1 (2008): 71–106.

Cosgrove, Denis. "Measures of America." In *Geography and Vision,* 87–103. London: I. B. Tauris, 2008.

Craddock, Susan. "Beyond Epidemiology: Locating AIDS in Africa." In *HIV and AIDS in Africa: Beyond Epidemiology,* edited by Ezekiel Kalipeni, Susan Craddock, Joseph Oppong, and Jayati Ghosh, 1–10. Malden, MA: Blackwell Publishing, 2004.

———. *City of Plagues: Disease, Poverty, and Deviance in San Francisco.* Minneapolis: University of Minnesota, 2000.

Craib, Raymond B. *Cartographic Mexico: A History of State Fixations and Fugitive Landscapes.* Durham, NC: Duke University Press, 2004.

Cronon, William. "A Place for Stories: Nature, History, and Narrative." *Journal of American History* 78, no. 4 (1992): 1347–76.

———. "The Trouble with Wilderness; or, Getting Back to the Wrong Nature." In *Uncommon Ground: Toward Reinventing Nature,* edited by William Cronon, 69–90. New York: W. W. Norton & Co., 1995.

Cueto, Marcos. "Appropriation and Resistance: Local Responses to Malaria Eradication in Mexico, 1955–1970." *Journal of Latin American Studies* 37 (2005): 533–59.

———. *Cold War, Deadly Fevers: Malaria Eradication in Mexico, 1955–1975.* Baltimore: Johns Hopkins University Press, 2007.

———. *El regreso de las epidemias. Salud y sociedad en el Perú del siglo XX.* Lima: Instituto de Estudios Peruanos, 2000.

———. *Excelencia científica en la periferia: Actividades científicas e investigación biomédica en el Perú 1890–1950.* Lima: GRADE, 1989.

———. "Laboratory Styles in Argentine Physiology." *Isis* 85 (1994): 228–46.

———, ed. *Missionaries of Science: The Rockefeller Foundation and Latin America.* Bloomington: Indiana University Press, 1994.

———. "The Rockefeller Foundation's Medical Policy and Scientific Research in Latin America: The Case of Physiology." In *Missionaries of Science: The Rockefeller Foundation and Latin America,* edited by Marcos Cueto, 126–48. Bloomington: Indiana University Press, 1994.

———. *The Value of Health: A History of the Pan American Health Organization.* Rochester, NY: University of Rochester Press, 2007.

Curto de Casas, Susana Isabel. "Geografía de los complejos patógenos en el territorio argentino." Doctoral thesis, Universidad de Buenos Aires, 1983.

Curto de Casas, S. I., Y. Verhasselt, R. Caracavallo, and R. Boffi. "Environmental Risk Factors for Diseases Transmitted by Vectors: A Case Study in North-Argentina." *GeoJournal* 44 (1998): 121–27.

Cutolo, Vicente Osvaldo. *Nuevo diccionario biográfico argentino (1750–1930).* Buenos Aires: Editorial ELCHE, 1978.

Dantur Juri, Maria Julia, W. R. Almirón, and G. L. Claps. "Population Fluctuation of Anopheles (Diptera: Culicidae) in Forest and Forest Edge Habitats in Tucumán Province, Argentina." *Journal of Vector Ecology* 35, no. 1 (2010): 28–34.

Dantur Juri, Maria Julia, Mario Zaidenberg, and Walter Almiron. "Distribución espacial de Anopheles pseudopunctipennis en las Yungas de Salta, Argentina." *Rev. Saúde Pública* 39, no. 4 (2005): 565–70.

Dantur Juri, Maria Julia, Mario Zaidenberg, Guillermo Claps, Mirta Santana, and Walter Almiron. "Malaria Transmission in Two Localities in North-Western Argentina." *Malaria Journal* 8, no. 1 (2009): 18.

Davis, Diana K. "Indigenous Knowledge and the Desertification Debate: Problematising Expert Knowledge in North Africa." *Geoforum* 36, no. 4 (2005): 509–24.

———. *Resurrecting the Granary of Rome: Environmental History and French Colonial Expansion in North Africa.* Athens: Ohio University Press, 2007.

de Imaz, Jose Luis. "Alejandro E. Bunge, economista y sociologo (1880–1943)." *Desarrollo Económico* 14, no. 55 (1974): 545–67.

De la Fuente, Ariel. *Children of Facundo: Caudillo and Gaucho Insurgency during the Argentine State-Formation Process (La Rioja, 1853–1870).* Durham: Duke University Press, 2000.

de Santillán, Diego A., ed. *Gran Enciclopedia Argentina.* Buenos Aires: Ediar, 1956.

Defant de Bravo, A. J., and A. M. Orce de Llobeta. "Reflectura y reflexiones sobre el pensamiento educativo de Juan B. Terán." In *La 'Generación del Centenario' y su proyección en el Noroeste Argentino (1900–1950). Actas de las IV Jornadas realizadas en San Miguel de Tucumán del 3 al 5 de octubre de 2001,* edited by Florencia Aráoz de Isas, 130–41. Tucumán: Fundación Miguel Lillo, Centro Cultural Alberto Rougés, 2002.

DeLaney, Jeane H. "Imagining El Ser Argentino: Cultural Nationalism and Romantic Concepts of Nationhood in Early Twentieth-Century Argentina." *Journal of Latin American Studies* 34, no. 3 (2002): 625–58.

Della Paolera, Gerardo, and Alan M. Taylor. *Straining at the Anchor: The Argentine Currency Board and the Search for Macroeconomic Stability, 1880–1935.* Chicago: University of Chicago Press, 2001.

Devoto, Fernando. *Nacionalismo, fascismo y tradicionalismo en la Argentina moderna: Una historia.* Buenos Aires: Siglo Veintiuno, 2002.

Driever, Steven L., and Rafael Espejo-Saavedra. *Spanish/English Dictionary of Human and Physical Geography.* Westport, CT: Greenwood Press, 1994.

Eidt, Robert C. *Pioneer Settlement in Northeast Argentina.* Madison: University of Wisconsin Press, 1971.

Elmhirst, Rebecca. "Space, Identity Politics and Resource Control in Indonesia's Transmigration Programme." *Political Geography* 18, no. 7 (1999): 813–35.

Ettling, J. *The Germ of Laziness: Rockefeller Philanthropy and Public Health in the New South.* Cambridge: Harvard, 1981.

Evans, Hughes. "European Malaria Policy in the 1920s and 1930s: The Epidemiology of Minutiae." *Isis* 80, no. 1 (1989): 40–59.

Fairhead, James, and Melissa Leach. *Misreading the African Landscape: Society and Ecology in a Forest-Savanna Mosaic.* Cambridge: Cambridge University Press, 1996.

Faran, Michael E., and Kenneth J. Linthicum. "A Handbook of the Amazonian

Species of Anopheles (Nyssorhynchus) (Diptera: Culicidae)." *Mosquito Systematics* 13, no. 1 (1981): 1–81.

Farley, J. "Mosquitoes or Malaria? Rockefeller Campaigns in the American South and Sardinia." *Parassitologia* 36 (1994): 165–73.

Ferguson, James. *The Anti-politics Machine: "Development," Depoliticization, and Bureaucratic Power in Lesotho.* Cambridge: Cambridge University Press, 1990.

Fernández, María Estela. "Salud y condiciones de vida. Iniciativas estatales y privadas en Tucumán. Fines del siglo XIX y comienzos del XX." In *Historias de enfermedades, salud y medicina,* edited by Adriana Alvarez, Irene Molinari, and Daniel Reynoso, 111–34. Mar del Plata: Universidad Nacional de Mar del Plata, 2004.

Formoso, Silvia Eugenia. "Padilla, Rougés y la cultura folklórica." In *La 'Generación del Centenario' y su proyección en el Noroeste Argentino (1900–1950). Actas de las IV Jornadas realizadas en San Miguel de Tucumán del 3 al 5 de octubre de 2001,* edited by Florencia Aráoz de Isas, 171–81. Tucumán: Fundación Miguel Lillo, Centro Cultural Alberto Rougés, 2002.

Foster, David William. *The Argentine Generation of 1880: Ideology and Cultural Texts.* Columbia: University of Missouri Press, 1990.

Franco Agudelo, Saul. *El paludismo en América Latina.* Guadalajara: Editorial Universidad de Guadalajara, 1990.

Fustinoni, Osvaldo. "El académico Gregorio Aráoz Alfaro (conferencia pronunciada por el Académico Osvaldo Fustinoni en el Círculo Médico de Córdoba, 1 Julio 1994)." *Boletín de la Academia Nacional de Medicina de Buenos Aires* 72 (1994): 469–90.

Gade, Daniel W. *Nature and Culture in the Andes.* Madison: University of Wisconsin Press, 1999.

Garcia, Susana V. "Ni solas ni resignadas: La participación femenina en las actividades científico-académicas de la Argentina en los inicios del siglo XX." *Cadernos Pagu* 27 (2006): 133–72.

Garcia Costa, Victor. *Alfredo Palacios: Entre el clavel y la espada. Una biografía.* Buenos Aires: Planeta, 1997.

Garrett, Victoria Lynn. "Dispelling Purity Myths and Debunking Hygienic Discourse in Roberto Arlt's 'El jorobadito.'" *Hispania* 93, no. 2 (2010): 187–97.

Gené, Marcela M. *Un mundo feliz: Imágenes de los trabajadores en el primer peronismo, 1946–1955.* Victoria, Buenos Aires: Universidad de San Andrés, 2005.

Gilles, Herbert Michael, D. A. Warrell, and Leonard Jan Bruce-Chwatt. *Bruce-Chwatt's Essential Malariology.* 3rd ed. London, Boston: Edward Arnold, 1993.

Gladwell, Malcolm. "The Mosquito Killer." *New Yorker,* July 2, 2001.

Gordillo, Gastón. *Landscapes of Devils: Tensions of Place and Memory in the Argentinean Chaco.* Durham, NC: Duke University Press, 2004.

Gregory, Derek. "Edward Said's Imaginative Geographies." In *Thinking Space,* edited by Mike Crang and Nigel Thrift, 302–48. London: Routledge, 2000.

Guy, Donna J. *Argentine Sugar Politics: Tucumán and the Generation of Eighty.* Tempe: Center for Latin American Studies, Arizona State University, 1980.

———. "Public Health, Gender, and Private Morality: Paid Labor and the Formation of the Body Politic in Buenos Aires." *Gender and History* 2 (1990): 298–317.

Harrison, Gordon A. *Mosquitoes, Malaria, and Man: A History of the Hostilities since 1880.* New York: Dutton, 1978.

Harrison, Mark. *Climates and Constitutions: Health, Race, Environment, and British Imperialism in India.* Oxford: Oxford University Press, 1999.

Hodges, Donald Clark. *Argentina, 1943–1987: The National Revolution and Resistance.* Albuquerque: University of New Mexico Press, 1988.

Hollander, Frederick A. "Oligarchy and the Politics of Petroleum in Argentina: The Case of the Salta Oligarchy and Standard Oil, 1918–1933." PhD diss., University of California, 1976.

Honigsbaum, Mark. *The Fever Trail: In Search of the Cure for Malaria.* New York: Farrar Straus & Giroux, 2002.

Humphreys, Margaret. *Malaria: Poverty, Race, and Public Health in the United States.* Baltimore: Johns Hopkins, 2001.

James, Daniel. *Resistance and Integration: Peronism and the Argentine Working Class.* Cambridge: Cambridge University Press, 1988.

Jankilevich, Angel. "Testimonio De Adolfo Alzugaray." *Hospital y Comunidad* 4, no. 4 (2001): 428–36.

Jansson, David R. "Internal Orientalism in America: W. J. Cash's *The Mind of the South* and the Spatial Construction of American National Identity." *Political Geography* 22, no. 3 (2003): 293–316.

Jepson, Wendy. "Of Soil, Situation, and Salubrity: Medical Topography and Medical Officers in Early Nineteenth-Century British India." *Historical Geography* 32 (2004): 137–55.

Johnson, Steven. *The Ghost Map: The Story of London's Most Terrifying Epidemic.* New York: Riverhead Books, 2006.

Juarez-Dappe, Patricia Isabel. *When Sugar Ruled: Economy and Society in Northwestern Argentina, Tucumán, 1876–1916.* Athens: Ohio University Press, 2010.

Kaika, Maria. *City of Flows: Modernity, Nature, and the City.* New York: Routledge, 2005.

Kerr, J. Austin, ed. *Building the Health Bridge: Selections from the Works of Fred L. Soper.* Bloomington: Indiana University Press, 1970.

Kirchner, John A. *Sugar and Seasonal Labor Migration: The Case of Tucumán, Argentina.* Chicago: Department of Geography, University of Chicago, 1980.

Koch, Tom. "The Map as Intent: Variations on the Theme of John Snow." *Cartographica* 39, no. 4 (2004): 1–14.

Kohn Loncarica, Alfredo G., Abel L. Agüero, and Norma Isabel Sánchez. "Nacionalismo e internacionalismo en las ciencias de la salud: El caso de la lucha antipalúdica en la Argentina." *Asclepio* 49, no. 2 (1997): 147–63.

Kropf, Simone Petraglia, Nara Azevedo, and Luiz Otávio Ferreira. "Biomedical Research and Public Health in Brazil: The Case of Chagas' Disease (1909–1950)." *Social History of Medicine* 16, no. 1 (2003): 111–29.

Lagos, Marcelo. *La cuestión indígena en el Estado y en la sociedad nacional. Gran Chaco, 1870–1920.* Jujuy: Unidad de Investigación en Historia Regional, Fac. de Humanidades y Ciencias Sociales, U. Nac. de Jujuy, 2000.

Lagos, Marcelo, María Silvia Fleitas, and María Teresa Bovi, eds. *A cien años del informe de Bialet Massé.* Jujuy: Unidad de Investigación en Historia Regional, Facultad de Humanidades y Ciencias Sociales, Universidad Nacional de Jujuy, 2004.

Leonard, Jonathan. "Investigaciones en el interior de la Argentina: La búsqueda de la salud emprendida por Salvador Mazza." *Boletín de la Oficina Sanitaria Panamericana* 113, no. 4 (1992): 301–13.

Lewis, Paul H. "Was Peron a Fascist? An Inquiry into the Nature of Fascism." *Journal of Politics* 42, no. 1 (1980): 242–56.

Livingstone, David N. *The Geographical Tradition: Episodes in the History of a Contested Enterprise.* Oxford, UK; Cambridge, MA: Blackwell Publishers, 1993.

Longobardi, Cesare. *Land-Reclamation in Italy: Rural Revival in the Building of a Nation.* Translated by Olivia Rossetti Agresti. London: P. S. King & Son, Ltd., 1936.

Loudet, Osvaldo. "Tres sabios médicos tucumanos. Eliseo Cantón, Gregorio Aráoz Alfaro, Tiburcio Padilla." *La Semana Médica* 159, no. 9 (1981): 289–98.

Luna, Félix. *Perón y su tiempo.* Buenos Aires: Editorial Sudamericana, 1984.

Manguin, S., D. R. Roberts, E. L. Peyton, E. Rejmankova, and J. Pecor. "Characterization of *Anopheles pseudopunctipennis* larval habitats." *J Am Mosq Control Assoc* 12, no. 4 (1996): 619–26.

Mariscotti, Mario A. J. *El secreto atómico de Huemul. Crónica del origen de la energía atómica en la Argentina.* Buenos Aires: Estudio Sigma S.R.L., 1996.

Martine, Eduardo H., and Raul A. Jorge. "Se acabó el chucho. Carlos Alberto Alvarado y la lucha contra anófeles." *Todo es Historia* 17, no. 198 (1983): 70–88.

Massey, Doreen. *World City.* Cambridge: Polity, 2007.

McGuinness, Aims. "Searching for 'Latin America': Race and Sovereignty in the Americas in the 1850s." In *Race and Nation in Modern Latin America,* edited by Nancy P. Appelbaum, Anne S. Macpherson, and Karin Alejandra Rosemblatt, 87–107. Chapel Hill: University of North Carolina Press, 2003.

McMichael, Anthony J. "Environmental and Social Influences on Emerging Infectious Diseases: Past, Present and Future." *Philosophical Transactions of the Royal Society of London Series B-Biological Sciences* 359, no. 1447 (2004): 1049–58.

Meade, Melinda S. "The Rise and Demise of Malaria: Some Reflections on Southern Settlement and Landscape." *Southeastern Geographer* 20 (1980): 77–99.

Meade, Melinda S., and Robert J. Earickson. *Medical Geography.* 2nd ed. New York: Guilford Press, 2000.

Miller, Marilyn G. *Rise and Fall of the Cosmic Race.* Austin: University of Texas Press, 2004.

Miller, Matt. "Dirty Decade: Rap Music and the U.S. South, 1997–2007." *South-*

ern Spaces, June 10, 2008, http://www.southernspaces.org/contents/2008/miller/1a.htm. Accessed July 1, 2009.

Miranda, Marisa, and Gustavo Vallejo, eds. *Darwinismo social y eugenesia en el mundo latino.* Buenos Aires: Siglo XXI de Argentina Editores, 2005.

Mitchell, Timothy. *Rule of Experts: Egypt, Techno-politics, Modernity.* Berkeley: University of California Press, 2002.

Mitman, Gregg. *The State of Nature: Ecology, Community, and American Social Thought, 1900–1950.* Chicago: University of Chicago Press, 1992.

Mitman, Gregg, and Ronald L. Numbers. "From Miasma to Asthma: The Changing Fortunes of Medical Geography in America." *History and Philosophy of the Life Sciences* 25 (2003): 391–412.

Monmonier, Mark S. *How to Lie with Maps.* 2nd ed. Chicago: University of Chicago Press, 1996.

Morón, Cecilio. "Endemias y epidemias en la historia de Salta." In *Los primeros cuatro siglos de Salta, 1582–1982,* 55–68. Salta: Universidad Nacional de Salta, 1982.

Moseley, William G., and Paul Laris. "West African Environmental Narratives and Development-Volunteer Praxis." *Geographical Review* 98, no. 1 (2008): 59–81.

Muchnik, Daniel. "Dengue y otras pestes," April 4, 2009, http://weblogs.clarin.com/detrasdeltelon/archives/2009/04/dengue_y_otras_pestes.html. Accessed July 25, 2010.

Nascimbene, Mario C. *El nacionalismo liberal y tradicionalista y la Argentina inmigratoria: Benjamín Villafañe (h.), 1916–1944.* Buenos Aires: Editorial Biblos, 1997.

Nash, Linda L. *Inescapable Ecologies: A History of Environment, Disease, and Knowledge.* Berkeley: University of California Press, 2006.

Nouzeilles, Gabriela. *Ficciones somáticas: Naturalismo, nacionalismo y políticas médicas del cuerpo (Argentina, 1880–1910).* Rosario: Beatriz Viterbo, 2000.

Occhipinti, Laurie. "Being Kolla: Indigenous Identity in Northwestern Argentina " *Canadian Journal of Latin American and Caribbean Studies* 27, no. 54 (2002): 319–45.

Oficina Sanitaria Panamericana. "Llamamiento regional a las armas, 1946–1958." *Boletín de la Oficina Sanitaria Panamericana* 113 (1992): 396–405.

Orlove, Benjamin S. "Mapping Reeds and Reading Maps: The Politics of Representation in Lake Titicaca." *American Ethnologist* 18, no. 1 (1991): 3–38.

Ortiz de D'Arterio, Julia Patricia. "Azúcar y mortalidad. Un análisis evolutivo de la mortalidad infantil y de menores de 15 años en el área cañera de la provincia de Tucumán." In *El complejo azucarero en Tucumán: Dinámica y articulaciones (CD-ROM),* edited by Alfredo S. C. Bolsi. Tucumán: Instituto de Estudios Geográficos, Universidad Nacional de Tucumán, 2002.

Otero, Hernán. *Estadística y nación: Una historia conceptual del pensamiento censal de la Argentina moderna, 1869–1914.* Buenos Aires: Prometeo Libros, 2006.

———. "La transición demográfica argentina a debate. Una perspectiva espacial de las explicaciones ideacionales, económicas y político-institucionales." In

El mosaico argentino: Modelos y representaciones del espacio y de la población, siglos XIX–XX, edited by Hernán Otero, 71–170. Buenos Aires: Siglo Veintiuno de Argentina Editores, 2004.

Packard, Randall M. *The Making of a Tropical Disease: A Short History of Malaria.* Baltimore: Johns Hopkins University Press, 2007.

———. " 'Malaria Blocks Development' Revisited: The Role of Disease in the History of Agricultural Development in the Eastern and Northern Transvaal Lowveld, 1890–1960." *Journal of Southern African Studies* 27, no. 3 (2001): 591–612.

Packard, Randall M., and Paulo Gadelha. "A Land Filled with Mosquitoes: Fred L. Soper, the Rockefeller Foundation, and the Anopheles gambiae Invasion of Brazil." *Parassitologia* 36 (1994): 197–213.

Páez de la Torre, Carlos. "Apenas ayer: Eucalyptus vs. paludismo. En 1877, el gobierno propició la plantación de esos árboles." *La Gaceta,* April 18, 1995, 13.

———. "Apenas ayer: Un gran médico. Hace cien años nació Tiburcio Padilla." *La Gaceta,* October 23, 1993, 13.

———. *Historia de Tucumán.* Buenos Aires: Plus Ultra, 1987.

Palmer, Steven. "Central American Encounters with Rockefeller Public Health, 1914–1921." In *Close Encounters of Empire: Writing the Cultural History of U.S.-Latin American Relations,* edited by Gilbert M. Joseph, Catherine C. LeGrand, and Ricardo D. Salvatore, 311–32. Durham: Duke University Press, 1998.

Paterlini de Koch, Olga. *Parque 9 de Julio.* Tucumán: Grafica Noroeste, 1992.

Peet, Richard, and Michael Watts. "Liberation Ecology: Development, Sustainability, and Environment in an Age of Market Triumphalism." In *Liberation Ecologies: Environment, Development, Social Movements,* edited by Richard Peet and Michael Watts, 1–45. London: Routledge, 1996.

Pelis, Kim. *Charles Nicolle, Pasteur's Imperial Missionary: Typhus and Tunisia.* Rochester, NY: University of Rochester Press, 2006.

Perdue, Peter C. "Where Do Incorrect Political Ideas Come From? Writing the History of the Qing Empire and the Chinese Nation." In *The Teleology of the Modern Nation-State: Japan and China,* edited by Joshua A. Fogel, 174–99. Philadelphia: University of Pennsylvania Press, 2005.

Pereira, Enrique. "Miguel Sussini." *Diccionario Biográfico Nacional de la Unión Cívica Radical* (2009), http://diccionarioradical.blogspot.com/search/label/Corrientes. Accessed September 12, 2009.

Pérgola, Federico. "Lepra, paludismo y otras endemias." *Todo es Historia,* no. 444 (2004): 48–58.

Personalidades de la Argentina. Diccionario Biográfico Contemporaneo. 3rd ed. Buenos Aires: Veritas–F. Antonio Rizzuto, 1948.

Peyton, E. L., Richard C. Wilkerson, and Ralph E. Harbach. "Comparative Analysis of the Subegenera Kerteszia and Nyssorhynchus of Anopheles (Diptera: Culicidae)." *Mosquito Systematics* 24, no. 1 (1992): 51–69.

Potash, Robert A. *The Army and Politics in Argentina.* Stanford, CA: Stanford University Press, 1969.

Prieto, Adolfo. *El discurso criollista en la formación de la Argentina moderna.* Buenos Aires: Siglo Veintiuno, 2006.

Quevedo, Emilio, and Francisco Gutiérrez. "Scientific Medicine and Public Health in Nineteenth-Century Latin America." In *Science in Latin America: A History,* edited by Juan José Saldaña, 163–96. Austin: University of Texas Press, 2006.

Quintero, Silvina. "La interpretación del territorio argentino en los primeros censos nacionales de población (1869, 1895, 1914)." In *El mosaico argentino: Modelos y representaciones del espacio y de la población, siglos XIX–XX,* edited by Hernán Otero, 267–97. Buenos Aires: Siglo Veintiuno de Argentina Editores, 2004.

Ramacciotti, Karina Inés. "La política sanitaria argentina entre 1946–1954: Las propuestas de Ramón Carrillo." *Taller* 6, no. 17 (2001): 35–55.

———. *La política sanitaria del peronismo.* Buenos Aires: Editorial Biblos, 2009.

———. "Las huellas eugénicas en la política sanitaria argentina (1946–1955)." In *Darwinismo social y eugenesia en el mundo latino,* edited by Marisa Miranda and Gustavo Vallejo, 311–50. Buenos Aires: Siglo XXI de Argentina Editores, 2005.

———. "Las sombras de la política sanitaria durante el peronismo: Los brotes epidémicos en Buenos Aires." *Asclepio* 58, no. 2 (2006): 115–38.

———. "Ramón Carrillo." In *Dictionary of Medical Biography,* edited by W. F. Bynum and Helen Bynum, 308–10. Westport, CT: Greenwood Press, 2007.

Ramacciotti, Karina Inés, and Adriana María Valobra. "'Plasmar la raza fuerte.' Relaciones de género en la campaña sanitaria de la Secretaría de Salud Pública de la Argentina (1946–1949)." In *Generando el peronismo. Estudios de cultura, política y género (1946–1955),* edited by Ramacciotti and Valobra, 19–64. Buenos Aires: Proyecto Editorial, 2004.

Ratier, Hugo E. *El Cabecita Negra.* Buenos Aires: Centro Editor de América Latina, 1972.

Reber, Vera Blinn. "Blood, Coughs, and Fever: Tuberculosis and the Working Class of Buenos Aires, Argentina, 1885–1915." *Social History of Medicine* 12 (1999): 73–100.

Reboratti, Carlos E. *El alto Bermejo: Realidades y conflictos.* Buenos Aires: La Colmena, 1998.

———. *La Quebrada: Geografía, historia y ecología de la Quebrada de Humahuaca.* Buenos Aires: Editorial La Colmena, 2003.

Ribot, Jesse. "A History of Fear: Imagining Deforestation in the West African Dryland Forests." *Global Ecology and Biogeography* 8 (1999): 291–300.

Rock, David. *Argentina, 1516–1987: From Spanish Colonization to Alfonsín.* Berkeley: University of California Press, 1987.

———. *Authoritarian Argentina: The Nationalist Movement, Its History, and Its Impact.* Berkeley: University of California Press, 1992.

Rodriguez, Julia. *Civilizing Argentina: Science, Medicine, and the Modern State.* Chapel Hill: University of North Carolina Press, 2006.

Rodríguez Ocaña, Esteban, Rosa Ballester Añón, Enrique Perdiguero, Rosa

María Medina Doménech, and Jorge Molero Mesa. *La acción médico-social contra el paludismo en la España metropolitana y colonial del siglo XX*. Madrid: Consejo Superior de Investigaciones Científicas, 2003.

Roe, Emery. "Development Narratives, or Making the Best of Blueprint Development." *World Development* 19 (1991): 287–300.

Romero, José Luis. *Breve historia de la Argentina*. Colección Tierra Firme. 1965. Reprint, Buenos Aires: Fondo de Cultura Económica, 1996.

———. *Las ideas políticas en Argentina*. 1956. Reprint, Buenos Aires: Fondo de Cultura Económica, 2001.

Romero, Simon. "In Bolivia, Untapped Bounty Meets Nationalism." *New York Times,* February 2, 2009.

Rosenzvaig, Eduardo. *Historia social de Tucumán y del azúcar*. Tucumán: UNT, 1986.

Rozendaal, Jan A. "Vector Control: Methods for Use by Individuals and Communities." Geneva: World Health Organization, 1997.

Russell, Edmund. *War and Nature: Fighting Humans and Insects with Chemicals from World War I to Silent Spring*. Cambridge: Cambridge University Press, 2001.

Sachs, Jeffrey, and Pia Malaney. "The Economic and Social Burden of Malaria." *Nature* 415 (2002): 680–85.

Salomon, O. Daniel, Mario Zaidenberg, Ricardo Burgos, Viviana Heredia, and S. Liliana Caropresi. "American Cutaneous Leishmaniasis Outbreak, Tartagal City, Province of Salta, Argentina, 1993." *Rev. Inst. Med. Trop. S. Paulo* 43 (2001): 105–8.

Sánchez, Norma Isabel. *La higiene y los higienistas en la Argentina (1880–1943)*. Buenos Aires: Sociedad Científica Argentina, 2007.

Sánchez de Maldonado, Sandra. "Creación y evolución de la Universidad de Tucumán (1914–1921)." In *La cultura en Tucumán y en el Noroeste Argentino en la primera mitad del siglo XX*. Tucumán: Fundación Miguel Lillo y Centro Cultural Alberto Rougés, 1997.

Sawers, Larry. *The Other Argentina: The Interior and National Development*. Boulder, CO: Westview Press, 1996.

Scenna, Miguel Angel. *Cuando murió Buenos Aires, 1871*. Buenos Aires: Ediciones La Bastilla, 1974.

Schvarzer, Jorge. "Los avatares de la industria nacional." In *Lo mejor de Todo es Historia,* edited by Félix Luna, 435–67. Buenos Aires: Taurus, 2002.

Scobie, James R. *Argentina: A City and a Nation*. New York: Oxford University Press, 1964.

Scobie, James R., and Samuel L. Baily. *Secondary Cities of Argentina: The Social History of Corrientes, Salta, and Mendoza, 1850–1910*. Stanford: Stanford University Press, 1988.

Scott, James C. *Seeing like a State: How Certain Schemes to Improve the Human Condition Have Failed*. New Haven, CT: Yale University Press, 1998.

Shumway, Nicolas. *The Invention of Argentina*. Berkeley: University of California Press, 1991.

Sierra Iglesias, Jobino Pedro. *Carlos Alberto Alvarado: Vida y obra.* Salta: Comisión Bicameral Examinadora de Obras de Autores Salteños, 1993.

———. *Salvador Mazza: Su vida, su obra.* San Salvador de Jujuy: Universidad Nacional de Jujuy, 1990.

———. *Vida y obra del Doctor Guillermo Cleland Paterson.* San Salvador de Jujuy: Universidad Nacional de Jujuy, 1996.

Skidmore, Thomas E., and Peter H. Smith. *Modern Latin America.* 5th ed. New York: Oxford University Press, 2001.

Snowden, Frank M. *The Conquest of Malaria: Italy, 1900–1962.* New Haven, CT: Yale University Press, 2006.

Solberg, Carl E. *Immigration and Nationalism, Argentina and Chile, 1890–1914.* Austin: University of Texas Press, 1970.

Spektorowski, Alberto. "The Ideological Origins of Right and Left Nationalism in Argentina, 1930–43." *Journal of Contemporary History* 29, no. 1 (1994): 155–84.

Spielman, Andrew, and Michael D'Antonio. *Mosquito: A Natural History of Our Most Persistent and Deadly Foe.* New York: Hyperion, 2001.

Stapleton, Darwin H. "Lessons of History? Anti-malaria Strategies of the International Health Board and the Rockefeller Foundation from the 1920s to the Era of DDT." *Public Health Reports* 119, no. 2 (2004): 206–15.

Stepan, Nancy Leys. *"The Hour of Eugenics": Race, Gender, and Nation in Latin America.* Ithaca, NY: Cornell University Press, 1991.

———. "The Only Serious Terror in These Regions: Malaria Control in the Brazilian Amazon." In *Disease in the History of Modern Latin America: From Malaria to AIDS,* edited by Diego Armus, 25–50. Durham, NC: Duke University Press, 2003.

Sufian, Sandra M. *Healing the Land and the Nation: Malaria and the Zionist Project in Palestine, 1920–1947.* Chicago: University of Chicago Press, 2007.

Sutter, Paul S. "Nature's Agents or Agents of Empire? Entomological Workers and Environmental Change during the Construction of the Panama Canal." *Isis* 98 (2007): 724–54.

Swift, Jeremy. "Desertification: Narratives, Winners, and Losers." In *The Lie of the Land,* edited by M. Leach and R. Mearns, 73–90. London: International African Institute, 1996.

Terán, Soledad. "La biblioteca de la Fundación Miguel Lillo y sus aportes al desarrollo geológico." In *La cultura en Tucumán y en el Noroeste Argentino en la primera mitad del siglo XX,* 117–21. Tucumán: Fundación Miguel Lillo y Centro Cultural Alberto Rougés, 1997.

Thompson, Kenneth. "Insalubrious California: Perception and Reality." *Annals of the Association of American Geographers* 59, no. 1 (1969): 50–64.

Tilley, Virginia Q. *Seeing Indians: A Study of Race, Nation, and Power in El Salvador.* Albuquerque: University of New Mexico Press, 2005.

Tomes, Nancy. *The Gospel of Germs: Men, Women, and the Microbe in American Life.* Cambridge: Harvard University Press, 1998.

Urteaga, Luis. "Miseria, miasmas y microbios. Las topografías médicas y el estudio del medio ambiente en el siglo XIX." *GeoCrítica, Cuadernos Críticos de Geografía Humana (Barcelona)* 29 (September 1980): 5–50.

Valencius, Conevery Bolton. *The Health of the Country: How American Settlers Understood Themselves and Their Land.* New York: Basic Books, 2002.

———. "Histories of Medical Geography." In *Medical Geography in Historical Perspective (Medical History, Supplement No. 20),* edited by Nicolaas A. Rupke, 3–28. London: Wellcome Trust Centre for the History of Medicine, 2000.

Vandergeest, Peter. "Mapping Nature: Territorialization of Forest Rights in Thailand." *Society and Natural Resources* 9 (1996): 159–75.

Vandergeest, Peter, and Nancy Lee Peluso. "Empires of Forestry: Professional Forestry and State Power in Southeast Asia, Part 1." *Environment and History* 12 (2006): 31–64.

Verhasselt, Yola, Susana Isabel Curto de Casas, Rodolfo U. Carcavallo, and Rolando Boffi. "Geografía de la salud. Algunos factores ambientales de riesgo para enfermedades transmitidas por mosquitos (Salvador Mazza, Salta, Argentina)." *GAEA, Anales de la Sociedad Argentina de Estudios Geográficos* 20 (1996): 297.

Wade, Peter. *Race and Ethnicity in Latin America.* Chicago: Pluto Press, 1997.

Walker, Peter A. "Political Ecology: Where is the Policy?" *Progress in Human Geography* 30, no. 3 (2006): 382–95.

Webb, James L. A. *Humanity's Burden: A Global History of Malaria.* Cambridge: Cambridge University Press, 2009.

Whiteford, Scott. *Workers from the North: Plantations, Bolivian Labor, and the City in Northwest Argentina.* Austin: University of Texas Press, 1981.

Winichakul, Thongchai. *Siam Mapped: A History of the Geo-Body of a Nation.* Honolulu: University of Hawaii Press, 1994.

Wood, Denis. "Every Map Shows This . . . But Not That." In *The Power of Maps,* 48–69. New York: Guilford Press, 1992.

Worster, Donald. *Nature's Economy: A History of Ecological Ideas.*, 2nd ed. Cambridge: Cambridge University Press, 1994.

Wurgat, Ramy. "Viaje al corazón de la epidemia de dengue de Argentina," April 22, 2009, http://tejiendoelmundo.wordpress.com/2009/04/22/viaje -al-corazon-de-la-epidemia-de-dengue-de-argentina/. Accessed July 25, 2010.

Zimmerer, Karl. "Ecology as Cornerstone and Chimera in Human Geography." In *Concepts in Human Geography,* edited by Carville Earle, Martin S. Kenzer, and Kent Mathewson, 161–88. Lanham, MD: Rowman & Littlefield Publishers, 1996.

Zimmermann, Eduardo A. *Los liberales reformistas: La cuestión social en la Argentina 1890–1916.* Buenos Aires: Editorial Sudamericana Universidad de San Andrés, 1995.

———. "Racial Ideas and Social Reform: Argentina, 1890–1916." *Hispanic American Historical Review* 72, no. 1 (1992): 23–46.

Index